MW01634240

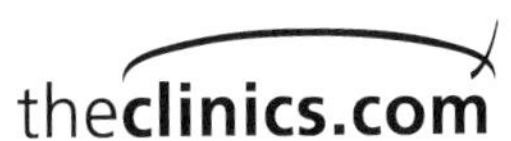

EMERGENCY MEDICINE CLINICS OF NORTH AMERICA

Emergency Medicine and the Public's Health

GUEST EDITORS
Jon Mark Hirshon, MD, MPH and
David M. Morris, MD, MPH

CONSULTING EDITOR
Amal Mattu, MD

November 2006 • Volume 24 • Number 4

SAUNDERS

An Imprint of Elsevier, Inc.
PHILADELPHIA   LONDON   TORONTO   MONTREAL   SYDNEY   TOKYO

W.B. SAUNDERS COMPANY
A Division of Elsevier Inc.

1600 John F. Kennedy Boulevard, Suite 1800 • Philadelphia, Pennsylvania 19103-2899

http://www.theclinics.com

**EMERGENCY MEDICINE CLINICS
OF NORTH AMERICA**
November 2006
Editor: Karen Sorensen

Volume 24, Number 4
ISSN 0733-8627
ISBN 1-4160-3883-3

The ideas and opinions expressed in *Emergency Medicine Clinics of North America* do not necessarily reflect those of the Publisher. The Publisher does not assume any responsibility for any injury and/or damage to persons or property arising out of or related to any use of the material contained in this periodical. The reader is advised to check the appropriate medical literature and the product information currently provided by the manufacturer of each drug to be administered to verify the dosage, the method and duration of administration, or contraindications. It is the responsibility of the treating physician or other health care professional, relying on independent experience and knowledge of the patient, to determine drug dosages and the best treatment for the patient. Mention of any product in this issue should not be construed as endorsement by the contributors, editors, or the Publisher of the product or manufacturers' claims.

Emergency Medicine Clinics of North America (ISSN 0733-8627) is published quarterly by Elsevier Inc., 360 Park Avenue South, New York, NY, 10010-1710. Months of issue are February, May, August, and November. Business and Editorial Offices: 1600 John F. Kennedy Boulevard, Suite 1800, Philadelphia, PA 19103-2899. Customer Service Office: 6277 Sea Harbor Drive, Orlando, FL 32887-4800. Periodicals postage paid at New York, NY, and additional mailing offices. Subscription prices are $193.00 per year (US individuals), $297.00 per year (US institutions), $259.00 per year (international individuals), $351.00 per year (international institutions), $237.00 per year (Canadian individuals), and $351.00 per year (Canadian institutions). International air speed delivery is included in all *Clinics'* subscription prices. All prices are subject to change without notice. POSTMASTER: Send address changes to *Emergency Medicine Clinics of North America*, Elsevier Periodicals Customer Service, 6277 Sea Harbor Drive, Orlando, FL 32887-4800. **Customer Service: 1-800-654-2452 (US). From outside of the US, call 1-407-345-4000. E-mail: hhspcs@harcourt.com.**

Emergency Medicine Clinics of North America is covered in *Index Medicus, Current Contents/Clinical Medicine, EMBASE/Excerpta Medica, BIOSIS, SciSearch, CINAHL, ISI/BIOMED,* and *Research Alert.*

Printed in the United States of America.

CONSULTING EDITOR

AMAL MATTU, MD, Associate Professor and Residency Director, Department of Emergency Medicine, University of Maryland School of Medicine, Baltimore, Maryland

GUEST EDITORS

JON MARK HIRSHON, MD, MPH, Acting Director, The Charles McC. Mathias, Jr. National Study Center for Trauma and EMS, University of Maryland School of Medicine, Baltimore, Maryland

DAVID M. MORRIS, MD, MPH, Attending Physician, Department of Emergency Medicine, MetroWest Medical Center, Framingham Union Hospital, Framingham, Massachusetts

CONTRIBUTORS

BRENT R. ASPLIN, MD, MPH, Department of Emergency Medicine, Regions Hospital, St. Paul, Minnesota; Department of Emergency Medicine, University of Minnesota, Minneapolis, Minnesota

BRUCE BECKER, MD, Associate Professor of Community Health, Department of Emergency Medicine, Brown Medical School, Providence, Rhode Island

STEVEN L. BERNSTEIN, MD, Department of Emergency Medicine, Albert Einstein College of Medicine, Montefiore Medical Center, Bronx, New York

LINDA C. DEGUTIS, DrPH, MSN, Associate Professor of Surgery and Public Health, Section of Emergency Medicine, Department of Surgery, and Department of Epidemiology and Public Health, Yale University School of Medicine, New Haven, Connecticut

GAIL D'ONOFRIO, MD, MS, Professor and Chief, Section of Emergency Medicine, Yale School of Medicine, New Haven, Connecticut

LOWELL W. GERSON, PhD, Professor Emeritus of Epidemiology, Northeastern Ohio Universities College of Medicine, Rootstown, Ohio; Senior Scientist, Emergency Medicine Research Center, Summa Health System, Akron, Ohio

PEGGY E. GOODMAN, MD, FACEP, Associate Professor of Emergency Medicine and Director, Violence Prevention Resources, Department of Emergency Medicine, Brody School of Medicine–East Carolina University, Greenville, North Carolina

JAMES A. GORDON, MD, MPA, Assistant Professor of Medicine, Harvard Medical School, Boston, Massachusetts; Attending Physician, Department of Emergency Medicine, Massachusetts General Hospital, Boston, Massachusetts

MARK GREVE, MD, Assistant Professor, Department of Emergency Services, Brown Medical School at Rhode Island Hospital, Providence, Rhode Island

LEON L. HALEY, JR, MD, MHSA, Associate Professor of Emergency Medicine, Emory University School of Medicine; Vice-Chair for Clinical Operations, Chief of Emergency Medicine, Grady Health System, Atlanta, Georgia

SHERYL L. HERON, MD, MPH, Associate Professor of Emergency Medicine and Associate Residency Director, Emory University School of Medicine, Atlanta, Georgia

JON MARK HIRSHON, MD, MPH, Acting Director, The Charles McC. Mathias, Jr. National Study Center for Trauma and EMS, University of Maryland School of Medicine, Baltimore, Maryland

YU-HSIANG HSIEH, PhD, Assistant Professor, Department of Emergency Medicine, The Johns Hopkins University School of Medicine, Baltimore, Maryland

DAVID KARRAS, MD, FACEP, FAAEM, Associate Professor, Department of Emergency Medicine, Temple University School of Medicine, Philadelphia, Pennsylvania

CATHERINE A. MARCO, MD, FACEP, Clinical Professor, Division of Emergency Medicine, Department of Surgery, Medical University of Ohio; Attending Physician, Department of Emergency Medicine, St Vincent Mercy Medical Center, Toledo, Ohio

DAVID M. MORRIS, MD, MPH, Attending Physician, Department of Emergency Medicine, MetroWest Medical Center, Framingham Union Hospital, Framingham, Massachusetts

DANIEL A. POLLOCK, MD, Healthcare Outcomes Branch Chief, Division of Healthcare Quality Promotion, National Center for Infectious Diseases, Centers for Disease Control and Prevention, Atlanta, Georgia; Clinical Associate Professor, Department of Emergency Medicine, Emory University School of Medicine, Atlanta, Georgia

KARIN V. RHODES, MD, MS, Director, Division of Health Care Policy Research, Department of Emergency Medicine, School Medicine & School of Social Policy and Practice, University of Pennsylvania, Philadelphia, Pennsylvania

RICHARD E. ROTHMAN, MD, PhD, Associate Professor, Director, Research Fellowship, Department of Emergency Medicine, The Johns Hopkins University School of Medicine, Baltimore, Maryland

MARK A. SAKS, MD, MPH, Clinical Instructor, Department of Emergency Medicine, Drexel University College of Medicine, Philadelphia, Pennsylvania

RAQUEL M. SCHEARS, MD, MPH, FACEP, Assistant Professor, Department of Emergency Medicine, Mayo Clinic/St. Mary's Hospital, Rochester, Minnesota

EDWARD STETTNER, MD, Assistant Professor of Emergency Medicine, Emory University School of Medicine, Atlanta, Georgia

KIRK A. STIFFLER, MD, Assistant Clinical Professor in Emergency Medicine, Northeastern Ohio Universities College of Medicine, Rootstown, Ohio; Associate Director, Emergency Medicine Research Center, Summa Health System, Akron, Ohio

SHAWN M. VARNEY, LT COL, USAF, MC, Emergency Department, 59 MDW/MCED, Lackland Air Force Base, Texas

ROBERT H. WOOLARD, MD, Professor, Department of Emergency Medicine, Brown Medical School, Providence, Rhode Island

SAMUEL YANG, MD, Assistant Professor, Department of Emergency Medicine, The Johns Hopkins University School of Medicine, Baltimore, Maryland

CONTENTS

> This issue of the *Emergency Medicine Clinics of North America* focuses on the spectrum of public health issues that significantly impact the practice of emergency medicine and which are faced by practicing emergency physicians on a daily basis. Topics include public health research in the emergency department; respiratory threats; emerging infectious diseases; emergency department overcrowding; end-of-life care; racial and ethnic disparities; issues of health promotion and disease prevention encompassing substance abuse, alcohol, and injury and violence; public health surveillance; and the problems of homeless and disadvantaged patients. This article gives a brief introduction to the important relationship between emergency medicine and public health.

> Emergency department (ED) crowding is becoming an increasing problem in EDs throughout the United States for a multitude of reasons, including an increase in patient volume and a decrease in available EDs. Crowding has an adverse impact on the ability to deliver quality and timely care and may contribute to adverse patient outcomes. Conceptually, factors that contribute to ED

crowding can be divided into three domains, which correspond to their "sites of action": input, throughput, and output. A number of measures have been developed to better quantify crowding and its effects. More research needs to be done to better understand the factors that contribute to crowding, the impact of this problem on patients and ED throughput, and how to alleviate this nation-wide crisis.

This article provides an overview of the role of the emergency department (ED) in the care of homeless and disadvantaged populations. It suggests that organized emergency medicine can have a significant impact on total community health by maintaining a universal "safety net" for the delivery of integrated health and human services. The epidemiology of social deprivation among ED patients is examined, with a particular focus on homelessness. Current research on the value of socio-medical integration in the ED setting is discussed, with emphasis on selected initiatives that have demonstrated feasibility, cost-effectiveness, and impact.

This article provides an overview of health promotion and disease and injury prevention concepts. It provides an emergency medicine perspective and reviews approaches that can be used in the emergency department. It discusses examples of innovative emergency medicine-based preventive activities including prevention in the prehospital setting. The article ends with a discussion of the importance of a system approach to prevention and suggests a role for a preventionist as a new member of the emergency medicine team.

Emergency medicine plays a significant role in injury prevention through the use of public health models that link injury data to prevention programming, research, and advocacy. The day-to-day experiences in the emergency department provide a picture of the injury problem in a given community and give the emergency practitioner a real-world basis for injury prevention efforts. This article covers the basics of injury prevention, including defining the problem, discussing data and conceptual aspects of injury prevention, and systematically identifying successful approaches to reducing the burden of injuries.

directives or communication with patients and surrogates. Resuscitative efforts are appropriate for many patients, but inappropriate for others. The goals of medicine remain the following: providing optimal health care, provision of the best possible symptom control, communication, empathy, and caring. As death approaches, provision of the best possible medical care, in accordance with the patient's wishes, can be rewarding for patients, families, and health care providers.

Respiratory infections are the most common communicable infectious diseases. EDs are the front line for patients with respiratory infections because of their acute nature and because the ED is the principal site of health care for those at highest risk. These diseases include influenza, tuberculosis, and measles, together accounting for 25% of infectious causes of death worldwide. There are emerging and biothreat agents that follow the same route of transmission, such as SARS and pneumonic plague. We discuss epidemiology, pathogenesis, diagnosis, and treatment of each agent. Emphasis is on the ED's role as a public health prevention arena, with attention to education and disease prevention, early identification of disease in patients at risk, and reduction of illnesses.

In recent years, multiple global forces have contributed to the emergence and widespread distribution of previously unknown disease entities. This article discusses Ebola virus, West Nile virus, and Hantavirus as representative emerging infectious diseases. Smallpox is discussed along with concerns about the safety of the smallpox vaccine, given the uncertain risk of bioterrorism and smallpox exposure. ED physicians must become familiar with the presentation, management, and public health impact of all of these entities, as well as understand the potential impact of other emerging infectious diseases.

The development of public health surveillance systems based on ED visits, in conjunction with other health and non-health-related data, is an important step to better understanding the health needs of the US population. There are multiple steps to develop a

FORTHCOMING ISSUES

RECENT ISSUES

GOAL STATEMENT

The goal of *Emergency Medicine Clinics of North America* is to keep practicing physicians up to date with current clinical practice in emergency medicine by providing timely articles reviewing the state of the art in patient care.

ACCREDITATION

The *Emergency Medical Clinics of North America* is planned and implemented in accordance with the Essential Areas and Policies of the Accreditation Council for Continuing Medical Education (ACCME) through the joint sponsorship of the University of Virginia School of Medicine and Elsevier. The University of Virginia School of Medicine is accredited by the ACCME to provide continuing medical education for physicians.

The University of Virginia School of Medicine designates this educational activity for a maximum of *15 AMA PRA Category 1 Credits™*. Physicians should only claim credit commensurate with the extent of their participation in the activity.

The Emergency Medicine Clinics of North America CME program is approved by the American College of Emergency Physicians for 60 hours of ACEP Category I Credit per year.

The American Medical Association has determined that physicians not licensed in the US who participate in this CME activity are eligible for *15 AMA PRA Category 1 Credits™*.

Credit can be earned by reading the text material, taking the CME examination online at http://www.theclinics.com/home/cme, and completing the evaluation. After taking the test, you will be required to review any and all incorrect answers. Following completion of the test and evaluation, your credit will be awarded and you may print your certificate.

FACULTY DISCLOSURE/CONFLICT OF INTEREST

The University of Virginia School of Medicine, as an ACCME accredited provider, endorses and strives to comply with the Accreditation Council for Continuing Medical Education (ACCME) Standards of Commercial Support, Commonwealth of Virginia statutes, University of Virginia policies and procedures, and associated federal and private regulations and guidelines on the need for disclosure and monitoring of proprietary and financial interests that may affect the scientific integrity and balance of content delivered in continuing medical education activities under our auspices.

The University of Virginia School of Medicine requires that all CME activities accredited through this institution be developed independently and be scientifically rigorous, balanced and objective in the presentation/ discussion of its content, theories and practices.

All authors/editors participating in an accredited CME activity are expected to disclose to the readers relevant financial relationships with commercial entities occurring within the past 12 months (such as grants or research support, employee, consultant, stock holder, member of speakers bureau, etc.). The University of Virginia School of Medicine will employ appropriate mechanisms to resolve potential conflicts of interest to maintain the standards of fair and balanced education to the reader. Questions about specific strategies can be directed to the Office of Continuing Medical Education, University of Virginia School of Medicine, Charlottesville, Virginia.

The authors/editors listed below have identified no professional or financial affiliations for themselves or their spouse/partner:
Brent R. Asplin, MD, MPH; Bruce Becker, MD; Steven L. Bernstein, MD; Gail D'Onofrio, MD, MS; Linda C. Degutis, DrPH, MSN; Lowell W. Gerson, PhD; Peggy E. Goodman, MD; James A. Gordon, MD, MPA; Mark Greve, MD; Leon L. Haley, Jr., MD, MHSA; Sheryl L. Heron, MD, MPH; Jon Mark Hirshon, MD, MPH (Guest Editor); Yu-Hsiang Hsieh, PhD; David Karras, MD, FACEP, FAAEM; Catherine A. Marco, MD, FACEP; Amal Mattu, MD, FAAEM, FACEP (Consulting Editor); David M. Morris, MD, MPH (Guest Editor); Daniel A. Pollock, MD; Karin V. Rhodes, MD, MS; Richard E. Rothman, MD, PhD; Mark A. Saks, MD, MPH; Raquel M. Schears, MD, MPH, FACEP; Karen Sorensen, Acquisitions Editor; Edward Stettner, MD; Kirk A. Stiffler, MD; Shawn Varney, Lt Col, USAF, MC; Robert H. Woolard, MD; and, Samuel Yang, MD.

Disclosure of Discussion of non-FDA approved uses for pharmaceutical products and/or medical devices:
The University of Virginia School of Medicine, as an ACCME provider, requires that all faculty presenters identify and disclose any "off label" uses for pharmaceutical and medical device products. The University of Virginia School of Medicine recommends that each physician fully review all the available data on new products or procedures prior to instituting them with patients.

TO ENROLL

To enroll in the Emergency Medicine Clinics of North America Continuing Medical Education program, call customer service at 1-800-654-2452 or visit us online at www.theclinics.com/home/cme. The CME program is available to subscribers for an additional fee of $195.00.

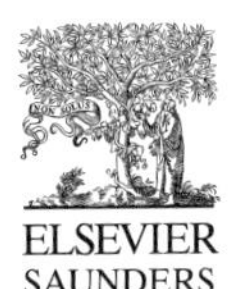

ELSEVIER
SAUNDERS

Emerg Med Clin N Am
24 (2006) xv–xvi

EMERGENCY
MEDICINE
CLINICS OF
NORTH AMERICA

Foreword

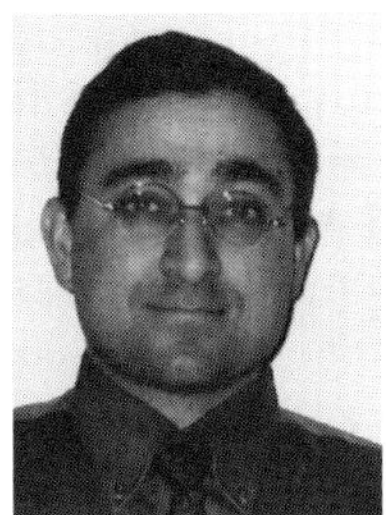

Amal Mattu, MD
Consulting Editor

The field of emergency medicine (EM) is intimately tied to the field of public health. On the surface, this statement seems contrary to the perception that most people have of EM as a specialty that focuses on the acute care and resuscitation of the individual. Non-urgent and primary care visits to the emergency department (ED) are often considered unwelcome or inappropriate. The media, also, has portrayed the ED as a place where every patient presents with a single acute, deadly illness, and where every patient's life hangs in the balance.

Although there are many ED patients who present with a single acute illness, it seems that the majority of patients actually do not fit this Hollywood stereotype. On the contrary, if you walk into any large ED, you are more likely to encounter the result of an imperfect health care system and society rather than the drama of Hollywood hype. Uninsured patients who have no primary care physician use the ED for their most basic medical care. Even many insured patients who are unable to see their physicians in a timely manner for simple ailments use the ED instead. Patients who abuse alcohol and other substances line the hallways of the ED. Victims of domestic violence sit in chairs awaiting counselors or transportation to shelters for protection. The ED, it turns out, is not just the site of care for individuals with single acute, deadly illnesses. It is also an important point of care for many patients with chronic or social problems, for patients who have nowhere else to turn for help.

Although the usual focus of ED care is on the individual patient, the ED is also a natural location in which to deliver and to monitor care of an entire

doi:10.1016/j.emc.2006.07.002   *emed.theclinics.com*

society. The ED is the first site at which most patients with communicable diseases present, the first site at which patients with outbreaks of "old" diseases present, and the first site at which patients with new emerging diseases present. Emergency medicine, therefore, presents a perfect opportunity to improve the health of a society by engaging in disease surveillance, primary care screening, and injury prevention counseling. There is no specialty in the field of medicine that serves as a more natural bridge between medicine and public health than EM. The two fields, although appearing on the surface to be disparate in philosophy, truly are bound together.

In this issue of the *Emergency Medicine Clinics of North America*, Drs. Jon Mark Hirshon and David Morris use their combined training in emergency medicine and public health to discuss this bridge. Various approaches to public health care in the ED are described by the editors and authors. At the same time, they are able to keep their focus on the concept that the ED is not the primary care clinic and does not have unlimited resources. The final article discusses future needs and trends in public health research.

The editors and authors are to be commended for creating this issue of *Clinics*. It represents a valuable addition to the series and should be considered must reading for anyone who desires to truly understand the incredible importance and unrealized potential of EM in our society.

Amal Mattu, MD
Department of Emergency Medicine
University of Maryland School of Medicine
Baltimore, MD, USA

E-mail address: amattu@smail.umaryland.edu

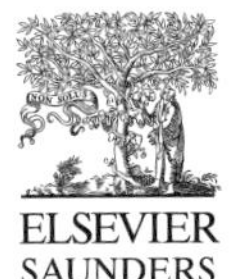
ELSEVIER
SAUNDERS

Emerg Med Clin N Am
24 (2006) xvii–xviii

EMERGENCY
MEDICINE
CLINICS OF
NORTH AMERICA

Preface

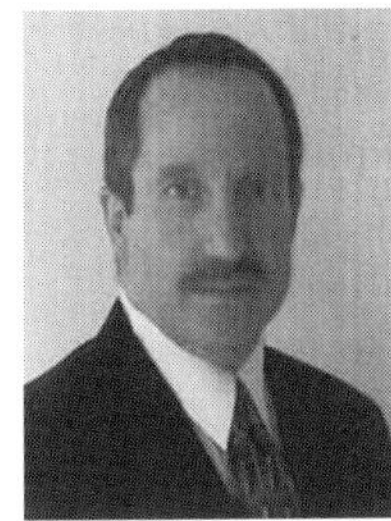 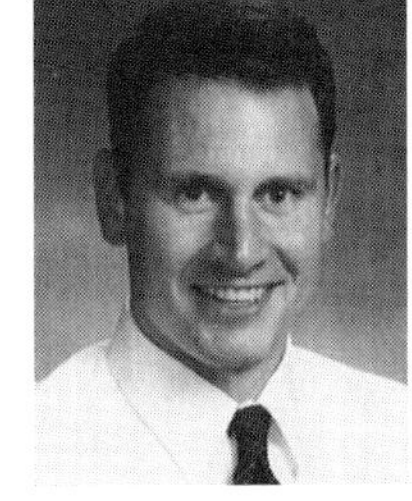

Jon Mark Hirshon, MD, MPH   David M. Morris, MD, MPH
Guest Editors

As clearly highlighted in the recent Institute of Medicine report titled *The Future of Emergency Care in the United States Health System*, emergency medicine and emergency departments (EDs) play a critical role within the American health system in providing needed care to millions of individuals every year. EDs are situated in a critical location at the interface of the American population and entry into hospitals and the medical care system. One cannot wear blinders and work in EDs; all of the health problems and many of the social problems of our society come to rest on our doorstep. Community members often view EDs as the main door into hospitals, and health professionals can conceptually understand the ED as a window on the health and social needs of our people.

This issue of the *Emergency Medicine Clinics of North America* focuses on the spectrum of public health issues that pertain to the practice of emergency medicine and that are faced by practicing emergency physicians every day. Topics include public health research in the ED; respiratory threats; emerging infectious diseases; ED overcrowding; end-of-life care; racial and ethnic disparities; issues of health promotion and disease prevention encompassing substance and alcohol abuse, injury, and violence; as well as public health surveillance, including the impacts of homeless and disadvantaged patients.

Understanding the interplay between medicine and public health is critical to addressing the health needs of Americans. This *Emergency Medicine Clinics* introduces and helps define many of the key public health issues impacting emergency practitioners. These issues are not abstractions, but are faced by us on a daily basis as we try to help the homeless to find needed

doi:10.1016/j.emc.2006.07.001   *emed.theclinics.com*

health care or look for ways to prevent a chronic drinker from driving while intoxicated. These articles discuss important modern societal problems that are part of the context in which we currently practice.

Jon Mark Hirshon, MD, MPH
The Charles McC. Mathias, Jr. National Study Center for Trauma and EMS
701 West Pratt Street, Room 524
Baltimore, MD 21201, USA

E-mail address: JHirs001@umaryland.edu

David M. Morris, MD, MPH
Framingham Union Hospital
115 Lincoln Street
Framingham, MA 01702, USA

E-mail address: Dmorris@quantech.net

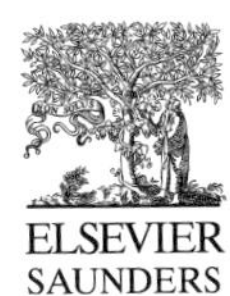
ELSEVIER
SAUNDERS

Emerg Med Clin N Am
24 (2006) 815–819

EMERGENCY
MEDICINE
CLINICS OF
NORTH AMERICA

Emergency Medicine and the Health of the Public: The Critical Role of Emergency Departments in US Public Health

Jon Mark Hirshon, MD, MPH[a],*,
David M. Morris, MD, MPH[b]

[a]Department of Emergency Medicine and Department of Epidemiology
and Preventive Medicine, University of Maryland School of Medicine,
The Charles McC. Mathias, Jr. National Study Center for Trauma and EMS,
701 West Pratt Street, Room 524, Baltimore, MD 21201, USA
[b]Department of Emergency Medicine, MetroWest Medical Center, Framingham Union
Hospital, Framingham, MA 01702, USA

Emergency departments (EDs) are situated in a critical location at the interface of the American population and the health care system. One cannot wear blinders and work in emergency medicine; all the health problems and many of the social problems of society come to rest on the doorstep. Community members often view EDs as the main door into hospitals, whereas health professionals can conceptually understand the ED as a window on the health and social needs of the people.

Understanding the interplay between medicine and public health is critical to addressing the health needs of Americans. This has been an issue previously recognized by the Institutes of Medicine [1,2]. Emergency physicians and their coworkers within and outside of EDs have the opportunity to improve the health of communities though understanding their health and social needs and developing appropriate and effective interventions.

What is public health?

Throughout history ill individuals have been separated from other people, although the concept of a 40-day isolation period (from Italian

---

* Corresponding author.
E-mail address: jhirs001@umaryland.edu (J.M. Hirshon).

doi:10.1016/j.emc.2006.06.012   *emed.theclinics.com*

quaranta giorni) originated in Venice in the fourteenth century as a means of addressing the problem of ships arriving with individuals potentially infected with the Black Death. Many local public health departments within the United States were started in response to outbreak events. For example, the Baltimore City Health Department was started over 200 years ago as a response to a yellow fever outbreak and to stop the spread of communicable diseases [3]. American public health on the national level dates back to the immigration laws of the 1800s. With large influxes of newcomers, physicians at Ellis Island in New York Harbor provided health inspections to all immigrants and looked for signs of contagious diseases, criminal behavior, and medical and psychiatric illness [4]. Since that time, multiple federal laws have been passed and federal agencies created to respond to infectious diseases and the importation of these diseases. These various actions helped lead to the development of the federal Public Health Service, and are part of the background that led to the creation of the current Centers for Disease Control and Prevention, which is part of the Department of Health and Human Services. The mission of the Centers for Disease Control and Prevention is "to promote health and quality of life by preventing and controlling disease, injury, and disability" [5]. It is recognized as the lead federal agency in this regard. There are many dimensions to improving the general health of Americans, from public water and sanitation works to social, behavioral, and environmental influences on patients [6]. The underlying theme in public health is health promotion and disease prevention, emphasizing efforts to reduce the amount of disease, morbidity, and mortality from disease and the burden of illness on the general population. This is a multidimensional task that includes general medical practices, individual practices, and the science of epidemiology.

The current public health system is designed to track acute and chronic illnesses, and to anticipate future threats, such as from influenza A H5N1, currently called avian flu. Surveillance of disease patterns and trends is essential to gaining understanding of treatment and prevention for populations and individuals. Identification of risk factors for illness and injury is vital, because these are the basis for intervention. Establishing a link between an exposure and disease outcome allows health care professionals to intervene to reduce the prevalence and morbidity and mortality of a disease [7].

What is emergency medicine?

Emergency medicine is a relatively young specialty that has evolved into a field of medicine that focuses on managing and evaluating critically ill and injured patients. Emergency medicine is designed to provide medical care to the general public 24 hours a day, 7 days a week, every day of the year. The ED has its front door open to insured and uninsured alike, with no preferential treatment. Medical acuity and urgency dictated the flow of patients, with the sick patients receiving immediate attention. All comers arriving to an ED are evaluated without a financial screen. Regardless of socioeconomic background, ethnicity, gender, or nationality, a person arriving to the ED is seen and treated. The practice of emergency medicine places emphasis on treating an individual and his or her physical manifestations of disease and injury [8].

How do emergency medicine and public health interface?

The current public health infrastructure concentrates on preventing adverse health outcomes and reducing risk for disease. The health of the population is the center of attention in public health, compared with the individual, which is the focus of emergency medicine. Public health interventions are often designed for long-term effect and may span months or years. In the ED, most interventions are implemented for immediate effect. Despite these differences, the health of the population is the common theme across these fields. The ED guarantees accessible health care and services for the general public including underserved and uninsured populations. As the safety net for health care the ED provides acute and urgent care to patients in rural and urban settings. The ED is typically located at the center of numerous epidemics including infectious disease, violence, and substance abuse. It is a logical place for public health and emergency medicine to partner together to protect and improve the health of the population [9].

Specific areas ready for collaboration

Many public health policies are meant to ensure access to health care for everyone. Problems related to ED crowding provide a unique opportunity to evaluate ongoing access to care in rural and urban communities. Analysis of ED volumes and obstacles facing patients from the waiting room to treatment to ultimate disposition is challenging. In-depth examination of ED crowding beyond established statistics of frequency of ED visits has potential to provide valuable insights into health care access [10].

Health promotion and disease prevention approaches should be implemented more uniformly in the ED. Emergency physicians are part of the continuum of health care and are in a unique place to establish meaningful communication to patients in acute crisis. Many patients lack other sources of routine health care, making the ED the central location for physicians to identify health problems and intervene effectively. Tertiary preventive care is a routine part of emergency care. Primary and secondary preventive services may not always be applicable to emergency services. There are select services that can be effectively administered in the ED, however, without impairing the sole responsibility of treating ill patients. Some examples include referral of children without primary care to continuity clinics, delivering educational messages on tobacco and alcohol use, updating tetanus, and screening for domestic violence [11].

The ED is the frontline for early identification of respiratory and infectious disease outbreaks. These diseases typically present in an acute nature, making the ED a principal site of health care. Reducing illness among patients with disease, and early identification and prevention of disease, are crucial practices in the ED.

High-risk groups susceptible to injury and violence are usually treated in the ED. Emergency physicians have a close look at patients who are victims of injury and violence. ED workers have an opportunity to identify risk factors for violence and injury, which can help guide public health policies to reduce their incidence and prevalence.

Summary

Understanding the interplay between medicine and public health is critical to addressing the health needs of Americans. This issue of the *Emergency Medicine Clinics of North America* focuses on the spectrum of public health issues that pertain to the practice of emergency medicine. Topics include public health research in the ED; respiratory threats; emerging infectious diseases; ED overcrowding; end-of-life care; racial and ethnic disparities; issues of health promotion and disease prevention encompassing substance abuse, alcohol, and injury and violence; and public health surveillance including the impacts of homeless and disadvantaged patients. This article creates a comprehensive review of important topics for emergency physicians to improve the understanding of the role that EDs and emergency medicine play in the health of the American public.

References

[1] Committee for the Study of the Future of Public Health; Division of Health Care Services. The future of public health. Institute of Medicine of the National Academies. Washington, DC: The National Academies Press; 1988.

[2] The future of the public's health in the 21st century. Committee on Assuring the Health of the Public in the 21st Century. Institute of Medicine of the National Academies. Washington, DC: The National Academies Press; 2002.

[3] Beilenson PL, Lambropoulos AS. Baltimore City Health Department: 200 years of progress and partnership. Md Med J 1993;42:729–33.

[4] Parascandola J. Doctors at the gate. PHS at Ellis Island. Public Health Rep 1998;113:83–6.

[5] CDC. About CDC. Available at: http://www.cdc.gov/aboutcdc.htm. Accessed July 19, 2006.

[6] Dolan JP, Adams-Smith WN. Health and society: a documentary history of medicine. New York: Seabury Press; 1978.

[7] Bernstrin E, Goldfrank LR, Kellemann AL, et al. A public health approach to emergency medicine: preparing for the twenty-first century. Acad Emerg Med 1994;1:277–86.

[8] Krome R. Twenty-five years of evolution and revolution: how the specialty has changed. Ann Emerg Med 1997;30:689–90.

[9] Clancy CM, Eisenberg JM. Emergency medicine in population-based systems of care. Ann Emerg Med 1997;30:800–3.

[10] Richardson LD, Hwang U. Access to care: a review of the emergency medicine literature. Acad Emerg Med 2001;8:1030–6.

[11] Rhodes KV, Gordon JA, Lowe RA. Preventive care in the emergency department, Part I: Clinical preventive services –are they relevant to emergency medicine? Society for Academic Emergency Medicine Public Health and Education Task Force Preventive Services Work Group. Acad Emerg Med 2000;7:1035–41.

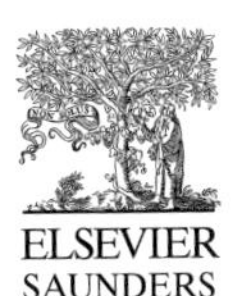
ELSEVIER
SAUNDERS

Emerg Med Clin N Am
24 (2006) 821–837

EMERGENCY
MEDICINE
CLINICS OF
NORTH AMERICA

Emergency Department Crowding: Old Problem, New Solutions

Steven L. Bernstein, MD*, Brent R. Asplin, MD, MPH

*Department of Emergency Medicine, Albert Einstein College of Medicine,
Montefiore Medical Center, 111 East 210th Street,
Bronx, NY 10467, USA*

In the 1990s, United States emergency departments (EDs) experienced explosive growth in patient visits, concurrent with a sharp decline in the number of hospital EDs. According to data from the National Hospital Ambulatory Medical Care Survey, annual ED visit volume rose 27% from 89.8 million to 113.9 million between 1992 and 2003 [1,2]. At the same time, the number of EDs fell 22%, from 5169 in 1988 to 4037 in 2002 [3]. Fig. 1 illustrates these trends. Over 15 years, the simple arithmetic demonstrates the basis for ED crowding. Although ED crowding is clearly related to ED volume, an ED can be busy without being crowded. Crowding refers to a condition when the needs of the patients in the ED (and patients in the waiting room) exceed the capacity of the department. Crowding is a function of patient volume, patient acuity, physical space, and on-duty staff. With increasing attention being paid to EDs as a vital component of the nation's health care safety net [4–7], ED crowding has moved to the top of the policy agenda in emergency medicine.

Origins of crowding

Early descriptions of ED crowding focused on the growth in the number of substance users, homeless, AIDS patients, and mentally ill in urban areas [8,9]. A 1993 report by the General Accounting Office attributed the growing volume of ED visits to these factors, noting that many of these patients were uninsured or had Medicaid and were using the ED for nonurgent conditions [9]. More visits by the elderly also were noted. This report and others

---

* Corresponding author.
E-mail address: sbernste@montefiore.org (S.L. Bernstein).

doi:10.1016/j.emc.2006.06.013   *emed.theclinics.com*

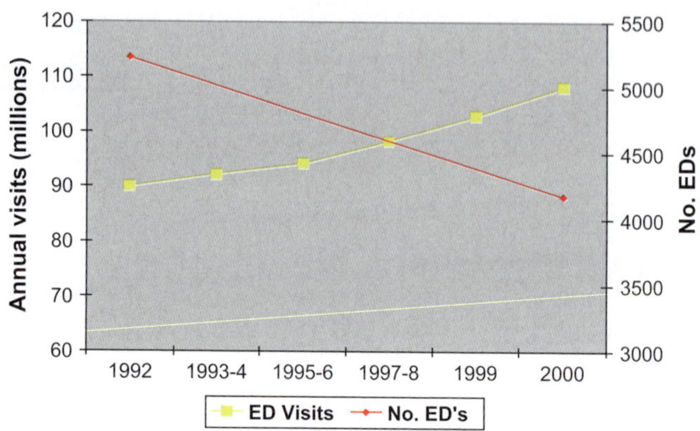

Fig. 1. Number of emergency departments, patient volume, 1992–2000.

focused attention on nonurgent, or unnecessary, visits by uninsured and underinsured patients as the root cause of ED crowding.

Modern concepts: 2003 Government Accounting Office report

In 2003 the Government Accounting Office revisited the issue of ED crowding [10]. In contrast to its 1993 study, this time the Government Accounting Office found that the single greatest contributor to ED crowding was the prolonged presence in the ED of patients already admitted to the hospital, for who no inpatient beds were available. These patients, known variously as boarders or holds, require considerable amounts of nursing time, physician time, and medical resources. They also, by virtue of occupying ED beds, prevent new patients from being seen and treated. Australian investigators refer to this phenomenon as "access block" [11,12]. It has become apparent that reduction of ED crowding necessitates more efficient management of boarders, including faster transfer to inpatient units. In addition, data now exist to suggest that low-acuity patients with nonurgent conditions contribute little, if at all, to the problems of crowding and ambulance diversion [13]. Nor does lack of insurance seem to be a powerful driver of ED usage: a 2003 report noted that two thirds of the increase in ED visits between 1996 and 1997 and 2000 and 2001 was accounted for by patients with private insurance or Medicare [14].

Financial implications of emergency department crowding

The 1980s and early 1990s were characterized by a relative lack of interest in addressing crowding by policy makers and hospital administrators. The perception that there were no financial implications to the hospital from a crowded ED may have permitted this lack of interest. In fact, a crowded

ED meant, on some level, that inpatient occupancy was high and "business was good." A 2002 study of a single hospital in New Jersey found that 34% of the gross revenue for inpatient services was contributed by patients admitted from the ED [15]. A 1994 study by Krochmal and Riley [16], however, showed that at a single hospital, inpatient length of stay was prolonged by a day or more for patients who spent at least 1 day in the ED. A more recent study of chest pain patients admitted to an urban teaching hospital showed no correlation between ED length of stay and total hospital length of stay, hospital costs, professional charges, and revenues. This study, however, demonstrated a modest opportunity cost of $204 per patient among those patients who waited 3 or more hours for an inpatient bed [17]. Although ED admissions provide a steady, reliable, and important revenue stream for hospitals, delays in transfer to inpatient beds represent lost revenue.

International dimensions of crowding

ED crowding has been studied and described most intensively from a North American perspective, but has been reported in Taiwan [18], Great Britain [19], Spain [20], and Australia [11,13]. These papers describe similar conditions: emergency care systems overwhelmed by demand for services, an inability to meet demands largely caused by delays in moving admitted patients to inpatient beds, and adverse quality outcomes.

Conceptual model: input-throughput-output

One early challenge for researchers and policymakers addressing ED crowding had been the lack of a theoretical framework. This problem was largely addressed with the publication in 2003 of the input-throughput-output conceptual model of ED crowding, described by Asplin and coworkers [21]. This model, reproduced in Table 1, posits a set of 38 measures of ED and hospital workflow that contribute to ED crowding at varying points in the patient flow process [22]. The measures are divided into three domains: input, throughput, and output, which corresponds to their "sites of action." The model explains ED crowding as resulting from increased numbers or acuity of arriving patients, inefficient ED operational processes, and downstream obstacles to moving patients out of the ED or some combination of these factors.

Measures of emergency department crowding

A fundamental difficulty in studying ED crowding is the lack of a universally accepted definition; there is no criterion standard [23]. The existing literature on ED crowding is characterized by confusion among causes of crowding, outcomes of crowding, measures of the phenomenon itself, and hospital-based measures [23]. Proposed markers of ED crowding are

Table 1
Consensus measures of ED crowding

Input measures	Throughput measures	Output measures
ED patient volume, standardized for bed hours	ED throughput time	ED boarding time
ED patient volume, standardized for annual average	ED bed placement time	ED boarding time components
ED ambulance volume, standardized for bed hours	ED ancillary service turnaround time	Boarding burden
ED ambulance volume, standardized for annual average	Summary workload, standardized for ED bed hours	Hospital admission source, standardized and adjusted
Patient source	Summary workload, standardized for nurse staff hours	ED admission transfer rate
Percentage of open appointments	Summary workload, standardized for physician staff hours	Hospital discharge potential
Percentage of patients who leave without treatment complete	ED occupancy rate	Hospital discharge process interval
Leave without treatment complete severity	ED occupancy	Inpatient cycling time
Ambulance diversion episodes	Patient disposition to physician staffing ratio	Hospital census
Ambulance diversion requests denied and forced openings		Hospital occupancy rate
Diverted ambulance patient description		Hospital supply and demand status forecast
Average EMS waiting time		Observation unit census
Patient complexity assessed at triage		ED volume/hospital capacity ratio
Patient complexity as percentage of ambulance patients		Agency nursing expenditures
Patient complexity as assessed by coding		

Abbreviations: ED, emergency department; EMS; emergency medical services.

Adapted from Solberg LI, Asplin BR, Weinick RM, et al. Emergency department crowding: consensus development of potential measures. Ann Emerg Med 2003;42:824–34; with permission.

numerous; they are summarized in Box 1. Many of these measures incorporate elements of the input-throughput-output model [21] and offer some use. Unfortunately, many of these measures are specific to a certain type of ED and cannot be applied across the wide variations in size, visit volume, acuity, and staffing capacity found in United States EDs.

A recent attempt to create a more uniform set of ED crowding measures involved a panel of 74 experts using a modified Delphi process [22]. The result was a list of 38 potential measures grouped into seven domains: (1) patient demand, (2) patient complexity, (3) ED capacity, (4) ED workload, (5) ED efficiency, (6) hospital capacity, and (7) hospital efficiency. The measures are listed in Table 1, along with their place within the input-throughput-output model.

An ideal measure of ED crowding is universal, reproducible, and consistently accurate across EDs of different sizes. It consists of data elements that are immediately available from existing sources or continuously monitored by existing information systems. An additional desirable feature of the measure is programmability into an ED's electronic patient tracking system, so that it could be used as a real-time measure of crowding. Such a measure provides an opportunity to study the relationships between ED crowding and quality, and ED crowding and adverse events [24].

Several candidate measures of ED crowding have been developed and tested, most at single institutions, two from multiple sites. Their generalizability is unclear. All, explicitly or implicitly, incorporate components of the input-throughput-output model. None have been prospectively validated or studied as real-time dashboard measures of crowding. These measures are all dynamic: their values may change from moment to moment. These omnibus scores are described next.

Emergency Department Crowding Score

This recently published score was developed at eight academic EDs in a prospective time series study [25]. The Emergency Department Crowding Score was developed by fitting an ordinal logistic model to variables identified from the input-throughput-output model, using physician and nurse assessment of crowding as the criterion standard. Variables found to be independently predictive of crowding were the number of boarders, the total number of ED patients, and the number of critical care patients. The Emergency Department Crowding Score was significantly associated with ED length of stay, mean boarding time, patients leaving without being seen, and diversion. The Emergency Department Crowding Score is scaled from 0 to 100; diversion and patients leaving without being seen become more likely when the score exceeds 65. The possible existence of a threshold Emergency Department Crowding Score, above which care and quality suffer, is an intriguing feature of this measure. The Emergency Department Crowding Score is currently being studied in real-time fashion at the principal investigator's ED.

Box 1. Definitions of ED crowding

1. ED factors
- Real-time computerized tracking of waiting times, treatment times, and current census of actual patients in the ED being treated or waiting to be seen
- Number of visits >120 per day
- Lack of capacity in observation area
- Response of nurses' and physicians' opinions of ED crowding and telling of being rushed
- ED bed ratio, acuity ratio, provider ratio, demand value
- Patients wait >30 minutes, or all ED beds filled >6 h/day, or patients placed in ED hallway, or physicians rushed
- Patients wait >30 minutes, patients wait >60 minutes, ED beds filled >6 h/day, patients placed in hallways >6 h/day, emergency physicians feel rushed >6 h/day
- Patients wait >60 minutes to see physician, ED beds full >6 h/day, patients placed in ED hallways >6 h/day, emergency physicians feel rushed >6 h/day, waiting room filled >6 h/day

2. Hospital factors
- When there are no in-hospital beds for patients admitted from the ED
- ED crowding occurs when ED patients are ready but unable to be admitted to either a floor or an ICU bed and are held in the ED
- Reduction of inpatient beds and a critical shortage of health care professionals
- When admitted ED patients cannot leave the department because all staffed inpatient and ICU hospital beds are occupied and no beds are available in neighboring facilities for transfer
- From boarding inpatients already admitted to the hospital for hours to several days
- When patients needing admission cannot leave the ED because of unavailability of inpatient beds
- When admitted ED patients cannot leave the department because all staffed inpatient and ICU beds in the hospital are occupied and no beds are available in neighboring facilities for transfer
- When acute care beds become filled
- When the delay in transfer of admitted patient to a hospital bed is longer than 4 h
- (Admitted) patients held overnight in the ED
- Too many sick patients, and too many admitted patients

3. External factors
- Periods of ambulance diversion

4. Combination of factors
- Patients wait >90 minutes, ED beds filled >6 h/day, >30% ED beds filled with admitted patients, patients in hallway >6 h/day, full waiting room >6 h/day
- Registered ED patients who leave without being seen, and frequency and duration of emergency medical services diversion
- Staff shortages, lack of available beds, poor operational process, increased number of patients who seek care, lack of universal access, shortage of inpatient beds, and hospital closures

5. Omnibus measures (see text for further discussion)
- Emergency Department Crowding Score
- Emergency Department Work Index
- National Emergency Department Overcrowding Score
- Real-time Emergency Analysis of Demand Indicators Scores

Adapted from Hwang U, Concato J. Care in the emergency department: how crowded is overcrowded? Acad Emerg Med 2004;11:1097–101; with permission.

Emergency Department Work Index

This index, also known as EDWIN, incorporates components of the input-throughput-output model (number and acuity of patients, ED staffing, and bed availability) into a composite index [26]. The index is defined as follows: $\text{EDWIN} = \sum n_{it} t_j / N_t (B - B_t)$, where n_i = the number of patients present in the ED in triage category i at time t; where t_j = the triage score (ordinal scale 1-5, 5 being most acute) for the jth patient; where N_t = the number of attending physicians on duty at time t; where B = the total number of beds or treatment bays available in the ED (a constant); and where B_t = the number of admitted patients (holds) in the ED at time t.

Once a patient is admitted, he or she is counted as a "hold," and is removed from the numerator, which is a sum of the triage categories of all active patients in the ED. The number of treatment bays (B) is derived from the ED's original blueprint. It omits beds creatively placed in hallways and corners by ED personnel. It also omits the second bed in a room designed for one patient that has been "doubled up."

The triage system used is the Emergency Severity Index, a five-level instrument that has high interobserver agreement, and is associated with resource use, hospitalization rates, and 6-month survival [27,28]. The Emergency Severity Index is modified slightly by reversing the ordinal ranking of triage categories: 1 is the least acute patient and 5 is the sickest. Hence, the units of EDWIN may be represented as "patient triage units per attending physician per available bed." Its numerator and denominator represent the ratio of ED workload (patient triage scores) to ED resources (staff and available beds).

EDWIN was developed and tested at a single ED [26]. This prospective, observational study measured agreement between nurse and physician perceptions of ED crowding and EDWIN, and studied the strength of association between EDWIN and a composite index of clinical end points. End points were defined as 72-hour return patients who are admitted, clinically important radiograph discordance between the emergency physician and radiologist, and cases referred to hospital quality improvement personnel in whom deviation from standard of care was found.

EDWIN showed excellent correlation with nurse and physician assessment of crowding, and was strongly predictive of ambulance diversion. EDWIN scores were also found to be slightly higher in patients with the composite end point than in patients without these outcomes. EDWIN was not higher in patients who left without being seen.

The data suggest that ED activity may be demarcated into three ordinal zones: (1) an active but manageable ED has an EDWIN score <1.5, (2) a busy ED has an EDWIN between 1.5 and 2, and (3) a crowded ED has a score >2. These active, busy, and crowded zones suggest an "ABC" paradigm to characterize ED activity. EDWIN remains to be tested at other institutions.

National Emergency Department Overcrowding Study

The National Emergency Department Overcrowding Study score is a five-question instrument that was developed at eight academic EDs and then validated against charge nurse and attending physician assessment of crowding [29]. The five data elements in the National Emergency Department Overcrowding Study score are: (1) number of ED patients divided by number of ED beds, (2) number of admitted patients in ED divided by number of hospital beds, (3) number of ED patients using a mechanical ventilator, (4) longest admit time for any ED patient, and (5) waiting room time of the last patient placed in an ED bed. Nomograms are used to assign points for the answers to these questions. The total number of points is then summed and referred to another nomogram to derive the final score, which is scaled from 0 to 200. This score showed good agreement with a composite outcome variable consisting of nurse and physician perceptions of crowding and the physician's sense of feeling rushed.

Real-Time Emergency Analysis of Demand Indicators scores

The Real-Time Emergency Analysis of Demand Indicators scores are a group of three measures of demand and capacity, developed for real-time use, which were measured against doctor and nurse perceptions of crowding [30]. The measures used are defined as follows:

$$\text{Bed Ratio} = (\text{number of patients in ED} + \text{predicted arrivals} - \text{predicted departures})/\text{ED spaces}$$

$$\text{Acuity Ratio} = \sum (\text{triage category})(\text{number in each category})/\text{number of patients}$$

$$\text{Provider Ratio} = \text{arrivals per hour}/\sum (\text{patients seen hourly by each physician})$$

$$\text{Demand Value} = (\text{Bed Radio} + \text{Provider Ratio}) \times (\text{Acuity Ratio})$$

During a 1-month study at a single ED, the investigators found poor agreement between the Real-Time Emergency Analysis of Demand Indicators scores and ED physician and nurse subjective assessments of crowding (kappas ranging from 0.02–0.21). Limitations of the study included poor response rate by providers (59%); possibly erroneous assumptions regarding predicted ED arrivals and discharges; and lack of real-time electronic calculation of the score.

Additional scores

A number of other crowding scores have been developed at single institutions in Boston [31], Spain [20,32], and Australia [33–37]. All incorporate some variables from the input-throughput-output model, such as total numbers of visits, total daily patient care time, and numbers of patients in various sections of the ED. These scores were tested against a variety of measures including 72-hour returns who were admitted, mortality rate, and diversion. None have been validated, scaled for use by EDs of different sizes, or used as real-time measures of crowding.

Recent policy and administrative interventions to alleviate crowding

The last 4 years have seen the first sustained policy, administrative, and clinical initiatives to cope with ED crowding. In part, this flurry of activity was spurred by the 2001 "Expert Meeting on ED Crowding and Ambulance Diversion," convened by the US Department of Health and Human Services [38]. These measures have met with some success, because episodes of ambulance diversion (defined as closing an ED to arriving ambulances) became less frequent in 2002 to 2003 than in previous years [39].

Hallway admissions

In 2000, New York State Commissioner of Health and former US Surgeon General Antonia Novello issued a directive to all acute care hospitals in the state, permitting the placement of admitted ED patients in "hallway" spaces of inpatient wards, if an inpatient room was unavailable [40]. Although not yet universally implemented, anecdotal evidence suggests this directive has allowed the two hospitals in this study to relieve some ED congestion, with no apparent adverse clinical outcomes.

Joint Commission on the Accreditation of Health Care Organizations

In 2003, the Joint Commission on the Accreditation of Health Care Organizations, a voluntary body that accredits and evaluates quality for hospitals and health care systems, issued landmark guidelines on crowding (available at www.jcaho.org). For the first time, the Joint Commission recognized the link between crowding and quality. Without mandating specific policies, these guidelines call for hospitals to have plans in place to handle crowded EDs, and to provide a level of service to admitted patients boarding in the ED comparable with that which they would receive on inpatient units. The guidelines are too recent to have had their impact assessed, but Joint Commission mandates typically result in substantial changes in hospital policy and procedure.

Urgent Matters

In 2002, the Robert Wood Johnson Foundation began a national program designed to identify practical solutions to ED crowding, and to assess its impact on the health care safety net. The program, Urgent Matters (www.urgentmatters.org), awarded 10 grants to health care systems throughout the country. Early results from Urgent Matters suggest that a combination of hospital-wide policies can reduce diversion and improve ED throughput; these include greater attention to inpatient discharge planning, faster turnaround from radiology and laboratory services, and greater coordination of care among EDs in a geographic region.

The 10 Urgent Matters hospitals used a variety of activities to alleviate crowding. Some examples of these strategies are given in Table 2. Because different institutions have different needs and capabilities, it is important for hospital leadership to understand which strategies are locally appropriate. Nonetheless, the Urgent Matters study team identified seven themes common to all sites [41]:

1. Hospital leadership must recognize that ED crowding is a hospital-wide problem, not an ED problem
2. Multidisciplinary teams are needed to design and implement change
3. An institutional champion for change is needed
4. Senior leadership must publicly support ED crowding reduction initiatives
5. Formal quality improvement tools, such as rapid cycle change, are needed
6. Routine and rigorous data collection is essential
7. Initiatives and data must be transparent to enhance buy-in from all stakeholders

A research agenda

The literature on ED crowding has developed substantially in 15 years. Early papers focused on qualitative definitions and descriptions of crowding. More recent work has sought to develop reproducible, quantifiable measures of crowding, link crowding to adverse quality outcomes, and propose policy and administrative interventions to alleviate crowding. The rapidly growing use of computerized clinical support systems in United States EDs will assist these efforts [42]. Fig. 2 shows the growth in the number of crowding papers in the English language medical literature from 1989 to 2004. The search examined English-language journals in Medline using "emergency department overcrowding" or "emergency department crowding" as keywords.

Four areas of focus have been cited for a research agenda in ED crowding [21,24]:

1. Development of valid and reliable measures of crowding
2. Understanding the causes of crowding
3. Exploring the link between crowding and quality of care
4. Testing interventions to alleviate crowding.

Substantial progress has been made in the development of metrics to quantify crowding, although a validated, omnibus measure is still lacking. Similarly, there is now a deeper understanding of the causes of crowding. There has been some progress in designing and testing interventions to reduce crowding [43,44], although important work in this area yet remains.

Additional insights into causes and potential solutions for ED crowding have been provided by concepts borrowed from the fields of econometrics and operations research [45]. Siddharthan and coworkers [46] used queuing theory to quantify the contribution of nonurgent visits to ED workload and waiting times. Bagust and coworkers [19] developed a discrete-event

Table 2
Strategies and innovations to address crowding

Category	Strategies and innovations
Patient flow coordination and facilitation	Implement a "bed czar" or patient flow manager by designating a specific position responsible for ensuring the timely transfer of ED patients to assigned inpatient beds
	Dedicate a nurse with admission-discharge-transfer duties who is specifically responsible for facilitating pending discharges to accelerate available beds for admits
	Develop accelerated triage and registration processes to triage more efficiently based on the patient's acuity and to reduce waiting times by reordering or combining triage and registration processes
Early discharge	Initiate preliminary discharge by designating patients for early discharge the next day
	Redesign rounding and discharge processes to focus on patients ready for discharge
	Create a discharge room or lounge for inpatients who have been discharged and are awaiting transportation, medications, or education
	Establish a discharge coordinator position to coordinate procuring information that is required to discharge the patient
	Implement financial (bonuses) and nonfinancial (movie tickets or cafeteria vouchers) incentives for physicians and nurses to promote efficient and early discharge of patients who are ready to go home
Boarding and inpatient bed assignment	Replace the traditional "push system" with a "pull system" in which the inpatient floors play an active role in pulling ED patients into available beds
Diversion management and reduction	Establish new protocols and monitoring systems to determine when the hospital is approaching maximum operating capacity and its threshold for diversion
	Develop a hospital-wide diversion response protocol to focus existing resources on facilitating all appropriate patient discharges in a more timely manner
	Create a community-wide diversion plan in collaboration with local hospitals and the community's emergency medical services unit to establish common protocol for hospitals going on and off diversion or bypass

Abbreviation: ED, emergency department.

Adapted from Wilson MJ, Nguyen K. Bursting at the seams: improving patient flow to help America's emergency departments. Washington: Urgent Matters/George Washington University Medical Center; 2004; with permission.

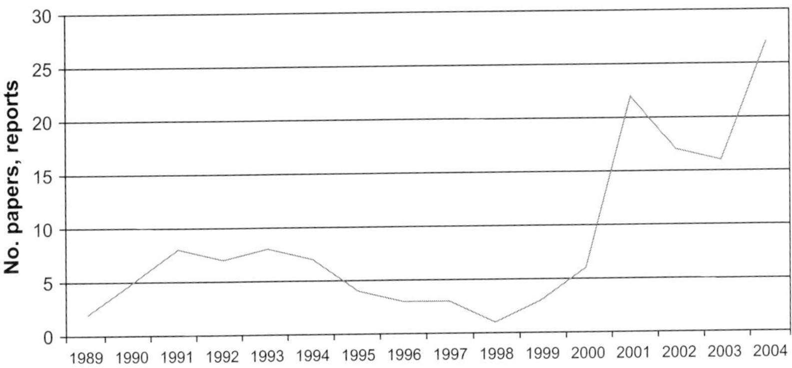

Fig. 2. Number of papers and reports on emergency department crowding, 1989–2004.

stochastic simulation model to demonstrate that prompt access to hospital beds for newly admitted patients is threatened when inpatient occupancy exceeds 85% to 90%. Litvak's studies of strategies to smooth artificial variability in scheduling elective surgical cases contributed substantially to the reduction in ED crowding at Boston Medical Center [41,47].

A critical piece of the research agenda in crowding is to explore the link between crowding and quality of care [24]. To date, there has been only anecdotal evidence, and some limited reports, of adverse quality outcomes resulting from crowding. Miro and coworkers [32] found an association between ED visit volume and mortality. Derlet [48,49] has reported cases of missed myocardial infarction, intracranial hemorrhage, and pediatric sepsis during periods of crowding. Schull and coworkers [50] found that time to administration of thrombolytic increased during periods of community-wide ambulance diversion. Sprivulis and coworkers [51] found an association between ED and inpatient bed occupancy and 7-day mortality for patients admitted through the ED.

The six dimensions of quality defined by the Institute of Medicine can provide a template for investigators: (1) safety, (2) patient centeredness, (3) timeliness, (4) efficiency, (5) effectiveness, and (6) equity [52]. The increasing focus on patient safety and quality of care, spurred by several Institute of Medicine reports, may drive the research agenda on ED crowding. Both federal agencies and nonprofit organizations have funded research in ED crowding, including the Agency for Healthcare Research and Quality, the Robert Wood Johnson Foundation, and the Kaiser Family Foundation. It seems likely that funders will continue to remain interested in crowding.

Some research questions that await study include:

- Is pain management delayed or omitted during periods of crowding?
- Are times to reperfusion longer for patients with acute myocardial infarction?

- Are patients with acute coronary syndrome less likely to receive aspirin or β-blockers, or will administration of these drugs be delayed?
- Do patients with infections requiring intravenous antibiotics wait longer to receive their initial dose?
- Do patients with asthma wait longer to receive their inhaled β-agonists or corticosteroids?
- Are medication errors and near misses more common during crowding?
- Do important imaging studies, like head CTs, take longer to perform?
- Are emergency physicians more likely to misread radiographs?
- Does patient satisfaction decrease during crowding?
- Are patient walkouts and departures against medical advice more common?
- Are patients more likely to make an unscheduled return visit within 72 hours if the initial visit occurred during a period of crowding?
- What kinds of interventions can alleviate crowding, improve quality and safety, and be generalized to other EDs?

The potential research agenda is rich; the burgeoning use of electronic health information systems should facilitate this work. United States EDs are increasingly computerized; between 2001 and 2003, 31% used electronic patient medical records and 40% used automated drug dispensing systems, higher than in outpatient departments and physician offices [42].

By exploring the real-time use of various crowding measures, researchers can fulfill the Agency for Healthcare Research and Quality's mission to translate research into practice and "improve the quality, safety, efficiency and effectiveness of health care for all Americans" [53]. Further, it allows the ongoing monitoring and evaluation of ED data "to understand trends and provide early warning of impending health care crises, particularly those which may disproportionately affect safety net populations" [6].

Summary

ED crowding is an administrative problem with important clinical consequences that has waxed and waned in severity for at least 15 years. The current state of knowledge recognizes input, throughput, and output contributors to crowding; on a national scale, output variables contribute the greatest delays. Substantial progress has been made in quantifying and measuring crowding. Recent work has begun to explore crowding's effects on patient safety and quality of care. In the last few years, analysis of ED operations through the lens of operations management has begun to yield administrative interventions that have ameliorated crowding in larger centers. Significant work remains to be done to correlate crowding with adverse outcomes and medical error and to explore the generalizability of these administrative interventions.

References

[1] Burt CW, McCaig LF. Trends in hospital emergency department utilization: United States, 1992–99. National Center for Health Statistics. Vital Health Stat 2001;13:1.

[2] McCaig LF, Burt CW. National Hospital Ambulatory Medical Care Survey: 2003 emergency department summary. Advance data from vital health and statistics; no 358. Hyattsville (MD): National Center for Health Statistics; 2005.

[3] American College of Emergency Physicians. Emergency medicine statistical profile. Available at: www.acep.org. Accessed June 23, 2006.

[4] Richardson LD, Hwang U. America's health care safety net: intact or unraveling? Acad Emerg Med 2001;8:1056–63.

[5] Richardson LD, Hwang U. Access to care: a review of the emergency medicine literature. Acad Emerg Med 2001;8:1030–6.

[6] Weinick RM, Burstin H. Monitoring the safety net: data challenges for emergency departments. Acad Emerg Med 2001;8:1019–21.

[7] Defending America's safety net. Dallas: American College of Emergency Physicians; 1999.

[8] Gallagher EJ, Lynn SG. The etiology of medical gridlock: causes of emergency department overcrowding in New York City. J Emerg Med 1990;8:785–90.

[9] Emergency departments: unevenly affected by growth and change in patient use. Washington: US General Accounting Office; 1993.

[10] Hospital emergency departments: crowded conditions vary among hospitals and communities. Washington: US General Accounting Office; 2003.

[11] Richardson DB. The access-block effect: relationship between delay to reaching an inpatient bed and inpatient length of stay. Med J Aust 2002;177:492–5.

[12] Fatovich DM, Nagree Y, Sprivulis P. Access block causes emergency department overcrowding and ambulance diversion in Perth, Western Australia. Emerg Med J 2005;22:351–4.

[13] Sprivulis P, Grainger S, Nagree Y. Ambulance diversion is not associated with low acuity patients attending Perth metropolitan emergency departments. Emerg Med Australasia 2005;17:11–5.

[14] Cunningham P, May J. Insured Americans drive surge in emergency department visits. Issue brief No. 70. Washington: Center for Studying Health System Change; 2003.

[15] Sacchetti A, Harris RH, Warden T, et al. Contribution of ED admissions to inpatient hospital revenue. Am J Emerg Med 2002;20:30–1.

[16] Krochmal P, Riley TA. Increased health care costs associated with ED overcrowding. Am J Emerg Med 1994;12:265–6.

[17] Bayley MD, Schwartz JS, Shofer FS, et al. The financial burden of emergency department congestion and hospital crowding for chest pain patients awaiting admission. Ann Emerg Med 2005;45:110–7.

[18] Hu SC. Clinical and demographic characteristics of adult emergency patients at the Taipei Veterans General Hospital. J Formos Med Assoc 1994;93:61–5.

[19] Bagust A, Place M, Posnett JW. Dynamics of bed use in accommodating emergency admissions: stochastic simulation model. BMJ 1999;319:155–8.

[20] Miro O, Antonio MT, Jimenez S, et al. Decreased health care quality associated with emergency department overcrowding. Eur J Emerg Med 1999;6:105–7.

[21] Asplin BR, Magid DJ, Rhodes KV, et al. A conceptual model of emergency department crowding. Ann Emerg Med 2003;42:173–80.

[22] Solberg LI, Asplin BR, Weinick RM, et al. Emergency department crowding: consensus development of potential measures. Ann Emerg Med 2003;42:824–34.

[23] Hwang U, Concato J. Care in the emergency department: how crowded is overcrowded? Acad Emerg Med 2004;11:1097–101.

[24] Magid DJ, Asplin BR, Wears RL. The quality gap: searching for the consequences of emergency department crowding. Ann Emerg Med 2004;44:586–8.

[25] Asplin BR, Rhodes KV, Flottemesch TJ, et al. Is this emergency department crowded? A multicenter derivation and evaluation of an emergency department crowding scale (EDCS) [abstract]. Acad Emerg Med 2004;11:484.

[26] Bernstein SL, Verghese V, Leung W, et al. Development and validation of a new index to measure emergency department crowding. Acad Emerg Med 2003;10:938–42.

[27] Wuerz R, Group ETS. Emergency Severity Index Triage category is associated with six-month survival. Acad Emerg Med 2001;8:61–4.

[28] Wuerz RC, Milne LW, Eitel DR, et al. Reliability and validity of a new five-level triage instrument. Acad Emerg Med 2000;7:236–42.

[29] Weiss SJ, Derlet R, Arndahl J, et al. Estimating the degree of emergency department over-crowding in academic medical centers: results of the National ED Overcrowding Study (NE-DOCS). Acad Emerg Med 2004;11:38–50.

[30] Reeder TJ, Burleson DL, Garrison HG. The overcrowded emergency department: a comparison of staff perceptions. Acad Emerg Med 2004;10:1059–64.

[31] Epstein SK. Development of an emergency department workscore to predict ambulance diversion [abstract]. Acad Emerg Med 2004;11:484.

[32] Miro O, Sanchez M, Milla J. Hospital mortality and staff workload [letter]. Lancet 2000;356:1356–7.

[33] Richardson DB. Association of daily patient care time with adverse events in patients who do not wait to be seen [abstract]. Acad Emerg Med 2004;11:461–2.

[34] Richardson DB. A new definition of emergency department overcrowding using point occupancy [abstract]. Acad Emerg Med 2004;11:462.

[35] Richardson DB. Prospective validation of point occupancy definition of overcrowding [abstract]. Acad Emerg Med 2004;11:462–3.

[36] Richardson DB, Bryant M. Daily patient care time is the best predictor of waiting time performance [abstract]. Acad Emerg Med 2004;11:461.

[37] Richardson DB, Bryant M. Confirmation of association between overcrowding and adverse events in patients who do not wait to be seen [abstract]. Acad Emerg Med 2004;11:462.

[38] Richardson LD, Asplin BR, Lowe RA. Emergency department crowding as a health policy issue: past development, future directions. Ann Emerg Med 2002;40:388–93.

[39] Brewster LR, Felland LE. Emergency department diversions: hospital and community strategies alleviate the crisis. Issue brief No. 78. Washington: Center for Studying Health System Change; 2004.

[40] State of New York Department of Health. Health Commissioner directs hospitals to take immediate steps to avert hospital emergency room overcrowding. Available at: http://www.health.state.ny.us/press/releases/2001/erover.htm. Accessed July 14, 2006.

[41] Wilson MJ, Siegel B, Williams M. Perfecting patient flow: America's safety net hospitals and emergency department crowding. Washington: National Association of Public Hospitals; 2005.

[42] Burt CW, Hing E. Use of computerized clinical support systems in medical settings: United States, 2001–03. Advance data from vital and health statistics; No. 353. Hyattsville (MD): National Center for Health Statistics; 2005.

[43] Regenstein M, Nolan L, Wilson M, et al. Walking a tightrope: the state of the safety net in ten US communities. Washington: George Washington University Medical Center, Robert Wood Johnson Foundation; 2004.

[44] Anonymous. Three strategies to reduce overcrowding and gridlock. Hosp Case Manag 2004;12:139–40.

[45] Buhaug H. Long waiting lists in hospitals. BMJ 2002;324:252–3.

[46] Siddharthan K, Jones WJ, Johnson JA. A priority queuing model to reduce waiting times in emergency care. Int J Health Care Qual Assur 1996;9:10–6.

[47] Management of Variability Program. Available at: http://www.bu.edu/mvp/research/overcrowding.html. Accessed July 8, 2005.

[48] Derlet RW, Richards JR. Emergency department overcrowding in Florida, New York, and Texas. Southern Medical Association Journal 2002;95:846–9.

[49] Derlet RW. Triage and ED overcrowding: two cases of unexpected outcomes. California J Emerg Med 2002;3:8–9.

[50] Schull MJ, Vermeulen M, Slaughter G, et al. Emergency department crowding and thrombolysis delays in acute myocardial infarction. Ann Emerg Med 2004;44:577–85.

[51] Sprivulis P, Silva JD, Jacobs I, et al. Hospital overcrowding is associated with increased seven-day emergency admission mortality: a new imperative for patient safety [abstract]. Presented at the American Society of General Internal Medicine Annual Scientific Meeting, New Orleans, 14 May 2005 and the Academy of Health Annual Research Meeting, Boston, 26 June 2005.

[52] Institute of Medicine. Crossing the quality chasm: a new health system for the 21st century. Washington: National Academy Press; 2001.

[53] Clancy CM. AHRQ's FY 2005 budget request: new mission, new vision. Health Serv Res 2004;39:xi–xviii.

Emerg Med Clin N Am
24 (2006) 839–848

EMERGENCY
MEDICINE
CLINICS OF
NORTH AMERICA

The Role of the Emergency Department in the Care of Homeless and Disadvantaged Populations

David M. Morris, MD, MPH[a],*,
James A. Gordon, MD, MPA[b]

[a]Department of Emergency Medicine, MetroWest Medical Center,
Framingham Union Hospital, Framingham, MA 01702, USA
[b]Department of Emergency Medicine, Massachusetts General Hospital,
Harvard Medical School, Boston, MA 02114, USA

Emergency departments (EDs) provide the only universal health care accessible to the general public in the United States, with well over 100 million patient visits per year [1,2]. Operating at the critical interface between the hospital and its community, EDs are designed to meet the demands of all patients. Whereas the specific needs of each community will vary, the fundamental approach to delivering emergency care remains the same—dedicated health professionals work 24 hours a day, 7 days a week to provide care to all patients, regardless of social circumstance. Because the ED functions as the ultimate health care "safety net," it can have a critical impact on homeless and other disadvantaged populations [3]. This chapter will review the epidemiology of social deprivation among ED patients, with a particular focus on understanding the nature of homelessness. It will then explore the value of an integrated approach to socio-medical care in the ED, and highlight successful ED-based approaches.

An overview of social deprivation among ED patients

Despite the development of outreach programs such as Health Care for the Homeless, many of the most disadvantaged individuals in our society rely on EDs for medical care [4–8]. A Los Angeles study of the homeless found that only 57% had any contact with medical care, and 23% of those

---
* Corresponding author. Department of Emergency Medicine, MetroWest Medical Center, Framingham Union Hospital, Framingham, MA 01702.
E-mail address: DMorris@quantech.net (D.M. Morris).

0733-8627/06/$ - see front matter © 2006 Elsevier Inc. All rights reserved.
doi:10.1016/j.emc.2006.06.011

used the local ED as their primary point of care [9]. In San Francisco, 40% of homeless and "marginally housed" individuals surveyed had used the ED in the past year, a rate three times higher than the national average compared with the general population [10]. One New York City (NYC) hospital even reported a 20% to 30% incidence of homelessness among its ED population. These patients—who averaged six ED visits per year—were more likely to be middle-aged men suffering from tuberculosis, HIV, depression, schizophrenia, alcoholism, poor dentition, or penetrating trauma [6].

While disadvantaged populations have significant medical needs, their critical social needs often go unaddressed in the health care setting, leading to a vicious cycle of poverty and illness. Alarming levels of hunger (up to 18%) have been seen in ED populations, leading to untenable tradeoffs, for example, between paying for medicine or food [11]. Some patients are even forced to "heat or eat" during the harsh winter months [12]; almost 10% of patients in one Michigan ED reported their gas or electric service had been turned off in the previous year [13]. Across three EDs in the same study, 31% of patients reported one or more serious social deprivations over the past year, including housing eviction; interruption of power or phone service; lack of food; no working refrigerator, stove, or telephone; and crowded or dilapidated housing.

Homelessness: a critical issue in emergency departments

Epidemiology of homelessness

A homeless person lacks a stable nighttime residence and usually lives in temporary accommodations. Temporary living accommodations include shelters, community institutions, and open places not intended for regular sleeping accommodations [14]. Homelessness is the consequence of a number of factors, including poverty and the lack of low-cost housing, the absence of social plans, and insufficient general health and public services [15,16].

The Urban Institute estimates that 3.5 million people, including 1.35 million children, are homeless during a given year [14,17]. These approximations likely underestimate the true prevalence of homelessness because complete data are very difficult to collect on this itinerant population. Data collection of persons using homeless shelters, for example, represents only a cross-section of the homeless population. A 2001 study of seven American cities reported that that 37% of all requests for emergency shelter were unmet owing to lack of resources [18]. Many rural areas of the United States lack homeless shelters, despite significant levels of need. The "hidden homeless" are often uncounted, comprising individuals who frequently stay in automobiles, campgrounds, public parks, or other "unofficial" residences. One study reported that automobiles provide the most common form of shelter for these individuals (59.2%) followed by makeshift housing such as tents, boxes, caves, or boxcars (24.6%) [19,20].

The homeless population is a heterogeneous group [6,19–21]. The Centers for Disease Control and Prevention estimated in 1991 that men were more likely than women to be homeless. Fifty-one percent of the homeless were 31 to 50 years old. Whereas white males account for 80% of the homeless, families with children comprised the fastest growing segment of the homeless population; overall, 39% of the US homeless population consisted of children younger than 18 years. Forty percent of the homeless had served in the armed forces, compared with 34% of the general male population. Over the subsequent 10 years, the demographics of the homeless population evolved. In 2003, the US Conference of Mayors reported the ethnic distribution of the homeless across 25 cities: 49% African American, 35% Caucasian, 13% Hispanic, 2% Native American, and 1% Asian [18].

Etiology of homelessness

Two trends are largely responsible for the rise of the homeless population over the past 30 years: (1) shortage of affordable housing and (2) an increase in poverty [22]. There is a gap between the number of people who need affordable housing and the number of housing units available. This has created a housing crisis for the poor. Approximately 2.2 million low-rent housing units disappeared from the market over a 20-year span between 1973 and 1993 [6,22]. These units were abandoned, demolished, converted into condominiums, or became unaffordable. In the mid-1990s, the median rental cost paid by low-income renters rose 21% [22], a rate greater than the rise in income levels [14]. This situation leaves many families on long waitlists for public housing. The average wait time for federal housing assistance rose from 26 months to 28 months between 1996 and 1998 [22]. Length of stay within homeless shelters has subsequently increased, especially as actual shelter space declines. In New York City during the 1990s, families stayed in shelters for an average of 5 months before relocating to housing [23]. Since then, the length of stay in a shelter has risen to a year [15].

Individuals living at poverty levels must constantly manage tensions about unforeseen illness, accidents, or missed paychecks, which could catapult a person into homelessness. Other factors influencing homelessness include domestic violence, mental illness, substance abuse, and lack of affordable health care [19,24]. In a study of 777 homeless parents in 10 US cities, 22% were homeless because of domestic violence and abusive relationships [25]. It is difficult to calculate the annual incidence of domestic violence and its true influence on homelessness. Most Americans stereotype homeless people as individuals with severe mental illness. In fact, about 22% of the single adult homeless population suffers from some form of severe and persistent mental illness, ranging from depression, bipolar disorder, and schizophrenia [26]. There is a complex relationship between substance abuse and homelessness such that there are disproportionately high rates of alcohol and drug abuse among the homeless [27–29]. The US Conference of Mayors found that 30% of the single male homeless population had problems with substance abuse, including alcohol, cocaine, and heroin [18]. Lack of affordable health care also contributes to the cause of homelessness [30]. Members of the working poor who develop serious illnesses or disabilities are prone to job loss and depletion of savings simply because they lack insurance. Uninsured medical care carries such a high price tag that the working poor may choose to defer needed health care. Such a delay can lead to complications of formerly simple medical illness, fostering late presentations of progressed disease states. Because of the lack of affordable health care, especially in consideration of the fact that 14% of all ED visits are made by uninsured patients [2], many working poor end up in the ED for basic medical and social care [13,21,31].

Health of the homeless

Poor health is closely associated with homelessness, and homeless individuals are much more likely to use the ED as a source of care [6]. By necessity, some subjugate their health care to competing needs for food, clothing, and shelter [11]. Not surprisingly, the homeless population has a particularly high mortality rate. In Philadelphia during 1994, the homeless had an age-adjusted mortality rate 3.5 times higher than the general population [32]. In New York City during 1990, the mortality rates of homeless individuals were 2 to 3 times that of the general population [33]. In Atlanta during 1987, the median age at death among homeless persons was 44 years [30]. The median age at death among the homeless in San Francisco during the period of 1985 to 1990 was 41 years [30]. Between 1988 and 1993, the Boston Health Care for Homeless Program reported a median death age of 47 years. Among the Boston cohort, the leading causes of death among homeless males age 18 to 24 years were homicide, traumatic injury, and acute poisoning from overdose. HIV and AIDS accounted for the leading cause of death among men and women age 25 to 44. Cancer and heart disease were the leading causes of death among men and women age 45 to 54 [34–36].

Health issues are compounded by homelessness. Environmental injuries such as exposure to the cold and heat are frequent reasons for ED visits. Homeless patients with frostbite and heat exhaustion generally present in later disease states. Cold winter nights prompt individuals to seek out the ED for food and shelter. Homelessness also precludes good nutrition, hygiene, and basic first aid, adding to the complex needs of the homeless. Exposure to the dirty environment of the street, coupled with inadequate clothing and nutrition, often predisposes homeless persons to skin and soft tissue infections. The homeless also suffer a greater risk of trauma from muggings, beatings, and rape [9,29,37].

Chronic medical problems are exacerbated by homelessness. Approximately 40% of homeless persons report at least one chronic health problem, including psychiatric and medical health issues [6]. These chronic illnesses frequently go unrecognized and untreated until late in their course. Even when health conditions are detected, lack of compliance and consistent follow-up often result in disease progression, disability, and premature death. Conditions that require meticulous treatment such as HIV, diabetes, psychiatric illness, and substance abuse are extremely difficult to treat and control among the homeless. One study examining diabetes management among residents of homeless shelters in Toronto revealed an increased risk of mortality and morbidity. Among 50 individuals surveyed, 72% reported experiencing difficulties with diabetes management and 44% had poor glucose control [38].

HIV and homelessness

Studies indicate that the prevalence of HIV among homeless persons ranges between 3% and 20% [39]. A Los Angeles study found that two thirds of people with AIDS had been homeless. Up to 50% of persons living with HIV and AIDS are expected to need housing assistance of some kind during their lifetime [40]. HIV infection exacerbated by homelessness leads to higher morbidity and mortality. Homeless people with HIV die from AIDS more commonly than other HIV-infected populations [39]. These patients also tend to have higher rates and more advanced forms of tuberculosis.

Homeless HIV patients face many barriers to optimal care. Injection drug use and lack of health insurance among homeless individuals have been shown to negatively effect health care use, level of medical care, and health status. Adherence to complex medical regimens may be more difficult if one does not have stable housing or access to basic subsistence needs such as food and clean clothing. Poor compliance among homeless HIV patients is a strong predictor of protease inhibitor failure and a contributing cause of medication resistance, which has grave personal and public health implications [41,42]. High-risk sexual behavior and drug use are prevalent among the homeless population, further complicating HIV prevention efforts [43–45].

Mental illness and homelessness

Approximately 20% to 25% of the single adult homeless population suffers from some form of severe and persistent mental illness. However, only 5% of the estimated 4 million people who have serious mental illness are homeless at any given point in time [26]. According to the Federal Task Force on Homelessness and Severe Mental Illness, only 5% to 7% of homeless persons with mental illness need to be institutionalized; most can live within the community with appropriate supportive housing options. Unfortunately, there are not enough community-based mental health treatment programs and affordable housing to accommodate the number of people disabled by mental illness in the United States. Homeless people with mental disorders remain homeless for longer periods of time and encounter more barriers to stability than other homeless populations. They tend to be in poorer physical health, are more frequently unemployed, and have more contact with the legal system compared with homeless individuals who do not suffer from a mental disorder [46].

Pediatric illness and homeless children

Homelessness is an independent risk factor for poor pediatric health status [47,48]. Homeless children experience an increased number of acute illnesses, and frequently present to the ED for health care [49,50]. The most common presentations include fever, ear infection, diarrhea, and asthma [51]. Rates of immunization among homeless children are consistently lower compared with their domiciled counterparts. In New York City, approximately 61% of homeless children studied had not received their proper immunizations, compared with 23% of all New York City 2 year olds. An estimated 38% of homeless children in the NYC shelter system have asthma —a rate four times that for all NYC children, and the highest prevalence of any pediatric population in the United States. Homeless children suffer from acute otitis media at a rate that is 50% greater than the national average [50,51]. They also live in less structured and safe environments, placing them at greater risk for injury, lead toxicity, anemia, malnutrition, iron and calcium deficiencies, and depression. These children are more likely to be exposed to domestic violence, mental illness, and substance abuse, resulting in academic and behavioral problems and developmental delays [47,48].

Integrating health and human services in the ED

A 2001 study of mortality among the homeless in Boston discovered that 21% of the homeless had contact with medical care within 1 month before death, and 21% had greater than six contacts [37]. For many of these disadvantaged patients, the ED is their primary or only health care site [13]. Clearly, the isolated provision of medical care in this setting is not enough to interrupt the cycle of poverty and illness.

However, since the ED is a high-cachment area for disadvantaged individuals, it is well positioned to serve as a community triage and coordinating entity for essential social and human services. Providing dedicated social work and case management services in the ED is essential. A system of "social triage" can build on the traditional social work approaches by institutionalizing social assessment and service referrals alongside medical diagnosis and treatment [3]. Project ASSERT (Alcohol, Substance Abuse, Service, Educate, Referral, Treatment Program) is one example of an ED program started in Boston, Massachusetts, designed to screen patients for social problems, like alcoholism, substance abuse, and domestic violence, and to coordinate referral and access to community services [52]. Simply coordinating primary care discharge referrals for children, for instance, has been shown to decrease recurrent ED visits [53]. Project ASSERT has now spread to other sites, serving as a model for integrating social services and health care in the ED. Other programs have automated the screening and referral process through computer-based "kiosks," strategically positioned user-friendly information booths for use in ED waiting rooms [54].

Although dedicated social outreach workers are vital to providing comprehensive care for disadvantaged ED patients, many hospitals struggle to pay for social work services [55]. Using volunteers and automated screening can help with costs, but cannot replace dedicated professionals. Recent studies suggest that creative social outreach not only makes a significant difference in the lives of patients, but can also pay for itself [56]. A multicenter trial of health insurance outreach among uninsured children presenting to the ED demonstrated that simply handing out blank insurance applications could nearly quadruple the odds of successful enrollment [57]. Adopted nationwide, this approach could lead to coverage for more than a quarter million additional children per year. Such enhanced enrollment, according to another Michigan study, could allow hospitals to retroactively recover payment for previously unfunded visits [58]. This funding stream could potentially supercede the cost of salaries for ED-based social outreach workers to care for our most disadvantaged patients.

Summary

Homelessness and social deprivation is widespread among ED patients. Organized emergency medicine can have a significant impact on total community health by maintaining a universal "safety net" for the delivery of integrated health and human services. Cost-effective approaches to socio-medical integration in the ED are not only feasible, but are critical to promoting the health and welfare of homeless and other disadvantaged populations.

References

[1] Fields WW, Asplin BR, Larkin GL, et al. The Emergency Medical Treatment and Labor Act as a federal health care safety net program. Acad Emerg Med 2001;8:1064–9.

[2] McCaig LF, Burt CW. National Hospital Ambulatory Medical Care Survey: 2002 emergency department summary. Adv Data Vital Health Stat.; no 340. Hyattsville, MD: National Center for Health Statistics, March 2004. Available at: http://www.cdc.gov/hchs/data/ad/ad340.pdf. Accessed July 7, 2005.

[3] Gordon JA. The hospital emergency department as a social welfare institution. Ann Emerg Med 1999;33:321–5.

[4] O'Toole SM, Withers JS. From the streets, to the emergency department, and back: a model of emergency care for the homeless. Top Emerg Med 1998;20(4):12–20.

[5] Stein JA, Andersen RM, Koegel P, et al. Predicting health services utilization among homeless adults: a prospective analysis. J Health Care Poor Underserved 2000;11(2):212–30.

[6] D'Amore J, Hung O, Chiang W, et al. The epidemiology of the homeless population and its impact on an urban emergency department. Acad Emerg Med 2001;8(11):1051–5.

[7] Lowenstein SR, Koziol-MeLain J, Thompson M, et al. Behavioral risk factors in emergency department patients: a multisite survey. Acad Emerg Med 1998;5:781–7.

[8] Weinberger M, Oddone EZ, Henderson WG. Does increased access to primary care reduce hospital admissions? N Engl J Med 1996;334:1441–7.

[9] Gallagher TC, Andersen RM, Koegel P, et al. Determinants of regular source of care among homeless adults in Los Angeles. Med Care 1997;35(8):814–30.

[10] Kushel MB, Perry S, Bangsberg D, et al. Emergency department use among the homeless and marginally housed: results from a community-based study. Am J Public Health 2002; 92:778–84.

[11] Kersey MA, Beran MS, McGovern PG, et al. The prevalence and effects of hunger in an emergency department patient population. Acad Emerg Med 1999;6(11):1109–14.

[12] Frank DA, Roos N, Meyers A, et al. Seasonal variation in weight-for-age in a pediatric emergency room. Pub Health Rep 1996;111(4):366–71.

[13] Gordon JA, Chudnofsky CR, Hayward RA. Where health and welfare meet: social deprivation among patients in the emergency department. J Urban Health 2001;78(1):104–11.

[14] National Coalition for the Homeless. Who is homeless? (NCH Fact Sheet #3). Washington, DC: National Coalition for the Homeless; 1999.

[15] National Coalition for the Homeless. Why are people homeless? (NCH Fact Sheet #1). Washington, DC: National Coalition for the Homeless; 1999.

[16] National Coalition for the Homeless. How many people experience homelessness? (NCH Fact Sheet #2). Washington, DC: National Coalition for the Homeless; 1999.

[17] Urban Institute. A new look at homelessness in America. Washington, DC: Urban Institute; 2001.

[18] US Conference of Mayors. A status report on hunger and homelessness in American cities: 2001. Washington, DC: US Conference of Mayors; 2001.

[19] Link BG, Susser E, Stueve A, et al. Lifetime and five-year prevalence of homelessness in the United States. Am J Public Health 1994;84(12):1907–12.

[20] Link BG, Phelan J, Bresnahan M, et al. Lifetime and five-year prevalence of homelessness in the United States: new evidence of an old debate. Am J Orthopsychiatry 1995;65(3): 347–54.

[21] Centers for Disease Control and Prevention. Characteristics and risk behaviors of homeless black males. MMWR 1991;40:865–8.

[22] Susser E, Moore R, Link B. Risk factors for homelessness. Epidemiol Rev 1993;15(2): 546–56.

[23] Shinn M, Weitzman BC, Stojanovic D, et al. Predictors of homelessness among families in New York City: from shelter request to housing stability. Am J Public Health 1998; 88(11):1651–7.

[24] Herman DB, Susser ES, Struening EL, et al. Are there risk factors for homelessness? Am J Public Health 1997;87(2):249–55.

[25] Zorza J. Woman battering: a major cause of homelessness. Clearinghouse Review 1991; 25(4):421–9.

[26] National Coalition for the Homeless. Mental illness and homelessness (NCH #5). Washington, DC: National Coalition for the Homeless; 1999.

[27] National Coalition for the Homeless. Addiction disorders and homelessness. Washington, DC: National Coalition for the Homeless; 1999.

[28] National Coalition for the Homeless. Health care and homelessness. Washington, DC: National Coalition for the Homeless; 1999.

[29] Broadhead WE, Kaplan BH, James SA, et al. The epidemiologic evidence for a relationship between social support and health. Am J Epidemiol 1983;117(5):521–37.

[30] Kushel MB, Vittinghoff E, Haas JS. Factors associated with health care utilization of homeless persons. JAMA 2001;285(2):200–6.

[31] Bollinger K, Goup A, Vigna G. Health care for the homeless: a public concern. J Louisiana S Med Soc 1993;145(7):321–3.

[32] Hibbs JR, Benner L, Klugman L, et al. Mortality in a cohort of homeless adults in Philadelphia. N Engl J Med 1994;331(5):304–9.

[33] Barrow SM, Herman DB, Cordova P, et al. Mortality among homeless shelter residents in New York City. Am J Public Health 1999;89(4):529–34.

[34] Cuddy R. Anonymous demise: mortality in the homeless. J Emerg Med 1997;15(3):373–4.

[35] Hwang SW, Lebow JM, Bierer MF, et al. Risk factors for death in homeless adults in Boston. Arch Intern Med 1998;158(13):1454–60.

[36] Hwang SW, Orav EJ, O'Connell JJ, et al. Causes of death in homeless adults in Boston. Ann Intern Med 1997;126(8):625–8.

[37] Hwang SW, O'Connell JJ, Lebow JM, et al. Health care utilization among homeless adults prior to death. J Health Care Poor Underserved 2001;12(1):50–8.

[38] Hwang SW. Mortality among men using homeless shelters in Toronto, Ontario. JAMA 2000;283(16):2152–7.

[39] National Coalition for the Homeless. HIV/AIDS and homelessness. Washington, DC: National Coalition for the Homeless; 1999.

[40] Kleinman LC, Freeman H, Perlman J, et al. Homing in on the homeless: assessing the physical health of homeless adults in Los Angeles County using an original method to obtain physical examination data in a survey. Health Serv Res 1996;31(5):533–49.

[41] Bamberger JD, Unick J, Klein P, et al. Helping the urban poor stay with HIV drug therapy. Am J Public Health 2000;90(5):699–701.

[42] Wagner JH, Justic AC, Chesney M, et al. Patient and provider adherence: toward a clinically useful approach to measuring antiretroviral adherence. J Clin Epidemiol 2001;12(S1): S91–8.

[43] Shuter J, Alpert PL, DeShaw MG, et al. Gender differences in HIV risk behaviors in an adult emergency department in New York City. J Urban Health 1999;76(2):237–46.

[44] Kelen GD, Shahan JB, Quinn TC. Emergency department-based HIV screening and counseling: experience with rapid and standard serologic testing. Ann Emerg Med 1999;33: 147–55.

[45] Rothman RE, Ketlogetswe KS, Dolan T, et al. Preventive care in the emergency department: should emergency departments conduct routine HIV screening? A systematic review. Acad Emerg Med 2003;10:278–85.

[46] Federal Task Force on Homelessness and Sever Mental Illness. Outcasts on Main Street: a report of the Federal Task Force on Homelessness and Mental Illness. Delmar, NY: National Resource Center on Homelessness and Mental Illness; 1992.

[47] Newacheck P. Poverty and childhood chronic illness. Arch Pediatr Adolesc Med 1994;148: 1143–9.

[48] Foltin GL. Critical issues on urban emergency medical services for children. Pediatrics 1995; 96(1 pt 2):174–9.

[49] Wise PH, Kotelchuch M, Wilson ML, et al. Racial and socioeconomic disparities in childhood mortality in Boston. N Engl J Med 1985;313:360–6.

[50] Wood D, Valdez RB, Hayashi T, Shen A. Health of the homeless children and housed poor children. Pediatrics 1990;(86):858–66.

[51] Weinreb L, Goldberg R, Bassuk E, Purloff J. Determinants of health and service use patterns in homeless and low-income housed infants and toddlers. Pediatrics 1998;(102): 554–62.

[52] Bernstein E, Bernstein J, Levenson S. Project ASSERT: an ED based intervention to increase access to primary care, preventive services, and the substance abuse treatment system. Ann Emerg Med 1997;30:181–9.

[53] Grossman LK, Rich LN, Johnson C. Decreasing nonurgent emergency department utilization by Medicaid children. Pediatrics 1998;102(1 pt 1):20–4.

[54] Rhodes KV, Lauderdale DS, Stocking CB, et al. Better health while you wait: a controlled trial of a computer-based intervention for screening and health promotion in the emergency department. Ann Emerg Med 2001;37:284–91.
[55] Gordon JA. Cost-benefit analysis of social services in the emergency department: a conceptual model. Acad Emerg Med 2001;8:54–60.
[56] Gordon JA. The science of common sense: integrating health and human services in the hospital emergency department [editorial/commentary]. Ann Emerg Med 2005;45(3):251–2.
[57] Gordon JA, Emond JA, Camargo CA. The State Children's Health Insurance Program (SCHIP): a multicenter trial of outreach through the emergency department. Am J Public Health 2005;95(2):250–3.
[58] Mahajan P, Stanley R, Ross K, et al. Evaluation of an emergency department-based enrollment program for uninsured children. Ann Emerg Med 2005;45(3):245–50.

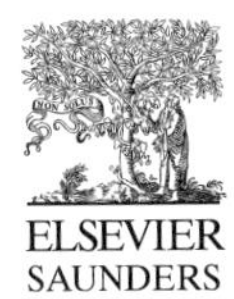

ELSEVIER
SAUNDERS

Emerg Med Clin N Am
24 (2006) 849–869

EMERGENCY
MEDICINE
CLINICS OF
NORTH AMERICA

Health Promotion and Disease Prevention in the Emergency Department

Kirk A. Stiffler, MD[a],*, Lowell W. Gerson, PhD[b]

[a]*Northeastern Ohio Universities College of Medicine, Akron City Hospital, 41 Arch Street, Suite 519, PO Box 2090, Akron, OH 44309–2090, USA*
[b]*Northeastern Ohio Universities College of Medicine, PO Box 95, Rootstown, OH 44272, USA*

There is a story about an unfortunate event at a postgraduate day picnic. The picnic ground was on the bank of a river swollen from the heavy spring run off. The residents' activities were interrupted when someone screamed "there is a car in the water." The car, actually a van, was spotted hung up on rocks about 20 ft off shore. Emergency medicine residents were first on the scene. Five of them jumped into the water and pulled five people (two adults and three children) from the van. All the victims were unresponsive. The emergency medicine residents, joined by a cardiology fellow, started life support. Someone called 911. Soon, a second vehicle appeared floating in the rapids, followed by a third and a forth. Looking up river it seemed that there was a car flotilla. By now almost all the residents joined in the rescue attempt: diving into the water, pulling victims from cars, and starting resuscitation. The residents were overwhelmed by so many victims, but they kept going from one to another doing what they had been trained to do. While all this was going on the sole preventive medicine resident ran up river and found that a bridge had washed out. She quickly erected a makeshift barricade and stopped traffic from plunging into the river. An ounce of prevention was worth a pound of cure.

Disease and injury prevention and health promotion

What is prevention and why should emergency medicine professionals care about it? Prevention is "actions aimed at eradicating, eliminating, or

---

* Corresponding author.
E-mail address: stifflek@summa-health.org (K.A. Stiffler).

0733-8627/06/$ - see front matter © 2006 Elsevier Inc. All rights reserved.
doi:10.1016/j.emc.2006.06.010

minimizing the impact of disease and disability. The concept of prevention is best defined in the context of levels, traditionally called primary, secondary, and tertiary prevention" [1]. Fig. 1 shows the natural history of disease or injury and the three levels of prevention.

Interventions that occur before the onset of the disease or injury are considered primary prevention. Some examples of popular primary prevention activities include measles-mumps-rubella vaccination or prophylactic aspirin to prevent myocardial infarction. Haddon's model for injury prevention, discussed elsewhere in this issue, calls this the pre-event phase [2]. The preventive medicine resident's environmental change, barricading the road, was primary prevention; it stopped the event from happening.

Prevention often is linked with health promotion. Health promotion interventions are those that modify human behavior to reduce or eliminate harmful factors. This can be achieved through health education, organizational change, political action, and economic interventions or a combination designed to facilitate environmental or behavioral adaptations that improve health. Health promotion is concerned with sociobehavioral processes. A vaccination is primary prevention; activities to convince people of the need for vaccination are health promotion.

Disease and injury prevention and health promotion in the emergency department

Primary prevention is possible in the emergency department (ED). The Society for Academic Emergency Medicine (SAEM) Public Health and Education Task Force did systematic reviews of 17 possible preventive behaviors. Six of the seventeen were primary prevention and health promotion activities. The task force recommended providing pneumococcal vaccination to reduce invasive pneumococcal disease in persons more than 65 years old [3]. They determined that fall prevention activities for older persons and counseling about smoke detectors were good candidates, but further study is needed. They concluded that there was not enough evidence to recommend for or against counseling about firearm storage and motorcycle helmet use, and that vaccination of pediatric patients is not recommended in the ED [3].

Secondary prevention is detecting the disease at a stage where early treatment is likely to improve outcomes. Pap smears for early detection of

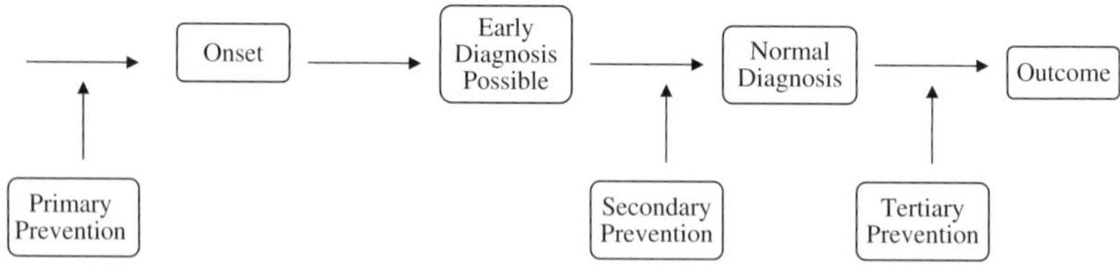

Fig. 1. Natural history of disease and three levels of prevention.

cervical cancer is an excellent example of a secondary preventive activity. The United States Preventive Services Task Force (USPSTF) strongly recommends Pap testing to detect cervical cancer in women who have been sexually active and have a cervix [4]. The SAEM Task Force reviewed Pap testing in the ED, a form of case finding. They concluded that there is not enough evidence to recommend for or against this intervention in women having a pelvic examination. They commented that follow-up procedures be established should a program be evaluated. The importance of this is demonstrated in a recent study of 41 medically indigent women being offered a Pap examination when having a clinically indicated pelvic examination in the ED. Only 2 of the 41 women they studied initiated contact for their test result. They had to track down the others but, despite extensive attempts, were unable to reach eight. It is noteworthy that five of the eight had abnormal results [5].

Tertiary prevention involves the care of established disease, and as such is not typically applied to the field of emergency medicine. The goals are to prevent complications and to return the patient to their normal function or to the highest level of function of which they are capable. Cardiac rehabilitation after a myocardial infarction is an example of tertiary prevention, and so is prescribing an appropriate antimicrobial in the ED.

Early diagnostic efforts (secondary prevention) are generically called "screening," but the logic underlying early detection activities in the ED may be clearer if one adopts Sackett and Holland's [6] distinction between screening and case-finding. Screening is the testing of volunteers from the general population to identify people with a high probability of having the disorder. Case-finding, however, is testing of patients who have sought medical care for a disorder that may be unrelated to their chief complaint.

Not every disorder makes a good target for screening. The disorder for which health care providers are screening should be important (ie, a disorder that significantly affects the public's health). It should have a high prevalence in the screened population. The natural history of the disease should have a period where early detection is possible and improves the chances for a good outcome. There has to be medical care available to treat the disorder and the patient has to be willing to undergo additional testing and use that care. The program should be cost-effective. The screening test to be used should be acceptable to the patient and should have high sensitivity (few false-negative results) and specificity (few false-positive results).

The assumption in case-finding is that the patient initiated the encounter and wants a comprehensive assessment of his or her health. Secondary prevention in the ED is more likely to be case-finding. Unlike a visit to a primary care physician with whom the patient has a therapeutic relationship, ED patients may not wish a comprehensive assessment of their health. Readers should not forget that ED patients are concerned mainly with the problem that prompted their ED visit that day, and that most ED testing is aimed toward establishing a diagnosis with regard to that acute problem.

Although the primary, secondary, and tertiary levels of prevention map out very nicely, the distinction may be more academic than real and it is recommended that readers focus more on what they hope to achieve with a preventive intervention than categorizing it. There is strong evidence to support screening adults for hypertension because hypertension is a risk factor for cerebrovascular disease, coronary heart disease, and renal disease (USPSTF) [7]. Is hypertension screening primary prevention? This view considers treating hypertension as preventing cerebrovascular disease, coronary heart disease, and renal disease before they start. Or, is screening for hypertension early detection of a disease process already underway? That is, is it secondary prevention? Or is the test for high blood pressure a diagnostic test, in which case it is part of disease management or tertiary prevention? The important point is that one can identify patients with elevated blood pressure while they are in the ED and refer them for follow-up.

Need for emergency department–based prevention

The first step in choosing an ED-based preventive strategy is defining the need, desire, and applicability of health promotion and disease prevention. The need becomes apparent because estimates from the Centers for Disease Control and Prevention report as many as 12 million years of potential life were lost before age 65. Causes noted in order of decreasing frequency from Centers for Disease Control and Prevention statistics include unintentional injuries (17.8%); neoplasms (15.2%); intentional injuries (12.6%); cerebrovascular diseases (11.2%); congenital anomalies (5.3%); and HIV infection (5.3%) [8]. Mokdad and colleagues [9] identify the actual causes of death in the United States (Table 1). Half of all deaths result from nine causes. The consequences of these behaviors are well known to emergency medicine professionals.

Table 1
Actual causes of death in the United States in 1990 and 2000

Actual cause	No. (%) in 1990*	No. (%) in 2000
Tobacco	400,000 (19)	435,000 (18.1)
Poor diet and physical inactivity	300,000 (14)	400,000 (16.6)
Alcohol consumption	100,000 (5)	85,000 (3.5)
Microbial agents	90,000 (4)	75,000 (3.1)
Toxic agents	60,000 (3)	55,000 (2.3)
Motor vehicle	25,000 (1)	43,000 (1.8)
Firearms	35,000 (2)	29,000 (1.2)
Sexual behavior	30,000 (1)	20,000 (0.8)
Illicit drug use	20,000 (<1)	17,000 (0.7)
Total	1,060,000 (50)	1,159,000 (48.2)

* The percentages are for all deaths.

Data from Mokdad AH, et al. Actual causes of death in the United States, 2000. JAMA 2004;291:1238–45.

ED patients and their friends and families want information about preventing disease and injury caused by these risk factors. Surveys, primarily of adult, noncritically ill patients and waiting room occupants, indicate this desire for information on various preventive health issues, including prostate examinations, mammography, cholesterol screening, and calcium supplementation [10,11]. This desire may not be universal for all patients or to all issues, however, with one study showing only a 5.9% acceptance rate for participation in a home safety survey study [12]. The authors cite in their discussion some of the many reasons why all programs may not succeed, including lack of education (both health care worker and patients); lack of trust; fear of wrongdoing on the part of the patient; and lack of credibility of educational attempts. Other reasons noted include lack of adequate time and funding and a perceived fragmentation of primary care [13].

Applicability of preventive services for emergency medicine has been systematically reviewed, with evidence from existing literature used to grade the intervention in terms of its potential use in EDs [14,15]. The SAEM Task Force reported that there was sufficient evidence to support instituting preventive programs for 6 of the 17 candidate interventions (chosen from the USPSTF): (1) alcohol screening and intervention; (2) HIV screening (for high-risk patients); (3) hypertension screening; (4) pneumococcal vaccination for patients greater than 65 years old; (5) smoking cessation counseling; and (6) social services needs assessment and referral to a primary care physician for children. Several other topics were rated as potentially useful to institute in the ED but more research is needed to delineate further their role in this setting. These activities included global social service needs assessment, Pap tests for sexually active women having pelvic examinations, referral for women not up-to-date in their Pap test, smoke detector counseling, and falls prevention for older patients.

The Joint Commission on Accreditation of Health Care Organizations (JCAHO) standards recognize the importance of prevention [16]. JCAHO guidelines include standards for preventive activities, particularly in the form of ED-based patient educational programs. JCAHO provides guidance on the applicability of these programs for ED use, the validity of content for ED populations, the awareness of patient's needs, and the safety of treatment information given out. They also recognize the importance of continued patient interaction and feedback, collaboration and cooperation with outside resources, patient responsibility, and ongoing care management issues to complete the prevention activity and gain the maximum benefit of the program.

Emergency department epidemiology

Returning to the residents' picnic, the downstream approach of rescue and resuscitation used by the emergency medicine residents and their colleagues soon overwhelmed their capacity to cope, a situation not unlike what is occurring in EDs across the county. The 2002 ED census was over 110 million visits, a growth of 23% in the decade from 1992 to 2002. At the same time the number of EDs decreased by 15% [17]. Simply stated, over-crowding results from too many patients visiting too few facilities. What can be done to reduce ED visits?

First one must ask, who visits the ED? Emergency departments are supposed to diagnose and manage acute illness and injury rapidly, but the ED has become much more than that. They have become a provider, often a primary care provider, for a large group of Americans who are at risk for disease and injury. This group is at risk because of their poor economic situation, because of their age, and because of their lifestyle.

ED patients often are economically disadvantaged and this puts them at risk. A total of 42 million Americans are uninsured [18]. The primary payers for over one third of ED visits is Medicaid, state children's health insurance, or self-pay [17]. Thirty-eight percent of ED patients report no access to primary care. The ED becomes their primary care physician. One third of visits for the medically indigent group's visits were classified as semi- or nonurgent. This is more pronounced in "safety net" hospitals, which are much more likely to be located in the south [19,20]. Significantly more visits to safety net hospitals (21.2%) are considered nonurgent compared with 16.9% in non–safety net hospitals. It is also worth noting, however, that 28% of visits by people with private insurance as the primary payer also are classified as semi- or nonurgent [19]. The uninsured are disproportionately members of racial and ethnic minority groups, which contribute to the health disparities that are well documented [18,21].

ED patients are at risk because of their age. Fifteen percent of visits are made by patients who are at least 65 years old [17]. The challenges of caring for older patients were a focus of the SAEM Geriatric Task Force [22]. Older patients require a model of care that considers more than the medical-surgical issues of the condition with which they present. Good care for elder patients recognizes the importance of considering the patient's mental status, physical function, and living environment. Siebens [23] refers to this comprehensive approach as the "domain management model." This comprehensive approach is tertiary prevention. It identifies potential problems that effect the ED management and the patient's future functioning. Failure to recognize this produces unnecessary return visits. McCusker and colleagues [24] report almost one of five older ED patients returns shortly after their visit (almost half within 6 months) and that those who do return are more likely to report social and functional problems.

ED patients are also at risk because of their lifestyle. A study that administered a version of the Behavioral Risk Factor Surveillance Survey in three urban EDs reported ED patients had higher than average rates of behaviors that placed them at risk of injury or disease. A total of 53% of the respondents did not wear seat belts regularly, 48% smoked, 23% had a positive

CAGE screen for alcoholism, 16% had not had their blood pressure checked in the past year, 15% had no working smoke detector, 11% had ridden in an automobile with an intoxicated driver, and 4% reported unsafe sexual practices. A total of 42% of women > 50 years old had not received a Pap test in the prior 2 years and 14% reported never having had a mammogram [25].

Injuries are the most common reason for an ED visit. Almost one of four ED patients, about 29 million visits, presents for an injury [17]. What would ED crowding look like if 10% of the injuries were prevented? Subtract a similar number of preventable cases of respiratory illness (13 million ED visits) and circulatory system diseases (4.6 million ED visits) and it would go a long way to reduce the crowding seen in EDs. What would the ED look like if no one smoked? The value of specific health promotion and disease and injury prevention activities are discussed elsewhere in this issue.

Professional associations' views

The ED population provides compelling evidence about why individual emergency medical professionals should care about prevention and promotion. Emergency medical professional societies have recognized the value of health promotion and disease prevention activities. Through this recognition they have identified many activities in which emergency medical professionals should become involved.

Rhodes and colleagues [15], writing for the SAEM Public Health and Education Task Force, identified four reasons for health promotion and disease-prevention activities. First, EDs are already doing some prevention, screening, and counseling (eg, ordering tetanus immunization as part of the treatment for laceration is tertiary prevention). Ordering tetanus-diphtheria vaccination adds primary prevention for diphtheria. Second, the ED is a major, and may be the only, source of preventive services for a highly vulnerable segment of the United States population. This lack of continuing medical care poses a special challenge as was seen previously in the case of the women with positive Pap smears. One must ask if it is reasonable to start a case-finding program without the promise of high-quality care as needed. Third, the ED encounter may be opportune because patients in the ED may experience a "teachable moment." Finally, unmet preventive health needs result in ED visits for more serious problems. Effective prevention may reduce crowding.

The American College of Emergency Physician has at least 27 policy statements that concern injury prevention. These statements range from specific recommendations about adult immunization to broad policy issues, such as worldwide nuclear disarmament (www.acep.org). The American College of Emergency Physician core content model of clinical practice includes prevention and education within the physicians' tasks [26].

The Emergency Nurses Association has position statements endorsing seven preventive topics: (1) alcohol screening and brief intervention, (2) elder abuse screen, (3) domestic violence, (4) firearm safety, (5) injury prevention, (6) burn prevention, and (7) substance abuse [27]. Although these position statements may not delineate any particular activities for emergency nurses, they stand as testament to the Emergency Nurses Association's belief in the value of promotional and preventive aspects of emergency care.

Preventive strategies in the emergency department

There are studies that detail the use of specific health promotion and disease prevention techniques, but reliable outcome data as to the effect of these interventions on society are lacking [28]. Many preventive techniques are currently in practice, including educational pamphlets, educational videos, paper and computerized discharge instructions, computer-guided tutorials, and even the presence of injury preventionists in the ED to address identified issues for trauma patients in real time. Each of these techniques is reviewed next.

Informal verbal communication

The simplest and most obvious strategy to convey health promotion and disease prevention information to the ED population is verbal interaction between caregivers and patients. There is little literature available reviewing the extent of use or impact of verbal communication for any given issue. It seems reasonable and easy to weave a prevention or health promotion strategy into the normal ED discussion with patients. For example, ED staff could warn a driver involved in an alcohol-related motor vehicle crash against further attempts at driving while under the influence of alcohol. Outcome studies assessing the impact of such informal educational attempts, however, were not found.

Written information and education

Written educational pamphlets and discharge instructions containing preventive content is an approach for dispensing information. Advantages of written informational pamphlets include low cost, ease of use, and time efficiency for ED staff. The prospective study of pamphlets by Berger and coworkers [29] to improve compliance for Pap smears, mammograms, and pneumococcal vaccinations concluded that a significant number of patients needed preventive services. The pamphlets were effective only in improving Pap smear compliance. The study had low follow-up rates. Among those they were able to contact, fewer than 65% of women had read the pamphlet and fewer than 10% of the men reported reading the pamphlet. The disadvantages of written educational materials outlined by the study of Berger and coworkers [29] included lack of ongoing interaction with the target population to assess the materials' impact, lack of interaction with staff to answer questions regarding the topic, and lack of opportunity for staff to initiate the interventions on patients' behalf.

The literacy level of the target population must be taken into consideration when using written information. Many studies have documented the poor correlation of patients' literacy level and the level at which discharge information from EDs is given to them [30–34]. Written information's effectiveness can only be as good as the readers' ability to comprehend the information. Asking patients to take the next step to initiate further outpatient care and preventive services may be beyond many peoples' ability. Poor comprehension leads to poor compliance with written instructions, as documented by Thomas and coworkers [35]. This study also demonstrated the correlation between passive instructions (the staff made no attempts to arrange follow-up) and poor compliance with recommendations. An alternative, potentially more successful strategy is for the staff to arrange a follow-up appointment before the patient leaves the ED.

Even if patients are able fully to understand the information given to them, the pamphlet's layout and attractiveness may also have a significant effect on its success. Berger and coworkers [29] speculate that the men's low rate of reading the informational pamphlet on Pap smears, mammograms, and pneumococcal vaccination may have been improved had the pneumococcal information been presented before the women's specific topics.

Others have explored novel methods of improving comprehension and retention of written information. Brooks [30] notes that awareness of literacy problems and tailoring language appropriately can benefit comprehension. Simplification of instructions and recommendations may lead to increased understanding, regardless of patient demographics [32]. Austin and colleagues [36] report that including illustrations within written information adds to a patient's understanding. Not all health care issues are amenable to graphic depiction. In practice, pictorial representation of many health preventive and promotional topics may prove somewhat difficult. Clinicians should take into consideration age-related changes in learning style and tailor information appropriately to improve comprehension. This was demonstrated in a randomized trial of geriatric-specific instructional materials for patients discharged from EDs [37].

Written information on health promotion and disease prevention that is simply handed out to an untargeted ED population is not a proved means by which to improve the overall health of the community. Furthermore, ensuring understanding of the information may not lead to as great an effect as hoped. Logan and coworkers [33] report that literacy itself could not fully account for all misunderstandings in ED discharge instructions. It seems that written information alone may have limited effect. No harm is typically caused by providing such information, yet lost opportunity during a patient encounter carries a cost. More interactive and proactive methods used in conjunction with written materials optimize individual outcomes, having a greater impact for the health of society.

Computerized information and education

With the increased availability and comfort level of the public with computer technology, health promotion and disease prevention topics can be dispensed easily to patients as they wait for treatment in EDs or immediately on discharge. Waiting time can be long in many departments and represent a captive time during which patients are susceptible to learning.

Rhodes and colleagues [38] studied the effect of a self-administered computer survey given in the waiting room. The computer generated individualized health information and recommendations based on the information patients' provided. They found that use of the computer survey led to the disclosure of a significant number of health risks and requests for information when compared with a control group who received usual care. Patients in the computer group were more likely to remember the advice given to them than were the controls. Computers also offer anonymity, which may improve detection rates of sensitive health issues and risk factors compared with personal interviewing [39]. These studies document the possible usefulness of the computer in eliciting sensitive and appropriate health risks, but do not document an outcome of improved personal or public health.

There have been attempts to assess behavioral outcomes related to computer-assisted recommendations. They showed limited success. Quan and coworkers [40] reported that only 41% of parents could recall a specific message pertaining to the use of swimming life vests given to them in the form of computerized discharge instructions when they left a pediatric ED. Additionally, only 35% said they would consider buying their child a life vest in the future. No verification of purchase was completed to document impact on behavior. Zonfrillo and coworkers [41] demonstrated a self-reported 10% behavior modification effect on parents given child restraint device information in the form of computerized discharge instructions after a visit to an ED.

Comfort levels and proficiency with computer technology for those at greatest risk need to be addressed before widespread use of this technique can be recommended. A goal of ED health promotion and disease prevention is to reach the population that typically cannot or does not access the health care system in any other way. This is the population that has less access to computers in their homes than other populations, which may lead to increased resistance against the use of the technology to achieve the stated goals.

Environmental education

ED waiting rooms may be an appropriate place to locate educational materials related to health promotion and disease prevention. These materials represent a passive means of communicating relevant information to patients and their families regarding health topics. These presentations could take many forms including simple written pamphlets, posters, and placards for high-visibility locations; closed-loop television programs; or on-demand streaming computer videos. The advantages of this approach include low additional overhead production costs and ease of use, without additional staffing requirements. Yet, one study evaluating this technique in a family practice waiting room setting showed no increase in the use of preventive services when compared with historical controls over a 4-month period [42]. Kleemeier and Hazzard evaluated a videotape on parenting tips in a pediatric waiting room versus the same videotape seen in a structured setting and found that unstructured learning was much less effective than structured learning [43]. Structured settings require additional resources. Further studies are needed, with particular attention to the unique needs of the ED population and the true impact of the presented material on patient behavior.

Behavioral change counseling and motivational interviewing

ED patients may be well served by brief sessions targeting specific health promotion and disease prevention topics incorporating their reason for visiting. One example is an intervention addressing driving and alcohol consumption in a patient being evaluated for injuries sustained during a motor vehicle collision. These sessions, referred to as "brief interventions" or "motivational interviewing," are designed to be interactive to motivate patients to change behavioral patterns [44]. They can be performed by various staff either already present in the ED or hired specifically for this task. Additional training for staff is required to direct effectively and proficiently brief motivational interview sessions to affect behavioral change. These techniques have been successfully implemented to address behavioral issues in other areas of medicine, particularly in addiction medicine [44–47].

Identification of appropriate issues to be addressed is the first step in using behavior change counseling. Typically, two approaches can be taken. The first takes advantage of the so-called "teachable moment" and addresses the issue directly related to the reason for the ED visit. Secondly, the ED staff can broadly address health promotion and disease prevention topics that are unrelated to the reason for the acute care visit. For example, mammography screening could be discussed with a woman seen in the ED for a laceration repair.

Once a particular topic is identified, trained personnel can approach each patient with provisional consent to discuss specific issues. The goal for the ED staff is to identify a discrepancy between the patients' current behaviors (ie, drinking and driving or avoidance of mammography) and their desired behavior (ie, not drinking and driving or obtaining screening mammography). Trained ED staff can direct conversations to help patients reflect on their behavior in a motivational, nonconfrontational fashion to promote healthy habits and favorable outcomes. Resistance can arise from many aspects of these interactions including patients' sense of threat, superiority, condemnation, coercion, or argumentation from the interviewer or staff [44]. Proper training of staff is critical in the application of brief motivational interviewing.

The motivational counseling technique has had varied levels of success. Behavior change counseling for adolescents has increased seatbelt and bicycle helmet use, but has not curtailed drinking and driving, riding with impaired driver, binge drinking, or weapon carrying rates [48]. Gentilello and coworkers [49] performed a randomized study of alcohol interventions in a trauma center to reduce the risk of injury recurrence. Understanding that alcohol is a leading risk factor for injury, they applied a brief intervention to a group of patients who screened positive for alcohol use as part of their trauma evaluation. They found those who received the intervention demonstrated a significant reduction in alcohol intake and a reduced risk of trauma recidivism in the year following the intervention compared with those who did not receive the brief intervention. Similarly encouraging results were found when brief interventions were used for tobacco abuse, both in adults and in adolescents [46,50].

Preventive services in the emergency department

Some EDs have moved beyond supplying preventive health information and have begun to provide disease prevention and health promotional services. These in-department programs have had varying degrees of success. They require extensive organization and cooperation with outpatient facilities to ensure proper follow-up of patients identified at risk and with disease. Simply identifying the appropriate patient for a service and providing that service or screen does not ensure cost-effective use of resources. Those patients identified and screened by EDs must receive definitive treatment to ensure maximal benefit to both the individual patient and the population as a whole.

One ED-based women's heath program assessed the feasibility of breast and cervical cancer screening in a public ED [51]. Patients were offered Pap tests and a clinical breast examination if 18 years or older, and a mammogram if over 40 years old. The Pap test and clinical breast examination were performed in the department on the day of the visit, whereas mammography was scheduled for a later date in the radiology department. Only 6% of the 1850 eligible women completed both screening tools for breast cancer and 20% completed Pap smears while in the ED. Follow-up rates were low (20% for breast screening and 50% for cervical screening). The authors report that the program's efficiency was limited because of low volume of screened patients and poor follow-up, despite high rates of cancer detection. As expected, greater organization, cooperation, and integration with outpatient facilities that are needed to provide testing and treatment is a limiting factor for these types of programs. A cost-effective analysis of this program showed that cervical screening was indeed cost-effective given detection and treatment rates, whereas breast cancer screening was not seen as favorable based on cost per life saved [52].

Project ASSERT, designed by Bernstein and coworkers [53], was implemented in a Boston ED to address substance abuse issues and access to primary care and preventive services for the ED population. The authors found no difference in ED use over the next 12 months despite this rather intensive educational effort. Reasons for this program's failure highlight the difficulties in educational program implementation. Educational programs must be highly tailored and validated for the targeted population, they must be closely monitored, and they must be continuously evaluated for overall effectiveness given their level of monetary and staffing requirements.

Shields and coworkers [54] studied an educational program for inner city children with asthma who used the ED for asthma treatment. The educational component included classroom instruction for parents on asthma and its appropriate management, and then subsequent follow-up telephone calls to provide additional reinforcement. This study, however, also failed to meets its goals.

Another area that is unique to emergency medicine is domestic violence prevention. Often, the ED is the only point of contact into the health care system for victims of this type of abuse. Although outcome and effectiveness data are lacking, it has been shown that the ED can formalize domestic violence initiatives to identify and begin treatment or at least initiate referral of domestic violence victims when they are seen in the ED for the acute event or injury [55]. All ED staff should be knowledgeable of community resources for domestic violence and willing openly to discuss these issues with any and all suspected victims.

Other areas that have been explored using ED-based programs include pediatric injury prevention, childhood literacy promotion, and poisoning prevention in children [56–58]. These programs have not all been successful, and there are limited outcome data.

Emergency medical services role in health promotion and disease prevention

Emergency medical services (EMS) has the opportunity, some say a responsibility, to contribute to the overall well-being of the community that it serves. This responsibility is increasingly being seen as primary injury prevention (ie, not only responding to injuries as they occur but becoming proactive in the prevention of the injuries commonly seen in the community). EMS is unique, as suggested by the EMS Agenda for the Future, because "EMS represents the intersection of public safety, public health, and health care systems" [59]. This perspective gives them the unique opportunity to identify many issues that may be positively influenced by simple EMS intervention, as delineated by Mann and Hedges [60]. These issues include elder abuse, child abuse, substance abuse, fire hazards, domestic violence, poisoning hazards, fall hazards, unsafe roadways, and infectious disease outbreaks.

There has been some research performed on the use of EMS in prevention. Gerson and coworkers [61] in Akron, Ohio, demonstrated the ability of EMS providers to identify and refer community-dwelling at-risk elderly to the community agency responsible for providing elder health and social services. Krumperman [62] showed similar ability of EMS to refer people at risk for injury to appropriate social service entities. Studies have examined other prevention roles of EMS. These include provision of home fire safety interventions in homes frequented by EMS personnel, geriatric injury prevention instructional programs, and pediatric injury prevention programs proposed to managed care organizations [63–65]. A rather extensive theoretical expansion for EMS has been undertaken by the Division of Emergency Medicine at Stanford University, called the "Accidents Aren't" Program [66]. This initiative provides a modular approach to the role of EMS in injury prevention, and allows communities to configure their primary injury prevention needs individually, while providing a foundation of knowledge on injury prevention techniques including instructor guidelines, training tools, and mnemonics to injury prevention approaches. All of these issues show promise in promoting the health of communities, but all require adequate additional work to establish whether or not they have a beneficial effect on the health of the individual and the community as a whole.

In addition to the expanding primary prevention role of prehospital care providers, EMS leaders should continually evaluate the impact and benefit of their overall effort [67,68]. Potential areas of study and progress are numerous: injury prevention for EMS providers, the outcome of injury prevention education for EMS providers, further injury data collection, organizational partnerships for the attainment of injury prevention, public relations techniques, and cooperation with other community organizations in injury prevention activities. Highlighting the opportunity for progress, a recent survey of paramedics demonstrated that many believe primary injury prevention to be an important aspect of their job, yet relatively few have received any significant training in it and even fewer actually practice injury prevention on a daily basis.

The shift from the traditional role of EMS in tertiary prevention toward a greater primary and secondary prevention role takes time, persistent effort, and additional training [69]. Patients themselves may also be reluctant to accept the expanded role of EMS. This was demonstrated by the preliminary study of an in-home prevention survey done in rural communities, in which only 5.9% of patients seen in an ED for injuries sustained in their homes participated in the study survey to asses the home environment for potential safety problems [12]. The shift toward a broader role of EMS providers in all levels of prevention takes time and resources. This transformation has tremendous potential for improving the health of communities. At the resident's picnic, a primary prevention task, such as barricading the road, could have prevented further victims from falling into the river.

Health promotion and disease prevention in emergency medicine: systems viewpoint

Classically, EDs and staff have not viewed themselves as preventionists. The SAEM Public Health and Education Task Force pointed out several reasons why emergency medicine can and should participate in prevention and screening activities [15]. Many factors support preventive medicine practices in the ED: existing prevention and health promotional services (eg, tetanus immunization); the role of the EDs as sole contact to the health care system for many patients; the susceptibility of ED patients to timely teaching and intervention (the teachable moment concept); and increasingly unmet needs of prevention.

The question of who provides such prevention and health promotion activities arises as a next logical step. Recent literature supports the concept that emergency medicine's efforts in health promotion and disease prevention should be integrated with a larger, more encompassing lead agency [70–73]. This agency is commonly thought to be analogous to but not necessarily equivalent to public health departments. Seamless integration of available community resources is vital to achieving a beneficial and cost-effective impact on the health of a community and its individuals. The concept of a public health outpost should be introduced, with a "health preventionist" staff member present in the ED at all times. Incorporating public health workers into existing emergency medicine infrastructures is a more comprehensive health care model, which can help bear the burden of providing for the entire health of a community. The cost of health promotion and disease prevention should be spread among governmental agencies, individual patients, health care insurers, hospitals and their agencies, and private industry.

A reasonable approach is an expansion of Bernstein and coworkers' Project Assert [74]. A designated health care worker who is a preventionist could support the primary prevention needs in the ED. This medical provider, with training as a health educator, would be responsible for addressing issues specifically revolving around patients' ED visits. Patient encounters provide several opportunities for identification of health needs, including initial screening at triage, issues identified by physicians and nurses during routine care, or established health promotional and disease and injury prevention programs. A medical preventionist could be responsible for brief counseling, informational distribution, scheduling of outpatient procedures and examinations, and referrals to other community agencies. Staffing of this position would ideally be 24 hours a day, fully to serve all patients reporting to the ED [75]. The ED census should determine optimum staffing pattern to provide the most cost-effective model of care.

A database compilation of all available community resources is a valuable tool for preventionists. Currently, many communities lack centralized organization of all available services, leaving some services underused and others overburdened. Experience and information technology from other industries may well provide answers to this issue.

It is worth noting that EDs and EMS systems of the future may become part of a region wide or nationwide public health surveillance system, as suggested by Hsiao and Hedges [76]. Garrison and coworkers [77] also propose a national strategy for ED surveillance of both injury and illness. They believe in a natural alliance of public health and emergency medicine that can identify, evaluate, and quickly respond to the health care needs of individual communities, while keeping track of overall health of the nation. Hirshon [78] outlined several reasons for a National Public Health Surveillance System, including better communication between health departments and EDs, quicker responses to rapidly developing public health emergencies, improved correlation of environmental events and ED visits, improved information on scope and nature of ED visits, improved infectious disease documentation and evaluation, improved hospital-based patient record systems, and better influence on public policy discussions and decisions.

Systematic collection of appropriate ED data is a major hurdle to overcome in establishing a region wide or nationwide network. Simply collecting hospitalization or mortality data misses a large proportion of injuries and illness that occur in the United States [79]. Additional data inclusive of ED visits and possibly even primary care visits must be collected. Once this type of information is available, communities could combine all available resources into one database. Databases could be used by health preventionists to initiate health promotion and disease prevention activities for ED patients. Integration into the community as a whole is crucial for the survival and effectiveness of these programs, and "the capacity of the ED to identify health problems in the population should not lead to the assumption that all problems can or should be solved in the ED" [71].

Finally, it is worth mentioning a social action approach to prevention. Emergency medicine professionals can bring their skills and knowledge to bear in a variety of issues relevant to emergency medicine. This can be accomplished through policy within professional organizations or through local efforts, such as testifying about relevant issues before legislative bodies. Additionally, emergency medical professionals can step out of the ED to promote public education or volunteer in public health sponsored preventive programs.

Summary

Health promotion and disease prevention can be incorporated into emergency medical tasks. Although some currently take place daily in the ED, others need greater efforts at implementation. Continuous screening and follow-up studies evaluating effectiveness, cost-efficiency, and community health impact are needed. The specialty of emergency medicine must heed two important issues regarding the implementation of prevention programs: adherence to the basic guidelines for effective preventive medicine programs and expectation of resistance to new programs.

Preventive medical services provided through EDs need to be cost effective in improving the health of individuals and the community in which they live. These services must address problems with a high incidence for the given population and they must have an acceptable and sensitive screening test to detect the problem. Health promotion activities, such as those aimed at sociobehavioral change, must be of proved value and benefit. Risk detection can be performed with routine questionnaire screening or may involve medical procedures scheduled at later dates. The health problem must be serious enough to warrant identification and timely intervention must be of proved benefit. Analysis of cost effectiveness must look beyond short-term costs associated with implementation and take into account long-term realizations including diseases or injuries avoided because of promotional and preventive activities.

Health promotion and disease prevention must frequently overcome resistance to fulfill its mission. Providing screening test or information about risk-taking behavior is only the first step. Effective mechanisms for follow-up and arrangement of further testing or intervention must be provided. For example, Rojas and coworkers [80] found many reasons for lack of adequate follow-up for women with abnormal mammograms. These included whether the patient was symptomatic at the time of the examination, whether the women were even told they needed follow-up, and whether the clinical examination was abnormal at time of mammogram. Shaw and coworkers [5] performed Pap screens in medically indigent women having a clinically indicated pelvic examination. The found that the ED patients were more likely to have a positive finding than were a control group of clinic patients. Noteworthy is that they were unable to reach 20% of patients for follow-up and almost two thirds of these had positive results. Other factors that must be overcome include physical constraints, such as location of provided services, and transportation problems, monetary and billing issues, and some patients' reluctance to experience uncomfortable procedures. Not to be forgotten is the resistance on behalf of the staff that is now being asked to provide a different, and in some cases additional, type of care to patients that may take them out of their comfort zone.

The ED has the potential to improve the public's health through various health promotion and preventive activities. The opportunity exists, but it has not been fully realized. With attention to the basic principles of preventive medicine, and evidenced-based objective evaluation of outcomes, many of the strategies for implementing health promotion and disease prevention activities can have a significant effect on the health of an entire population.

References

[1] Last JM, Spasoff R, Harris SS, et al. A dictionary of epidemiology. 4th edition. New York: Oxford University Press; 2001.

[2] Haddon W Jr., Baker, SP. Injury control, in preventive and community medicine. In: Clark D, editor. Little Brown; 1981. p. 109–40.

[3] Irvin CB. Public health preventive services, surveillance, and screening: the emergency department's potential. Acad Emerg Med 2000;7:1421–3.

[4] Department of Health and Human Services, Agency for Healthcare Research and Quality. United States Preventive Services Task Force. Screening for cervical cancer. Available at: http://www.ahrq.gov/clinic/uspstf/uspscerv.htm. Accessed August 15, 2006.

[5] Shaw J, G.K., Polifrone C, Williams J. Feasibility of ED based cervical cancer screening in a community setting. Presented at the CREOG (Council on Resident Education in Obstetrics & Gynecology) and APGO (Association of Professors of Gynecology & Obstetrics) annual meeting. Salt Lake City, 2005.

[6] Sackett DL, Holland WW. Controversy in the detection of disease. Lancet 1975;2: 357–9.

[7] Department of Health and Human Services, Agency for Healthcare Research and Quality. United States Preventive Services Task Force. High blood pressure screening. Available at: http://www.ahrq.gov/clinic/uspstf/uspshype.htm. Accessed August 15, 2006.

[8] Years of potential life lost before ages 65 and 85—United States, 1989–1990. MMWR Morb Mortal Wkly Rep 1992;41:313–5.

[9] Mokdad AH, Marks JS, Stroup DF, Gerberding JL. Actual causes of death in the United States, 2000. JAMA 2004;291:1238–45.

[10] Llovera I, Ward MF, Ryan JG, Latouche T, Sama A. A survey of the emergency department population and their interest in preventive health education. Acad Emerg Med 2003;10: 155–60.

[11] Rodriguez RM, Kreider WJ, Baraff LJ. Need and desire for preventive care measures in emergency department patients. Ann Emerg Med 1995;26:615–20.

[12] Moore E, McComas J. Acceptance of an injury-prevention program in rural communities: a preliminary study. Prehospital Disaster Medicine 1996;11:309–11.

[13] Fleisher GR, Crain EF, Li M, Rodewald LE, Hodge D 3rd, Avner JR, Isaacman D. The role of the emergency department in primary care. Pediatr Emerg Care 1992;8:98–104.

[14] Babcock Irvin C, Wyer PC, Gerson LW. Preventive care in the emergency department, Part II: Clinical preventive services–an emergency medicine evidence-based review. Society for Academic Emergency Medicine Public Health and Education Task Force Preventive Services Work Group. Acad Emerg Med 2000;7:1042–54.

[15] Rhodes KV, Gordon JA, Lowe RA. Preventive care in the emergency department, Part I: Clinical preventive services–are they relevant to emergency medicine? Society for Academic Emergency Medicine Public Health and Education Task Force Preventive Services Work Group. Acad Emerg Med 2000;7:1036–41.

[16] Joint Commission on Accreditation of Healthcare Organizations. Accreditation manual for hospitals. Oakbrook Terrace (IL): JCAHO; 1996.

[17] McCaig LF, Burt CW. National Hospital Ambulatory Medical Care Survey: 2002. Advance data from vital and health statistics; no. 340. Hyattsville, MD: National Center for Health Statistics. 2004.

[18] Cohen JJ. Disparities in health care: an overview. Acad Emerg Med 2003;10:1155–60.

[19] Burt CW, Arispe IE. Characteristics of emergency departments serving high volumes of safety-net patients: United States, 2000. Vital Health Stat 13. 2004; May;(155):1–16.

[20] Lewis Me, Altman S. America's health care safety net: intact but endangered. Washington: National Academy Press, 2000.

[21] Healthy People 2010. Available at: http://www.healthypeople.gov/. Accessed August 15, 2006.

[22] Sanders AB, W.D., Jones JS, Richmond K, Kidd P. Geriatric emergency care model in emergency care of the elder person. In: Sanders AB, editor. Geriatric Emergency Medicine Task Force. St. Louis, MO: Beverly Cracom Communications; 1996.

[23] Siebens H. The domain management model: a tool for teaching and management of older adults in emergency departments. Acad Emerg Med 2005;12(2):162–8.

[24] McCusker J, Cardin S, Bellavance F, Belzile E. Return to the emergency department among elders: patterns and predictors. Acad Emerg Med 2000;7:249–59.

[25] Lowenstein SR, Koziol-McLain J, Thompson M, Bernstein E, Greenberg K, Gerson LW, Buczynsky P, Blanda M. Behavioral risk factors in emergency department patients: a multi-site survey. Acad Emerg Med 1998;5:781–7.

[26] Hockberger RS, Binder LS, Graber MA, et al. The model of the clinical practice of emergency medicine. Ann Emerg Med 2001;37:745–70.

[27] Emergency Nurses Association. Position statements available at: http://www.ena.org/about/position/. Accessed: August 15, 2006.

[28] Gerson LW, Larkin GL, Degutis LC. Injury prevention research: quo vadis? Acad Emerg Med 2004;11:672–3.

[29] Berger P, Luskin M, Krishel S. Preventive health pamphlets in the emergency department. J Emerg Med 1998;16:691–4.

[30] Brooks DA. Techniques for teaching ED patients with low literacy skills. J Emerg Nurs 1998; 24:601–3.

[31] Chacon D, Kissoon N, Rich S. Education attainment level of caregivers versus readability level of written instructions in a pediatric emergency department. Pediatr Emerg Care 1994;10:144–9.

[32] Jolly BT, Scott JL, Feied CF, Sanford SM. Functional illiteracy among emergency department patients: a preliminary study. Ann Emerg Med 1993;22:573–8.

[33] Logan PD, Schwab RA, Salomone JA 3rd, et al. Patient understanding of emergency department discharge instructions. South Med J 1996;89:770–4.

[34] Spandorfer JM, Karras DJ, Hughes LA, Caputo C. Comprehension of discharge instructions by patients in an urban emergency department. Ann Emerg Med 1995;25:71–4.

[35] Thomas EJ, Burstin HR, O'Neil AC, Orav EJ, Brennan TA. Patient noncompliance with medical advice after the emergency department visit. Ann Emerg Med 1996;27:49–55.

[36] Austin PE, Matlack R 2nd, Dunn KA, et al. Discharge instructions: do illustrations help our patients understand them? Ann Emerg Med 1995;25:317–20.

[37] Hayes KS. Randomized trial of geragogy-based medication instruction in the emergency department. Nurs Res 1998;47:211–8.

[38] Rhodes KV, Lauderdale DS, Stocking CB, et al. Better health while you wait: a controlled trial of a computer-based intervention for screening and health promotion in the emergency department. Ann Emerg Med 2001;37:284–91.

[39] Rhodes KV, Lauderdale DS, He T, et al. "Between me and the computer": increased detection of intimate partner violence using a computer questionnaire. Ann Emerg Med 2002;40:476–84.

[40] Quan L, Bennett E, Cummings P, et al. Do parents value drowning prevention information at discharge from the emergency department? Ann Emerg Med 2001;37:382–5.

[41] Zonfrillo MR, Mello MJ, Palmisciano LM. Usefulness of computerized pediatric motor vehicle safety discharge instructions. Acad Emerg Med 2003;10:1131–3.

[42] Mead VP, Rhyne RL, Wiese WH, et al. Impact of environmental patient education on preventive medicine practices. J Fam Pract 1995;40:363–9.

[43] Kleemeier CP, Hazzard AP. Videotaped parent education in pediatric waiting rooms. Patient Educ Couns 1984;6:122–4.

[44] Lawendowski LA. A motivational intervention for adolescent smokers. Prev Med 1998; 27(5 Pt 3):A39–46.

[45] Berg-Smith SM, Stevens VJ, Brown KM, et al. A brief motivational intervention to improve dietary adherence in adolescents. The Dietary Intervention Study in Children (DISC) Research Group. Health Educ Res 1999;14:399–410.

[46] Colby SM, Monti PM, Barnett NP, et al. Brief motivational interviewing in a hospital setting for adolescent smoking: a preliminary study. J Consult Clin Psychol 1998;66:574–8.

[47] Monti PM, Colby SM, Barnett NP, et al. Brief intervention for harm reduction with alcohol-positive older adolescents in a hospital emergency department. J Consult Clin Psychol 1999; 67:989–94.

[48] Johnston BD, Rivara FP, Donovan DM, et al. Behavior change counseling in the emergency department to reduce injury risk: a randomized, controlled trial. Pediatrics 2002;110(2 Pt 1): 267–74.

[49] Gentilello LM, Rivara FP, Donovan DM, et al. Alcohol interventions in a trauma center as a means of reducing the risk of injury recurrence. Ann Surg 1999;230:473–80 [discussion: 480–3].

[50] Rollnick S, Butler CC, Stott N. Helping smokers make decisions: the enhancement of brief intervention for general medical practice. Patient Educ Couns 1997;31:191–203.

[51] Mandelblatt J, Freeman H, Winczewski D. Implementation of a breast and cervical cancer screening program in a public hospital emergency department. Cancer Control Center of Harlem. Ann Emerg Med 1996;28:493–8.

[52] Mandelblatt J, Freeman H, Winczewski D, et al. The costs and effects of cervical and breast cancer screening in a public hospital emergency room. The Cancer Control Center of Harlem. Am J Public Health 1997;87:1182–9.

[53] Bernstein E, Bernstein J, Levenson S. The effect of a patient education program on emergency room use for inner-city children with asthma. Ann Emerg Med 1990;80:36–8.

[54] Shields MC, Griffin KW, McNabb WL. The effect of a patient education program on emergency room use for inner-city children with asthma. Am J Public Health 1990;80:36–8.

[55] Hotch D, Griffin KW, McNabb WL. An emergency department-based domestic violence intervention program: findings after one year. J Emerg Med 1996;14:111–7.

[56] Ellerby P, Ward PM. Development of a pediatric injury prevention program for emergency departments. J Emerg Nurs 1989;15:224–8.

[57] Nagamine WH, Ishida JT, Williams DR, et al. Child literacy promotion in the emergency department. Pediatr Emerg Care 2001;17:19–21.

[58] Woolf AD, Saperstein A, Forjuoh S. Poisoning prevention knowledge and practices of parents after a childhood poisoning incident. Pediatrics 1992;90:867–70.

[59] National Highway Traffic Safety Administration. EMS historical perspective: emergency medical services agenda for the future. Washington: National Highway Traffic Safety Administration; 1995.

[60] Mann NC, Hedges JR. The role of prehospital care providers in the advancement of public health. Prehosp Emerg Care 2002;6(2 Suppl):S63–7.

[61] Gerson LW, Schelble DT, Wilson JE. Using paramedics to identify at-risk elderly. Ann Emerg Med 1992;21:688–91.

[62] Krumperman KM. Filling the gap. EMS social service referrals. Journal of Emergency Medical Services 1993;18(25):27–9.

[63] El Sanadi N. Geriatric injury prevention: a new role for EMS personnel? Emerg Med Serv 1996;25 51–3, 67.

[64] Moody-Williams JD, Athey J, Barlow B, et al. Injury prevention and emergency medical services for children in a managed care environment. Ann Emerg Med 2000;35:245–51.

[65] Pirrallo RG, Rubin JM, Murawsky GA. The potential benefit of a home fire safety intervention during emergency medical services calls. Acad Emerg Med 1998;5:220–4.

[66] Yancey AH II, Martinez R, Kellermann AL. Injury prevention and emergency medical services: the "Accidents Aren't" program. Prehosp Emerg Care 2002;6:204–9.

[67] Kinnane JM, Garrison HG, Coben JH, Alonso-Serra HM. Injury prevention: is there a role for out-of-hospital emergency medical services? Acad Emerg Med 1997;4:306–12.

[68] Garrison HG, Foltin GL, Becker LR, et al. The role of emergency medical services in primary injury prevention. Consensus workshop. Arlington, Virginia, August 25–26, 1995. Ann Emerg Med 1997;30:84–91.

[69] Jaslow D, Ufberg J, Marsh R. Primary injury prevention in an urban EMS system. J Emerg Med 2003;25:167–70.

[70] Gordon JA. The hospital emergency department as a social welfare institution. Ann Emerg Med 1999;33:321–5.

[71] Clancy CM, Eisenberg JM. Emergency medicine in population-based systems of care. Ann Emerg Med 1997;30:800–3.

[72] Micik S, Miclette M. Injury prevention in the community: a systems approach. Pediatr Clin North Am 1985;32:251–65.

[73] Bernstein E, Goldfrank LR, Kellerman AL, et al. A public health approach to emergency medicine: preparing for the twenty-first century. Acad Emerg Med 1994;1:277–86.

[74] Bernstein E, Bernstein J, Levenson S. Project ASSERT: an ED-based intervention to increase access to primary care, preventive services, and the substance abuse treatment system. Ann Emerg Med 1997;30:181–9.

[75] Soskis CW. Emergency room on weekends: the only game in town. Health Soc Work 1980;5: 37–43.

[76] Hsiao AK, Hedges JR. Role of the emergency medical services system in regionwide health monitoring and referral. Ann Emerg Med 1993;22:1696–702.

[77] Garrison HG, Runyan CW, Tintinalli JE, et al. Emergency department surveillance: an examination of issues and a proposal for a national strategy. Ann Emerg Med 1994;24:849–56.

[78] Hirshon JM. The rationale for developing public health surveillance systems based on emergency department data. Acad Emerg Med 2000;7:1428–32.

[79] Injury prevention: meeting the challenge. The National Committee for Injury Prevention and Control. Am J Prev Med 1989;5(3 Suppl):1–303.

[80] Rojas M, Mandelblatt J, Cagney K, et al. Barriers to follow-up of abnormal screening mammograms among low-income minority women. Cancer Control Center of Harlem. Ethn Health 1996;1:221–8.

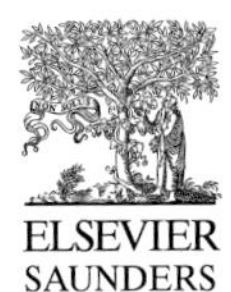

EMERGENCY
MEDICINE
CLINICS OF
NORTH AMERICA

Emerg Med Clin N Am
24 (2006) 871–888

Injury Prevention

Linda C. Degutis, DrPH, MSN[a,b,*], Mark Greve, MD[c]

[a]*Section of Emergency Medicine, Department of Surgery, Yale University School of Medicine, 464 Congress Avenue, New Haven, CT 06520, USA*
[b]*Department of Epidemiology and Public Health, 2 Church Street South, New Haven, CT 06519, USA*
[c]*Department of Emergency Medicine, Brown Medical School at Rhode Island Hospital, 593 Eddy Street, Providence, RI, USA*

Injuries, a major public health problem, are the leading cause of death for people in the United States between the ages of 1 and 44 and the fourth leading cause of death overall. An injury occurs when there is a transfer of energy from an injury-causing agent or vehicle to the host. This energy may be mechanical, chemical, or thermal.

Injuries, poisoning, and adverse effects of medical treatment accounted for approximately 35.5% of emergency department (ED) visits in 2002, with the total number of ED visits for injury amounting to approximately 39.2 million visits, or 13.8 visits per 100 persons. The leading causes of injury-related ED visits were falls, motor vehicle crashes, and being struck by or striking against an object [1].

Injuries fall into two categories of intent: unintentional and intentional. Unintentional injuries, which account for approximately two thirds of injury deaths, are those that occur as the result of circumstances in which the harmful outcome is not planned, such as most motor vehicle crashes, falls, and occupational injuries. Intentional injuries, or violent injuries, may be inflicted by others, or self-inflicted as with suicide.

To prevent injuries and the events that lead to them, it is necessary to have a basic understanding of the epidemiology of injury, and the contributions of various types of injury events to mortality and morbidity. Injuries are a major cause of death in young people, and one of the leading causes of deaths for all age groups. According to data from the Centers for Disease Control and Prevention, motor vehicle crashes are the single leading cause of death for people between the ages of 1 and 34. As illustrated in Fig. 1,

* Corresponding author.
E-mail address: linda.degutis@yale.edu (L.C. Degutis).

doi:10.1016/j.emc.2006.06.015   *emed.theclinics.com*

<table>
<tr><td colspan="12" align="center">Age Groups</td></tr>
<tr><td>Rank</td><td><1</td><td>1-4</td><td>5-9</td><td>10-14</td><td>15-24</td><td>25-34</td><td>35-44</td><td>45-54</td><td>55-64</td><td>65+</td><td>Total</td></tr>
<tr><td>1</td><td>Congenital Anomalies 5,621</td><td>Unintentional Injury 1,717</td><td>Unintentional Injury 1,096</td><td>Unintentional Injury 1,522</td><td>Unintentional Injury 15,272</td><td>Unintentional Injury 12,541</td><td>Unintentional Injury 16,766</td><td>Malignant Neoplasms 49,843</td><td>Malignant Neoplasms 95,692</td><td>Heart Disease 563,390</td><td>Heart Disease 685,089</td></tr>
<tr><td>2</td><td>Short Gestation 4,849</td><td>Congenital Anomalies 541</td><td>Malignant Neoplasms 516</td><td>Malignant Neoplasms 560</td><td>Homicide 5,368</td><td>Suicide 5,065</td><td>Malignant Neoplasms 15,509</td><td>Heart Disease 37,732</td><td>Heart Disease 65,060</td><td>Malignant Neoplasms 388,911</td><td>Malignant Neoplasms 556,902</td></tr>
<tr><td>3</td><td>SIDS 2,162</td><td>Malignant Neoplasms 392</td><td>Congenital Anomalies 180</td><td>Suicide 244</td><td>Suicide 3,988</td><td>Homicide 4,516</td><td>Heart Disease 13,600</td><td>Unintentional Injury 15,837</td><td>Chronic Low. Respiratory Disease 12,077</td><td>Cerebro-vascular 138,134</td><td>Cerebro-vascular 157,689</td></tr>
<tr><td>4</td><td>Maternal Pregnancy Comp. 1,710</td><td>Homicide 376</td><td>Homicide 122</td><td>Congenital Anomalies 206</td><td>Malignant Neoplasms 1,651</td><td>Malignant Neoplasms 3,741</td><td>Suicide 6,602</td><td>Liver Disease 7,466</td><td>Diabetes Mellitus 10,731</td><td>Chronic Low. Respiratory Disease 109,139</td><td>Chronic Low. Respiratory Disease 126,382</td></tr>
<tr><td>5</td><td>Placenta Cord Membranes 1,099</td><td>Heart Disease 186</td><td>Heart Disease 104</td><td>Homicide 202</td><td>Heart Disease 1,133</td><td>Heart Disease 3,250</td><td>HIV 5,340</td><td>Suicide 6,481</td><td>Cerebro-vascular 9,946</td><td>Alzheimer's Disease 62,814</td><td>Unintentional Injury 109,277</td></tr>
<tr><td>6</td><td>Unintentional Injury 945</td><td>Influenza & Pneumonia 163</td><td>Influenza & Pneumonia 75</td><td>Heart Disease 160</td><td>Congenital Anomalies 451</td><td>HIV 1,588</td><td>Homicide 3,110</td><td>Cerebro-vascular 6,127</td><td>Unintentional Injury 9,170</td><td>Influenza & Pneumonia 57,670</td><td>Diabetes Mellitus 74,219</td></tr>
<tr><td>7</td><td>Respiratory Distress 831</td><td>Septicemia 85</td><td>Septicemia 39</td><td>Chronic Low. Respiratory Disease 81</td><td>Influenza & Pneumonia 224</td><td>Diabetes Mellitus 657</td><td>Liver Disease 3,020</td><td>Diabetes Mellitus 5,658</td><td>Liver Disease 6,428</td><td>Diabetes Mellitus 54,919</td><td>Influenza & Pneumonia 65,163</td></tr>
<tr><td>8</td><td>Bacterial Sepsis 772</td><td>Perinatal Period 79</td><td>Benign Neoplasms 38</td><td>Influenza & Pneumonia 72</td><td>Cerebro-vascular 221</td><td>Cerebro-vascular 583</td><td>Cerebro-vascular 2,460</td><td>HIV 4,442</td><td>Suicide 3,843</td><td>Nephritis 35,254</td><td>Alzheimer's Disease 63,457</td></tr>
<tr><td>9</td><td>Neonatal Hemorrhage 649</td><td>Chronic Low. Respiratory Disease 55</td><td>Chronic Low. Respiratory Disease 37</td><td>Benign Neoplasms 41</td><td>Chronic Low. Respiratory Disease 191</td><td>Congenital Anomalies 426</td><td>Diabetes Mellitus 2,049</td><td>Chronic Low. Respiratory 3,537</td><td>Nephritis 3,806</td><td>Unintentional Injury 34,335</td><td>Nephritis 42,453</td></tr>
<tr><td>10</td><td>Circulatory System Disease 591</td><td>Benign Neoplasms 51</td><td>Cerebro-vascular 29</td><td>Cerebro-vascular 40</td><td>HIV 178</td><td>Influenza & Pneumonia 373</td><td>Influenza & Pneumonia 992</td><td>Viral Hepatitis 2,259</td><td>Septicemia 3,651</td><td>Septicemia 26,445</td><td>Septicemia 34,069</td></tr>
</table>

Source: National Vital Statistics System, National Center for Health Statistics, CDC.
Produced by: Office of Statistics and Programming, National Center for Injury Prevention and Control, CDC.

Fig. 1. Ten leading causes of death by age group, United States, 2003. SIDS, sudden infant death syndrome. (*From* National Vital Statistics System, National Center for Health Statistics, Centers for Disease Control and Prevention, Atlanta.)

injury events contribute to the 10 leading causes of death in all age groups. Falls are the most common cause of injuries that require treatment in the ED, as illustrated in Fig. 2. It is interesting to note that there is only one age group (15–24 year olds) for which falls are not the leading cause of injury-related ED visits. Although falls are the most frequently occurring cause for the other age groups, the etiology of fall events differs for various age groups. The chart also illustrates the fact that unintentional injury events are the most common types of injury events that result in ED visits. Intentional injury events appear as a leading cause only for selected groups, because assaults are the sixth leading cause of injury-related ED visits for 15 to 54 year olds, and the sixth leading cause overall.

Defining the injury problem

Before prevention efforts are undertaken, it is important to define the problem that is being addressed. Decisions need to be made about whether the focus is on a local, regional, state, or national level, and what types of data are needed to define the injury-related issues. Mortality data, which are the most readily available, do not provide a complete picture of the burden of injuries, but can aid in defining the problem. Other data sets may contain data restricted to particular injury types or injury events. Developing a collaborative relationship with an injury epidemiologist or injury researchers at a school of public health aids in the identification of data sets and problem definition.

Multiple data sources can be used to aid in this effort. Although case studies or anecdotes can provide specific examples of injury events, it is essential to understand the bigger picture of how injuries affect the population of a community or state. Injury surveillance systems provide data about the incidence, causes, and effects of injuries and may be used to evaluate the effectiveness of injury preventive programs. A number of data systems provide national data or estimates for specific types of injury events or specific injuries. Many of these are now readily accessible through the Internet, and can be queried for specific information. In addition, they provide state level data, which can be useful in documenting the need for intervention. Table 1 lists some of the commonly used databases, and describes their content and accessibility.

The Centers for Disease Control and Prevention's basic outline for injury surveillance programs includes seven elements [2]. (1) Simplicity is often considered the most important aspect of a successful program and pertains to the general structure and the ease of operation of a program. (2) Flexibility of a system allows it to be applied to different environments and adapt to changes within a given health care environment. (3) The acceptability of a system is the general speed and enthusiasm by which a program is adapted by the providers. (4) A sensitive program ideally allows the recognition of

Rank	Age Groups										
	<1	1-4	5-9	10-14	15-24	25-34	35-44	45-54	55-64	65+	Total
1	Unintentional Fall 126,459	Unintentional Fall 870,950	Unintentional Fall 676,444	Unintentional Fall 659,923	Unintentional Struck by/Against 951,581	Unintentional Fall 702,946	Unintentional Fall 765,275	Unintentional Fall 684,042	Unintentional Fall 490,737	Unintentional Fall 1,638,883	Unintentional Fall 7,410,159
2	Unintentional Struck by/Against 33,023	Unintentional Struck by/Against 390,945	Unintentional Struck by/Against 449,222	Unintentional Struck by/Against 622,615	Unintentional MV-Occupant 902,186	Unintentional Overexertion 701,783	Unintentional Overexertion 656,122	Unintentional Overexertion 393,539	Unintentional Struck by/Against 185,922	Unintentional MV-Occupant 193,068	Unintentional Struck by/Against 4,490,051
3	Unintentional Fire/Burn 13,193	Unintentional Other Bite/Sting 126,710	Unintentional Cut/Pierce 135,098	Unintentional Overexertion 288,074	Unintentional Fall 794,288	Unintentional Struck by/Against 671,811	Unintentional Struck by/Against 609,021	Unintentional Struck by/Against 385,139	Unintentional MV-Occupant 179,527	Unintentional Struck by/Against 190,501	Unintentional Overexertion 3,286,856
4	Unintentional Other Bite/Sting 10,926	Unintentional Foreign Body 106,331	Unintentional Pedal Cyclist 118,046	Unintentional Cut/Pierce 170,062	Unintentional Overexertion 758,312	Unintentional MV-Occupant 609,636	Unintentional MV-Occupant 515,768	Unintentional MV-Occupant 332,260	Unintentional Overexertion 175,009	Unintentional Overexertion 156,231	Unintentional MV-Occupant 2,988,064
5	Unintentional MV-Occupant 9,336	Unintentional Cut/Pierce 87,836	Unintentional Other Bite/Sting 96,330	Unintentional Pedal Cyclist 142,085	Unintentional Cut/Pierce 492,172	Unintentional Cut/Pierce 461,058	Unintentional Cut/Pierce 394,133	Unintentional Cut/Pierce 272,953	Unintentional Cut/Pierce 142,911	Unintentional Cut/Pierce 115,708	Unintentional Cut/Pierce 2,278,105
6	Unintentional Poisoning 8,814	Unintentional Poisoning 78,828	Unintentional MV-Occupant 79,531	Unintentional Unk./Unspecified 129,388	Other Assault[A] Struck by/Against 445,965	Other Assault[A] Struck by/Against 271,774	Other Assault[A] Struck by/Against 228,208	Other Assault[A] Struck by/Against 102,941	Unintentional Other Bite/Sting 57,805	Unintentional Other Bite/Sting 70,093	Other Assault[A] Struck by/Against 1,270,224
7	Unintentional Foreign Body 8,776	Unintentional Overexertion 74,530	Unintentional Overexertion 76,811	Unintentional MV-Occupant 115,920	Unintentional Unk./Unspecified 174,572	Unintentional Other Bite/Sting 121,398	Unintentional Other Specified 129,831	Unintentional Other Bite/Sting 94,895	Unintentional Other Specified 37,399	Unintentional Unk./Unspecified 47,825	Unintentional Other Bite/Sting 880,910
8	Unintentional Unk./Unspecified 6,916	Unintentional Fire/Burn 62,073	Unintentional Foreign Body 54,164	Other Assault[A] Struck by/Against 114,891	Unintentional Other Bite/Sting 126,498	Unintentional Other Specified 110,163	Unintentional Other Bite/Sting 115,409	Unintentional Other Specified 93,356	Unintentional Other Transport 34,315	Unintentional Other Transport 44,759	Unintentional Unk./Unspecified 742,188
9	Unintentional Inhalation/Suff. 6,452	Unintentional MV-Occupant 50,331	Unintentional Dog Bite 51,882	Unintentional Other Transport 65,375	Unintentional Other Transport 125,085	Unintentional Unk./Unspecified 109,749	Unintentional Poisoning 97,480	Unintentional Poisoning 74,802	Unintentional Unk./Unspecified 28,358	Unintentional Poisoning 31,073	Unintentional Other Transport 594,127
10	Unintentional Overexertion 6,336	Unintentional Unk./Unspecified 48,293	Unintentional Unk./Unspecified 48,079	Unintentional Other Bite/Sting 60,780	Unintentional Other Specified 111,000	Unintentional Other Transport 95,680	Unintentional Unk./Unspecified 92,403	Unintentional Foreign Body 57,803	Other Assault Struck by/Against 26,969	Unintentional Foreign Body 28,723	Unintentional Foreign Body 577,622

[A] The 'Other Assault' category includes all assaults that are **not** classified as sexual assault. It represents the majority of assaults.

Data Source: National Electronic Injury Surveillance System All Injury Program operated by the Consumer Product Safety Commission

Chart developed by the National Center for Injury Prevention and Control, CDC

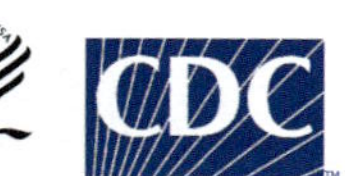

health issues before they become problematic. (5) These programs should have a high positive predictive value. Although this can be problematic in many other disease states, it is generally not in injury surveillance where diagnosis is typically less debatable. (6) The data should be representative of the true incidences of disease over an entire population. (7) Lastly, a good surveillance system should provide timely data so that interventions can be put into effect to prevent further injury.

The medical record can serve as one of the building blocks for injury surveillance. Hospital data may be more accurate, reliable, and cost-effective to collect than other forms of data gathering [3–5]. Hospital datasets do have limitations and biases, however, and cannot stand alone. Trauma registries have inherent biases in that they generally include only the most seriously injured patients, and the criteria for inclusion in the trauma registry differ from one institution to another. Not every state collects ED data on a statewide basis. The use of ED data for injury surveillance has been problematic for a number of reasons: data systems, data definitions, timeliness of data availability, and quality and completeness of data available are central issues of ED information.

Medical records are not standardized and are primarily oriented at documentation of patient assessment and treatment of disease. Although some data elements that are essential components of an injury surveillance system are included in the medical record (demographic information, diagnosis, immediate outcome), other essential information may be missing or incomplete. Some examples are details of the injury event; protective device used; and contributing factors, such as alcohol or other drug use. ED practitioners are trained to elicit medical histories and treat disease. Data elements that are essential for injury surveillance may be missing, however, from ED medical charts. Certain components of injury surveillance data are not included within these medical charts because the information may not pertain to the medical treatment of an ED patient.

Comprehensive injury surveillance encompasses a broad spectrum of injury data and sources. Household and health surveys are considered by some to be as vital a component to monitoring as ED-based surveillance [4]. It is not currently feasible for every patient who presents to every ED across the country to be included in a national injury surveillance database. Sampling is a major strategy that is used in deriving injury prevalence estimates. There are advantages to sampling, because it significantly reduces time and staffing constraints in already financially burdened hospitals and public health systems. When compiled fastidiously, sample data compares

Fig. 2. National estimates of the 10 leading causes of nonfatal injuries treated in hospital emergency departments, United States, 2002. The "other assault" category includes all assaults that are not classified as sexual assault. It represents most assaults. (*From* the National Electronic Injury Surveillance System All Injury Program, Consumer Product Safety Commission.)

Table 1
National injury data sources

Data source	Location and owner	Content	Queriability	Data levels
Fatality Analysis Reporting System	National Highway Traffic Safety Administration, ftp://ftp.nhtsa.dot.gov/FARS/	Data from fatal motor vehicle crashes occurring on public roads	On-line query system	National, can get state level information
National Electronic Injury Sampling System	Consumer Product Safety Commission, http://www.cpsc.gov/library/neiss.html	Data from a statistical sample of emergency departments around the country	On-line query system	National estimates
National Hospital Ambulatory Hospital Medical Care Survey	National Center for Health Statistics, http://www.cdc.gov/nchs/about/major/ahcd/ahcd1.htm	Data from a national sample of visits to hospital emergency departments and ambulatory care departments	Downloadable data files in multiple formats including SPSS, SAS, Stata	National data
National Hospital Discharge Data System	National Center for Health Statistics, http://www.cdc.gov/nchs/about/major/hdasd/nhds.htm	Data from a national sample of approximately 500 hospitals	Downloadable from website	National data

| National Trauma Data Bank | American College of Surgeons, http://www.facs.org/trauma/ntdb.html | Data submitted voluntarily to the American College of Surgeons from hospital-based trauma registries | On-line analysis and queries; downloadable files | National data |
| Web-based Injury Statistics Query and Reporting System | Centers for Disease Control and Prevention, National Center for Injury Prevention and Control, http://www.cdc.gov/ncipc/wisqars/default.htm | US injury mortality data and data for injuries treated in emergency departments | On-line queries; downloadable files; downloadable charts and maps | National data, state data |

favorably with total population data [6]. A relatively new, but important, development in injury surveillance is the expansion of the National Electronic Injury Surveillance System database [7]. This database was originally developed to record consumer product-related injuries. It is a national probability sample of hospitals in the United States and its territories. The National Electronic Injury Surveillance System has recently been undergoing an expansion to include all injury visits to hospitals included in the database.

The electronic medical record may help in solving some of the difficulties of data collection in EDs [8]. This type of medical record reflects standardized data points rather than written histories. This ensures consistency in what is recorded, and it is hoped improves completeness of records. Data points can be added on an ad hoc basis for the purposes of evaluation of particular programs or interventions. Data are accessible in a timelier manner because data may be entered and available on a real-time basis, reducing lag time and sampling errors [9]. Common data definitions are an essential component of these databases. The Centers for Disease Control and Prevention has developed the Data Elements for Emergency Department Systems, which defines data elements that can be used in ED data systems. Coding systems that allow for classification of injuries and external causes of injuries, such as the International Classification of Diseases, are also essential elements in developing data systems [10]. These efforts have proved to be valuable in injury surveillance [11] and in disease surveillance, such as surveillance of adverse drug events [12] and respiratory syndromes [13].

Injury surveillance data can be used for many applications. Data can be used to develop incidence-based cost models, to identify at-risk populations and those with high injury rates, to identify the burden of specific types of injury events or types of injuries in a community, or to assess the effectiveness of existing intervention programs. The data can drive the development of local and national priorities. ED surveillance should not be relied on as the sole form of data, but rather as a vital component of a multidiscipline effort [14].

Basic concepts of injury prevention

Understanding the sequence of events leading to an injury, or a series of common injury events, is made easier through the use of a matrix developed by Dr. William Haddon, a pioneer in injury research in the United States [15]. Haddon's matrix defines injury events in three phases: (1) pre-event, (2) event, and (3) postevent. These phases are cross-tabulated with contributing factors: human (host); agent (vehicle); and environment (physical and social-cultural-economic). By using the Haddon matrix, it is possible to examine the factors that contribute to a single injury event and its outcomes or to explore common factors in multiple injury incidents. Table 2 illustrates an analysis of a pedestrian-motor vehicle collision using the Haddon matrix. A 78-year-old woman exited a city transit bus at the bus stop and proceeded

Table 2
Haddon matrix analysis of a pedestrian-motor vehicle collision

	Human factors	Agent	Environment	
			Physical	Sociocultural
Pre-event phase	Pedestrian: age, osteoporosis, decreased visual acuity Driver: age, limited driving experience; distracted by other occupants of the motor vehicle	Condition of tires and brakes; visibility of vehicle (lights, vehicle color)	Weather: rain, poor visibility Road: no crosswalk, stop sign or traffic signal near bus stop	Drivers' licensing: lack of graduated licensure law for new drivers
Event phase	Energy tolerance of body tissues; height	Mass of vehicle; bumper height and design	Road surface slippery	
Postevent phase	Degree of blood loss and ability to compensate; comorbidities; fracture healing		Ambient temperature; rain; other vehicles in the area	Access to 911; availability of emergency treatment; rehabilatation availability and insurance coverage

to cross the street in front of the bus. As she passed the driver's side of the bus, she was struck by a car traveling at 40 mph. The driver of the vehicle was a 16-year-old boy who had recently obtained his driver's license. There were four occupants of the motor vehicle. The event occurred on a rainy weekday afternoon.

This example illustrates the various opportunities for intervention, both to prevent the injury event from occurring in the first place, and to mitigate the impact of the event once it has occurred. Interventions may include primary, secondary, and tertiary approaches, and can also be classified as individual, population-based, or environmental strategies. Not all approaches and strategies are equally effective or appropriate to all situations.

Haddon also proposed 10 strategies for the prevention of injury, which range from primary prevention to tertiary prevention (Table 3). Many of the countermeasures are environmental strategies, which involve a modification of the physical or sociocultural environment to prevent a potential injury-causing event from occurring or leading to an injury. Others focus on separation of the person at-risk of injury from the agent of injury, whereas the final strategy involves the mitigation of harm that has already occurred.

Table 3
Haddon's ten injury prevention countermeasures

Countermeasure	Examples
Prevent the initial creation of the hazard.	Do not allow production of dangerous products certain types of weapons; vehicles that are unsafe, such as three-wheeled all-terain vehicles
Reduce the amount of energy contained in the hazard.	Limit the horsepower of a vehicle engine; decrease muzzle velocity of a firearm
Prevent release of a hazard that already exists.	Prohibit sales of fireworks; store firearms and ammunition in locked cabinets
Modify the rate of or spatial distribution of the hazard.	
Separate, in time or space, the hazard from that which is to be protected.	Construct playgrounds away from busy streets; minimum legal drinking age
Separate the hazard from that which is to be protected by a material barrier.	Use fencing around swimming pools
Modify relevant basic qualities of the hazard.	Impact absorbing steering columns in cars; placement of material guards on machinery
Make what is to be protected more resistant to damage from the hazard.	Use protective clothing and devices, such as bicycle helmets and goggles
Begin to counter the damage already done by the hazard.	Provide emergency treatment
Stabilize, repair, and rehabilitate the object of the damage.	Provide acute care and rehabilitation services for injury victims

Adapted from Haddon W. Energy damage and the ten counter measure strategies. Journal of Trauma-Injury Infection and Critical Care 1973; 13:321–31.

Environmental strategies

Environmental strategies focus on changes in both the physical and sociocultural environment. In the example of the elderly pedestrian, physical environment changes that may have decreased the risk of the event include moving the bus stop to a location that is near a crosswalk with either traffic signals or a stop sign, or installing these near the bus stop. In the sociocultural environment, the enactment and enforcement of a graduated driver's licensure law, that does not allow new drivers to transport passengers, could lead to decreased risk of distraction for the driver. Environmental strategies are equally important in other types of injury events. Playgrounds that have energy-absorbing surfaces decrease fall-related injuries in children, whereas removing loose rugs in bathrooms and hallways can decrease falls in the elderly. Many aspects of road design have contributed to a safer environment for occupants of motor vehicles. The placement of Jersey barriers on highways to prevent traffic from crossing into other lanes and to ease re-entry to the road in the case of a vehicle that leaves the road is another example of an environmental strategy. Methods of decreasing the likelihood that a firearm can be fired by someone other than the owner are product-related examples of environmental approaches to injury prevention. Smart guns, which sense the fingerprint of the owner, or trigger lock devices, which prevent a gun from being fired, are examples of these devices. Many of these interventions are relatively low-cost, and simple to implement.

Policy strategies, which involve changes to existing laws and regulations or introduction of new laws, may be more challenging but are effective. Seatbelt and child safety seat laws have saved thousands of lives. Motorcycle helmet laws, however, have an interesting history. Between 1966 and 1975, all states except for California passed laws that required motorcyclists to wear protective helmets. There were federal highway-funding incentives for the passage of these laws. Many of these laws were repealed, and with this, a natural experiment occurred. With the repeal of these laws, deaths in motorcycle crashes increased by 55%. Louisiana was the first state to re-enact a motorcycle helmet law, and saw a decrease in fatalities of 30% in the first year after the law's passage. As of 2005, only 25 states have laws that require all motorcycle riders to wear helmets [16]. Another policy intervention is the passage of graduated driver's licensing. Graduated driver's licensing laws for new drivers have also proved to be effective in decreasing motor vehicle crashes and their consequences in young drivers. There is little uniformity in these laws across states, and not all states have passed graduated driver's licensing. These laws share some common provisions, including a period of time during which the new driver cannot drive without an adult licensed driver in the vehicle (permit period); nighttime restrictions on driving; and restrictions on passengers in the vehicle driven by a newly licensed driver.

Educational strategies

Often, educational strategies are advocated as a method of preventing injury. It is important to keep in mind that the more action that is required on the part of the individual, the less likely it is that a change will occur. Programs may highlight injury risk, such as slide shows or videos illustrating motor vehicle crashes and resulting injuries that are presented to high school students, and education of parents about the need for child restraints based on observation in the ED. Education alone, however, is not sufficient to change behavior, which is truly the required action when one expects individuals to take responsibility for preventing injury. For example, a parent may be well-informed about the importance of using a child safety seat for his or her child every time the child is in the car. The parent may go against this knowledge and better judgment, however, and allow the child to ride on his or her lap and help "drive" during a five-block ride to the store. Although well-educated about the risks to the child, the parent did not change his or her behavior. What would make the parent change this behavior? Robertson [17] points out that education includes four assumptions, either explicit or implicit:

1. Persons informed of risk will retain the information and take recommended action to reduce the risk.
2. Persons skilled in a given hazardous endeavor are less likely to be injured than those less skilled.
3. The educator has the means available to teach information or skills, and to cause behavior change related to emotions, attitudes, and values.
4. The training of people to perform a hazardous activity will not result in an increase in the activity to the point that any injury-reducing effect of the training is more than offset by increased injuries resulting from use of the new skill.

A key point is the need to change emotions, attitudes, and values. If these are successfully changed, then behavior change is possible. Prochaska and coworkers [18] describe six distinct stages of behavior change:

1. Precontemplation: there is no intent to change; the individual does not perceive that his or her behavior is a problem.
2. Contemplation: there is an awareness that a problem exists, and some thought that change is necessary, but no commitment to change; pros and cons of the problem are being weighed, solutions are being thought about.
3. Preparation: there is intent to take action; some small changes in behavior have occurred.
4. Action: there is a change in behavior or environment to overcome the problem.
5. Maintenance: there is effort directed toward preventing relapse, and toward consolidating gains that have been achieved.

6. Termination: change has taken place, and does not require continued effort.

This model of behavior change is important to remember in designing injury-prevention programs and strategies. It is useful in both individual and group settings, and can help in providing a framework for the design of educational interventions.

Counseling is one individual approach that may lead to behavior change. In the ED setting, counseling may reinforce the importance of seatbelt or child safety seat use or may involve brief interventions for harmful drinking. By determining how ready someone is to change, a brief intervention can be tailored to the individual's particular situation and willingness to change.

Advocacy and policy change

Emergency medicine practitioners can be some of the strongest advocates for policy change, because they have credibility, and can bring their clinical experiences forward to illustrate the importance of implementing policy that prevents injury. Knowing the data, and translating it so that it is understandable to policymakers, the media, and the public are valuable skills that emergency practitioners bring to this strategy for injury prevention. The data, paired with stories from people who have been affected by injuries, are powerful tools in advocating for policy change. Professional organizations have been strong advocates and partners in the policy development and advocacy process. Grass roots organizations frequently partner with skilled and experienced organizations when advocating policy reform. Given this, it is also important for emergency practitioners to seek out opportunities to learn advocacy skills and gain knowledge of the policy and political process. Advocacy on a local, state, or national level involves knowing the issue at hand, understanding the viewpoints of both advocates and opponents, and having the time and commitment to educate policymakers about the issue. Advocates often become discouraged when a policy is not changed the first time a change is proposed. It is unusual for policy changes to occur rapidly, unless a high-profile event highlights the need for a change. In addition to advocating for laws that decrease injury risk or affect the direct care of injured patients, emergency practitioners can take the lead on advocating for funding for injury prevention programs and injury research. Injuries are responsible for the greatest number of potential productive life years lost, yet prevention programs are underfunded in comparison with prevention and treatment research of other diseases. Emergency medicine practitioners have many opportunities to influence policy, and in so doing, to decrease the toll that injuries take on the community.

Measuring effectiveness

One of the most challenging aspects of injury prevention is documenting the effectiveness of prevention. It is very difficult to measure the specific number of incidents that have not occurred because of a particular strategy, but it is possible to use historical data and trend data to determine where changes have occurred. For example, alcohol-impaired driving has been a significant problem in the United States. In the 1980s, a number of strategies were adopted to decrease alcohol-related motor vehicle crashes and fatalities. These included increasing the minimum legal drinking age to 21 years in all states; strengthening state laws regulating driving while intoxicated through grass-roots advocacy, primarily by Mothers Against Drunk Driving; and public awareness campaigns highlighting the problem of driving while intoxicated, its consequences, and the potential for punishment for drivers caught driving drunk. Increasing the minimum legal drinking age has led to a decrease in alcohol-related motor vehicle fatalities in adolescents, whereas other changes in the law and enforcement have decreased the overall rate of alcohol-related fatalities. During this time period, there were also advances in trauma care, including the development of trauma systems in many states; improved access to 911; and a trend toward staffing of EDs by physicians trained and board-certified in emergency medicine. The strategies, although broad and population-based, allowed for an individual approach with respect to treatment of injury and mitigation of injuries that did occur.

Evaluation of local programs and efforts can be measured using existing injury surveillance and data systems, often in concert with additional data acquired as part of an evaluation strategy. Untested or unstudied programs should have evaluation plans built into their implementation, so that it is possible to determine effectiveness of a program in preventing injury, and the cost-benefit of the program. Collaboration with public health researchers who are familiar with program evaluation can be invaluable in this process. Programs successfully applied in one area may not work in another [19], which emphasizes the need for outcome research.

Emergency medicine and injury prevention

The ED can serve as a setting for interventions and a resource for data about injuries and the effectiveness of intervention strategies. Emergency medicine practitioners play an important role in all aspects of injury prevention. The ED visit provides a unique window of opportunity for intervention with individual patients. The experiences of emergency practitioners are invaluable in highlighting injury problems for policymakers and identifying the highest priority injury issues for intervention. The ED serves as a barometer of the health of the community, and a primary interface between the community and the health care system. Emergency medicine practitioners serve on the front line of this interface; they can provide care in the hospital setting and collaborate on prevention programs in the community. This may require a paradigm shift for many emergency physicians, but there are strategies that can be used in adapting to this dual role [20].

Screening and risk assessment

This is an opportunity to identify those who may most likely benefit from interventions and resources. Two examples of this are screening for domestic violence [21] and for problem drinking [22]. This is congruous with the role of health care provider to screen for disease on all health care encounters. Whether checking an ECG or a finger stick, clinicians regularly take on this role based on risk factors. This is simply an extension to include injury as another disease process.

Health information

Clinicians can improve the public understanding of injury prevention and inform the public of services available. This can be as simple as providing pamphlets and hanging posters in waiting rooms [23]. Discharge instructions are one of the most basic ways in which one can provide patients with information. By referring to outpatient resources and ensuring that their instructions include injury prevention information, one can ensure better awareness and compliance.

Health education and skill development

Important interventions in the ED include assisting patients in their efforts at changing behaviors and reducing risk. Simple interventions can be as straightforward as identifying the presence of firearms in the home and recommending to parents that they be stored locked and unloaded. This quick and basic interaction can reduce morbidity and mortality [24].

Community action

Opportunities to reduce injuries are not limited to the ED. By extending influence into the community clinicians can achieve greater awareness and success. By targeting at-risk populations clinicians can focus their efforts better. There is a need to understand the community and take a collaborative approach. It is important to recognize that the people who live in the community understand the community and its norms, although the ED staff sees the effects of specific community factors (eg, environment, social norms, risk-taking behaviors in youth). The shared knowledge and cooperation of the ED staff and the community can be leveraged to decrease injuries through environmental change, policy change, and program development.

Social marketing

Awareness campaigns can range from local to national. One national media campaign was very successful: in television advertisements, two mannequins named Vince and Larry preached, "You can learn a lot from a dummy." Americans listened: seat belt usage went from 14% to 79%, saving 85,000 lives and $3.2 billion [25].

Organizational development

Integration of injury prevention as a component of health care is needed. Injury prevention must be a part of the core mission of EDs and emergency medicine. Additionally, hospital administration and health policy administrators should be involved in conceptualizing this preventative aspect of health care so that clinicians can act together in injury prevention efforts.

Economic and regulatory activities

As health care advocates, clinicians should maintain a proactive role in promoting awareness and change. These efforts aim to create a social environment that promotes health. In an environment where potentially conflicting interests of industry and government threaten health care, it is imperative that emergency medicine maintains a strong and active role in not only education but also policy efforts. Perhaps one of the more famous examples of this is Dr. Robert Sanders' tireless efforts at passing child seatbelt legislation in 1977. Numerous other examples exist: Dr. Murray Katcher's work in advocating for lowered temperature settings on hot water heaters to prevent scald burns; Dr. Barbara Barlow's work in improving playgrounds in Harlem; and Dr. Arthur Kellerman's work on helmet laws in Georgia.

Summary

Emergency medicine plays a significant role in injury prevention through the use of public health models that link injury data to prevention programming, research, and advocacy. The day-to-day experiences in the ED provide a picture of the injury problem in a given community and give the emergency practitioner a real-world basis for injury prevention efforts. Successful injury prevention requires understanding of the problem of injury in general; identification of the injury issues in one's own community; partnerships with public health, law enforcement, community members, and policy makers; and ongoing program evaluation of interventions that are undertaken.

References

[1] McCaig LF, Burt CW. National hospital ambulatory medical care survey: 2002 emergency department summary. Advance Data Number 340. US Department of Health and Human Services, Centers for Disease Control and Prevention, National Center for Health Statistics, Hyatsville, MD: March 18, 2004.

[2] Klaucke DN, Buehler JW, Thacker SB, et al. Guidelines for evaluating surveillance systems. Morbidity and Mortality Weekly Report 1988;37(S-5):1–18.

[3] Petridou E, Dessypris N, Frangakis CE, et al. Estimating the population burden of injuries: a comparison of household surveys and emergency department surveillance. Epidemiology 2004;15:428–32.

[4] Mulder S. Recording of home and leisure accidents: differences between population surveys and A&E department surveillance systems. International Journal for Consumer Safety 1997; 4:165–78.

[5] Mann NC, Knight S, Olson LM, et al. Underestimating injury mortality using statewide databases. J Trauma 2005;58:162–7.

[6] Morrison A, Stone DH. Injury surveillance in accident and emergency departments: to sample or not to sample? Inj Prev 1998;4:50–2.

[7] National Electronic Injury Surveillance System. Available at: http://www.cpsc.gov/library/neiss.html. Accessed February 20, 2005.

[8] Chan JT, Cameron PA. A pragmatic approach to timely disease surveillance in the emergency department. Emerg Med J 2003;20:443–6.

[9] Davidson SJ, Zwemer FL Jr, Nathanson LA, et al. Where's the beef? The promise and the reality of clinical documentation. Acad Emerg Med 2004;11:1127–34.

[10] Pollock DA, Adams DL, Bernardo LM, et al. Data elements for emergency department systems, release 1.0 (DEEDS): a summary report. DEEDS Writing Committee. J Emerg Nurs 1998;24:35–44.

[11] Conn JM, Annest JL, Gilchrist J, et al. Injuries from paintball game related activities in the United States, 1997–2001. Inj Prev 2004;10:139–43.

[12] Budnitz DS, Pollock DA, Mendelsohn AB, et al. Emergency department visits for outpatient adverse drug events: demonstration for a national surveillance system. Ann Emerg Med 2005;45:197–206.

[13] Townes JM, Kohn MA, Southwick KL, et al. Investigation of an electronic emergency department information system as a data source for respiratory syndrome surveillance. J Public Health Manag Pract 2004;10:299–307.

[14] Stone DH, Morrison A, Smith GS. Emergency department injury surveillance systems: the best use of limited resources? Inj Prev 1999;5:166–7.

[15] Haddon W. Options for the prevention of motor vehicle crash injury. Isr J Med 1980;16: 45–68.

[16] National Highway Traffic Safety Administration. Motorcycle helmets: the facts of life. Campaign Safe and Sober. Available at: http://www.nhtsa.dot.gov/people/injury/alcohol/Archive/safesobr/OPlanner/protection/cycle.html. Accessed February 23, 2005.

[17] Robertson LS. Injuries: causes, control strategies, and public policy. Lexington (MA): Lexington Books; 1983.

[18] Prochaska JO, Norcross JC, DiClemente CC. Changing for good. New York: William Morrow; 1994.

[19] Ozanne-Smith J, Day L, Stathakis V, Sherrard J. Controlled evaluation of a community based injury prevention program in Australia. Inj Prev 2002;8:18–22.

[20] Bensberg M, Kennedy M. A framework for health promoting emergency departments. Health Promot Int 2002;17:179–88.

[21] Shattuck SR. A domestic violence screening program in a public health department. J Community Health Nurs 2002;19:121–32.

[22] D'Onofrio G, Nadel ES, Degutis LC, et al. Improving emergency medicine residents'
     approach to patients with alcohol problems: a controlled educational trial. Ann Emerg
     Med 2002;40:50–62.
[23] Ytterstad B. The Harstad Injury Prevention Study. A decade of community-based traffic
     injury prevention with emphasis on children. Postal dissemination of local injury data can
     be effective. Int J Circumpolar Health 2003;62:61–74.
[24] Borowsky IW. The role of the pediatrician in preventing suicidal behavior. Minerva Pediatr
     2002;54:41–52.
[25] National Center for Statistics and Analysis of the National Highway Traffic Safety Admin-
     istration. Available at: http://www-nrd.nhtsa.dot.gov/departments. Accessed November 10,
     2006.

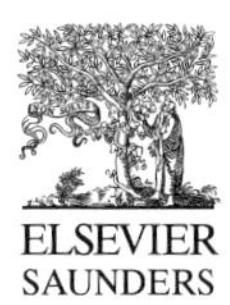

ELSEVIER
SAUNDERS

Emerg Med Clin N Am
24 (2006) 889–903

EMERGENCY
MEDICINE
CLINICS OF
NORTH AMERICA

The Relationship Between Intimate Partner Violence and Other Forms of Family and Societal Violence

Peggy E. Goodman, MD, FACEP

Department of Emergency Medicine, Brody School of Medicine–ECU, 3ED317, Greenville, NC 27834, USA

Intimate partner violence (IPV) is a significant individual and public health problem. In many cases the emergency department (ED) or emergency medical services provide these patients' first-line medical assessment. In the past IPV was usually treated by law enforcement as a private matter for a couple. It is now clearly recognized that IPV has significant medical ramifications and that the problem extends to the health and safety of the general public. Others involved in this private matter potentially include any current or former partners of each member of the couple; children of the current or prior relationships; and other family members, friends, or co-workers assisting either the perpetrator or victim of abuse. A variety of relationships, either heterosexual or homosexual, can occur, affecting not only the type of incident, but type of response involved.

The general public is also at risk because incidents occur not only at the victim's residence, but also in the workplace, and on other public or private property (eg, in a parking lot, a commercial establishment, or government building). Because abuse victims often seek medical attention only in the case of significant injury or other acute condition, it is vital that emergency physicians be aware not only of the medical issues involved, but also the greater public health and sociolegal ramifications of IPV.

Epidemiology

IPV affects multiple aspects of society, including the home; workplace; school; public and private property; the economy; and the health care, legal, and social service communities. In the United States, approximately 5.3

E-mail address: goodmanp@ecu.edu

doi:10.1016/j.emc.2006.06.014   *emed.theclinics.com*

million incidents occur annually, affecting approximately 1.8 million patients, predominantly women, with an annual prevalence of 3%, and a lifetime prevalence of 25% to 30% [1].

In the United States in 2001, 85% of reported nonlethal violent IPV events were against women; in 2000, 1247 women and 440 men were killed by intimates (current and former spouses, boyfriends, and girlfriends) [2]. Firearms were used in most cases; in 2002, 51% of homicides were committed with handguns, 16% with other guns, 13% with knives, 5% with blunt objects, and 16% with other weapons. Almost two thirds of intimate incidents (60% of IPV, 63% of sexual assaults) occurred between 6:00 PM and 6:00 AM [3]. This is particularly significant in emergency medicine because of the decreased availability of resources during these hours [4]. Approximately one fourth of the incidents of violent crime occurred at or near the victim's home, and 76% occurred within 5 miles of home. Other common locations included streets other than those near the victim's home (17%); school (14%); or at a commercial establishment (7%). A total of 19% reported they were at work or traveling to or from work when the crime occurred [3].

Women aged 16 to 24 experience the highest per capita rates of intimate violence, 19.6 victimizations per 1000 women. Risk factors for IPV among both men and women are being black; being young (16–24); being divorced or separated; and living in rental housing [3,5]. Risk factors for increased injury include attitudes of patriarchy or entitlement; exposure as a witness or victim to abuse as a child; unemployment; and alcohol use by the perpetrator. A total of 75% of all incidents and 67% of violent incidents involved a perpetrator who had been drinking, compared with 31% of incidents by strangers [2,6].

Costs to society

When evaluating the annual cost of IPV to society, the main costs are direct (ie, money spent on goods and services) and indirect (ie, loss of goods or services). Direct costs include those spent on health care expenses, law enforcement and court costs, and other public health and safety expenditures. Based on the National Violence Against Women Survey, which looked solely at health care costs, in 1995 (the last year for which data was collected) nearly 2 million IPV-related injuries (including physical assault and sexual assault) were inflicted on women aged 18 or older. Of these, 550,000 required medical attention, a quarter of which required admission to the hospital. An additional 18.5 million mental health care visits occurred after cases of physical assault, sexual assault, or stalking. These health care interventions cost 4.1 billion dollars in 1995. An additional 1.8 billion dollars per year of lost work and productivity, in the household and in the workplace, was incurred [1]. Because of the fragmented distribution of law enforcement and correctional costs among many local, state, and federal jurisdictions, estimates of these costs are not readily available.

Intimate partner violence

IPV is defined as current or former, emotional, psychologic, physical, or sexual abuse between current or former partners of an intimate relationship, regardless of gender or marital status.

Sexual assault, pregnancy, and intimate partner violence

Between 300,000 and 700,000 adult women are victims of sexual assault annually in the United States, with a lifetime prevalence of 13% to 25% [7]. Women in abusive relationships report a 40% to 50% incidence of nonconsensual intercourse [7–9]. Men constitute 5% to 10% of noninstitutional (ie, not incarcerated) victims and postmenopausal women constitute 2% to 3% of sexual assault victims. In 78% of the cases the victim knows the assailant. In assaults against both men and women the perpetrator defines himself as heterosexual. Fewer than one in five rapes are reported to the police because victims feel ashamed, guilty, may not define the occurrence as a sexual assault, or do not think the medical or legal system will be responsive. Men are even less likely to report having been sexually assaulted because of the greater stigma attached.

Lack of reproductive autonomy in an abusive relationship increases the risk of unplanned or unwanted pregnancy, with an approximate IPV prevalence of 3.9% to 8.3%, accounting for more than 324,000 women per year. This makes it more common than gestational diabetes (1.4%–6.1%) and as common as pre-eclampsia (6%–8%), two conditions routinely screened for during pregnancy.

IPV is the leading cause of maternal mortality and other adverse outcomes, such as preterm delivery, fetal distress, antepartum hemorrhage and preeclampsia, low birth weight, miscarriage, or elective termination of pregnancy. Continued high-risk behaviors by the pregnant woman, such as tobacco or alcohol use, and limited access to health care during the pregnancy also result in poor outcomes.

Same-sex relationships and intimate partner violence

Although most studies and resources concentrate on heterosexual relationships, defining the male as the perpetrator and the female as victim, it is important to remember that particularly with emotional and lethal abuse, women abusing men and abuse between members of homosexual couples often occur, with an estimated prevalence of 25% to 33% [10]. There is also the added social stigma regarding homosexual relationships; risks of outing by a current or former partner; and, in general, fewer resources available for victims. Seven states define domestic violence in a way that specifically excludes same-sex victims, and because of sodomy laws, same-sex victims may be forced to confess to a criminal act to prove that they are domestic partners [11].

Elder abuse

Elder abuse also needs to be evaluated in the context of IPV. Dependent and physically or cognitively impaired individuals are more susceptible to abuse, and some chronic abuse cases last many years without detection. Physical abuse accounts for 14.6% of elder abuse, 12.3% are caused by financial exploitation, and 55% of reported cases are caused by neglect. Caregivers' characteristics are strong predictors of abuse. Psychiatric illness, psychosocial stressors, emotional or financial dependency on the elder, history of abuse, social isolation, inexperience in caregiving, and disinclination to provide care are predictors, although alcohol abuse by the caregiver is the most predictive factor for elder abuse. Spouses perpetrate 15%, with adult children causing 30% to 33%, and other relatives accounting for 9% to 20% of elder abuse [7,12].

Elder abuse can be difficult to detect because victims may feel humiliated or responsible for their abuse, may fear retaliation or eviction from their homes with placement in a nursing home, or they may not want to take legal recourse against a family member. In some cases, medical conditions, such as aphasia or dementia, may make it difficult to elicit a history when abuse has occurred. In other cases, friable skin, balance problems, or osteoporosis may make trivial injuries more likely, even in the absence of abuse. It is important to proceed conscientiously and document well, to avoid misdiagnosis based on potential false-positive and false-negative indicators of abuse.

Child abuse

Children under the age of 12 resided in more than 50% of households in which IPV occurs, and child abuse has been estimated to occur in 30% to 60% of the homes with IPV [13]. Each year at least 3 to 10 million children are exposed to physical and verbal spousal abuse. This statistic is considered a significant underestimate because these data do not include situations where parents are divorced or children are under 3 years of age. Studies of children living in two-parent households report 16% to 20% incidence of physical partner violence [14]. Although pediatricians routinely screen children for abuse, they do not necessarily screen the parents for abuse; when performed, this type of screening revealed that 2% to 6% of children are in homes with current or recent IPV, and 14% to 22% are in homes with a history of past abuse [15].

It is well recognized that witnessing IPV harms children. Studies looking at children's exposure to IPV demonstrate that a child's reaction to IPV may vary according to a number of factors, including [16]:

- With which parent the child resides, and any custody arrangements that result
- Age of the child when he or she witnesses abuse
- Proximity to the violence (whether they are physically in the lap of a parent, in the path of a thrown object, in the same or another room)
- Temperament of the child
- Frequency, severity, and chronicity of the violence
- Support structure available to the child in the family, community, and school

Exposure to IPV may result in emotional distress, behavior regression, somatic complaints, and behavior modeled on the actions they see. These children are less socially competent and more fearful and anxious than other children, with a greater incidence of sleep, attention, and learning disorders. As with cases of divorce, they sometimes feel responsible for the household dysfunction, and respond with guilt or anger toward one or both parents.

Because it is well recognized that living in an abusive home is detrimental, there are attempts to improve identification of these families at risk. Management of cases in which a child who is not physically abused witnesses violence is sometimes controversial. Some states interpret this as potential or imminent danger to the child, requiring reporting as "suspicion of abuse." This sometimes results in charges of "failure to protect" against a victim who does not remove a child from a known abuse situation. Few states have primary statutes addressing children that witness IPV. In some states "witnessing abuse" is a loose enough term to refer to a child living in the same residence or within hearing distance, whereas other states' laws specify that the child must physically be in the same room or location and be able visually to witness the event. When granting custody, some jurisdictions are more likely to decide for the abuser, who tends to have the more stable home environment, with home ownership and greater financial resources than the victim, and presumably with less likelihood of uprooting the child from familiar surroundings, friends, and school. In many cases a no-win situation is created for the abuse victim, who must choose between remaining in the abusive environment or removing the child from the home, which can be perceived as disruptive to their lifestyle. Increased coordination among the legal and social service communities has been implemented to address these issues, with inconsistent results [17].

Pet abuse

Animal abuse, defined as intentional distress, suffering, or pain or death of an animal separate from food, hunting, or husbandry, is being increasingly recognized as a marker for family violence. Nearly three quarters of families with school-aged children have at least one companion animal. These pets play different roles in child development, including the development of trust, compassion, empathy, and responsibility. In some studies, children's relationships with pets were ranked higher than human relationships in supporting child development [18].

A total of 70% to 75% of women reporting domestic violence also reported that their partner had threatened, hurt or killed one or more of their pets, with actual harm occurring in 57% of cases [19]. In surveys of women going to domestic violence safe houses, 46% to 71% reported that their partner had threatened, hurt, or killed one or more of their pets, and 7% to 32% reported that one or more of their children hurt or killed family pets. A survey in 2002 by the Humane Society of the United States showed that 56% of animal cruelty cases were caused by intentional injury; adults were responsible for 76%, teenagers for 20%, and children for 4% of these cases. A total of 95% to 96% of the perpetrators of intentional animal cruelty are male [20]. When college students were surveyed about animal abuse, 17.7% reported abusing an animal; almost 11% reported the first incident before age 6, 40% were between ages 6 and 12, and 48% reported first abusing animals while in their teenage years. This looked only at cases of deliberate physical abuse, not neglect or psychologic abuse of the animal, such as teasing or prolonged confinement [21].

Cruelty to animals seems to be one of the earliest symptoms of conduct disorder in children. This is noted in children as young as 6.5 years, earlier than bullying, cruelty to people, vandalism, or setting fires. This underlines the importance of early education and intervention in children. A number of motivations have been suggested for animal abuse including retaliation against other people by hurting their pets or abusing animals in their presence, expression of aggression, development of one's own aggressiveness or bolstering self-esteem, transference of hostility toward a more vulnerable target, sadism, curiosity, peer pressure, relief of boredom or depression, sexual gratification, posttraumatic play, re-enactment of violent episodes, or manipulation of another individual. Some studies show that animal abuse was 88% higher in families where physical child abuse is present than in families without physical child abuse; children who are neglected, rejected, or subject to hostility are more likely to commit animal abuse, and pets rarely survive past the age of 2 years in violent households because they are either killed, die from neglect, or run away to escape the abuse [22]. These runaway pets are less likely to be properly immunized against rabies and other diseases, and are more likely to fear humans, responding to contact in either a defensive or aggressive fashion.

Currently, there is no national tracking of animal cruelty and only two states require reporting of animal abuse by veterinarians, although some are now recommending cross-reporting of animal abuse and child or elder abuse. All states have anticruelty laws, but they vary widely; in many cases animal abuse is still charged as property damage rather than intentional infliction of pain. Some victims of abuse are reluctant to leave home because of the need to leave an animal behind with the abuser; the Humane Society of the United States' "Safe Haven" program lists veterinarians and other groups willing to provide emergency safe shelter for these victims' pets.

Workplace violence

Another significant interface between IPV victims and society is in the workplace. A total of 75% of abuse victims report harassment by their abuser while at work. Approximately 1 million women are stalked each year [23], with approximately one fourth missing work as a result of the stalking, averaging 11 days of absence [24].

Representatives from the business community described the effects of IPV in the workplace as absenteeism, inability to focus, poor self-esteem, low productivity, and low morale. When employers take steps to prevent IPV, there are improvements in performance, productivity, health, work-site safety, job retention, and other outcomes related to employee well-being [25]. For women, homicide was the second leading cause of death on the job in 2003 [26].

School violence

Childhood behavior disorders and abnormal socialization from IPV exposure also carry over to the schoolyard. Children exposed to interparental violence are more likely to be aggressive toward others. Bullying affects approximately 7% to 35% of children and adolescents in the United States, Canada, Europe, Australia, and Japan. Violent homes are among the highest risk factor for the development of antisocial behavior; children exposed to domestic violence show more aggression toward both peers and those who are weaker. These boys and girls are more likely to commit delinquent acts and become victims of abuse at school. Although boys are more likely to develop conduct disorders, girls show more internalization, such as depression, anxiety, and eating disorders. Children who see more forms of violence are more likely to be involved in direct physical bullying and use violence as a method of conflict resolution than children exposed primarily to verbal insults and threats, who are more likely to use verbal threat and intimidation. One study showed evidence that 48.3% of all students reported bullying others at some point within the past 3 months and 59% of them had been victims of bullying. Boys were significantly more likely to use physical force or use name calling, whereas girls were more likely to be excluded or isolated by their peer group. Girls who are exposed to parental violence are 3.5 times more likely to bully others than girls not exposed to IPV [27].

Emergency department screening for abuse

Universal screening for family violence is recommended by most medical organizations [28], but often falls short in practice. Some of the reasons given by health care providers include lack of time, uncertainty about which patients to screen, concerns that patients might be offended by screening, discomfort with the issue, uncertainty about what steps to take if someone needs intervention and referral, liability concerns, and failure to acknowledge that family violence is a medical issue or one they should address in their patient population [29,30].

Patient barriers to disclosure include embarrassment, shame, feeling responsible for being victimized, fear of judgment, fear for their or their children's safety, and protectiveness of the abuser because of status in the community or because of economic dependence. Victims may also distrust the medical and legal systems, which have been nonresponsive in the past, and fear that disclosure may result in the escalation of violence. Cultural and religious factors, affecting what behaviors are considered abusive, deciding to receive assistance, or whether there will be a responsive support system may also impact reporting.

Screening evaluations as short as three or four questions reveal many cases of current or prior IPV. The Partner Violence Screen (Box 1) [31] or HITS screen ("How often does your partner *H*urt, *I*nsult, *T*hreaten or *S*cream at you"?) [32] can each be easily incorporated into a patient history. Studies show that patients are not offended when asked about IPV, particularly when they know that it is a general health care question and that they are not being targeted because of some behavior or other characteristic that makes them "look like a battered woman." They may be even more likely to disclose with self-administered questionnaires than with direct questioning [33]. Because same- sex violence and violence toward men by women does occur, universal screening of all adults is recommended. Screening of children for abuse tends to fall under other guidelines with greater protections

---

Box 1. Partner Violence Screen

1. Have you been hit, kicked, punched, or otherwise hurt by someone within the past year? If so, by whom?
2. Do you feel safe in your current relationship?
3. Is there a partner from a previous relationship who is making you feel unsafe now?

From Feldhaus KM, Koziol-McLain J, Amsbury HL, et al. Accuracy of 3 brief screening questions for detecting partner violence in the emergency department. JAMA 1997;277:1357–61; with permission.

for the children, although even in these cases the parent also should be screened. A wide variety of screening tools and suggested interventions exist depending on the practice setting, patient population, and resources available [34,35].

In 1996 and again in 2004, the US Preventive Services Task Force reviewed studies to make evidence-based recommendations regarding the risks and benefits of family violence screening and intervention. They concluded that there are no studies that determine the accuracy of screening tools; there was "fair to good" evidence that interventions reduce harm to children, limited evidence as to whether interventions harm women, no studies that examined the effectiveness of interventions in older adults, and no studies directly addressing the harm of screening and interventions for family and IPV. The US Preventive Services Task Force reported that they had insufficient evidence to recommend for or against screening of parents or guardians for the physical abuse or neglect of children, of women for IPV, or of older adults or their caregivers for elder abuse [36,37].

Most clinicians who have reviewed the task force recommendations point out that there is no gold standard for screening and that different medical specialties and geographic locations have unique patient populations and screening challenges. In addition, outcomes research in this field has inadequate funding, and data collection and sharing are often limited, particularly with restrictions imposed by the new Health Insurance Portability and Accountability Act of 1996 (HIPAA) requirements, and safety concerns for the victim often limit the ability to follow-up effectively to determine outcomes.

The long-reaching effects of child and partner abuse resulting in poor health outcomes should be screened for and addressed even when clear evidence of the effectiveness is not necessarily forthcoming [38–41].

Medical manifestations of abuse

Medical or psychologic manifestations account for 80% of abuse incidents. Although physical injuries are often more dramatic on initial medical evaluation, medical and psychologic manifestations of abuse are more insidious and are likely to have more severe long-term effects. Although few specific conclusions can be made, it seems that abuse victims have higher incidences of neuropsychiatric illness, such as anxiety disorders, sleep disorders, substance abuse, chronic pain syndromes, depression, chronic fatigue, and posttraumatic stress disorder. Other frequent presentations to the ED or physicians' offices include gastrointestinal symptoms, such as anorexia, eating disorders, ulcers, chronic abdominal pain, or irritable bowel syndrome; cardiac symptoms, such as hypertension, chest pain, palpitations, and hyperventilation; and gynecologic problems, such as sexually transmitted diseases, HIV, vaginal bleeding, vaginal infections, fibroids, decreased libido, genital irritation, dyspareunia, chronic pelvic pain, urinary tract infection, and infertility [42,43]. Patients with chronic illness, such as asthma, angina, or hypertension, may present to the ED with "poorly controlled" disease or "noncompliance," which may be caused by stress-related exacerbations of their disease or deliberate withholding of their medications by their abuser.

The most common injuries noted were soft tissue injuries including contusions, abrasions, and lacerations. These are often found on areas of the body that are hidden by makeup or clothing: within the scalp line; in central areas, such as the breasts, abdomen, or perineum (particularly in a pregnant patient); or in areas suggesting defensive injuries (ie, the forearm). A perforated eardrum, significant dental loss or injury in someone young whose dentition otherwise seems to be good, and evidence of pulled hair are suggestive of intentional injury [44,45]. Fractures and dislocations are most common on the arms and hands, particularly in defensive locations caused by warding off blows from the abuser.

Nonlethal strangulation may seem deceptively benign, with 20% reporting only pain; 42% with no visible injury; and the remaining 38% with generally "minor-appearing" contusions, abrasions, ligature marks, or finger impressions. Strangulation symptoms can also be subtle, such as hoarseness; difficulty swallowing; dizziness; and syncope, which may be incorrectly attributed to anxiety or hysteria rather than the development of traumatic laryngeal edema or neurologic sequelae from transient anoxia or traumatic brain injury [46–48].

Long-term negative health consequences of IPV, such as poor health status, poor quality of life, and high use of health services even in the absence of acute injury, are significant and well studied. When childhood abuse as a predictor of adult disability and death is studied, there are higher incidences of alcohol, tobacco, and other drug use; early sexual activity with sexually transmitted diseases and unintended pregnancy; depression; suicidality; anxiety; posttraumatic stress disorder; chronic pain; and other physical complaints [49–53].

The risk of death from IPV is also substantial; several studies looking at homicide rates also look at ED use. In general, approximately 5% to 10% of women who present to an ED are seeking care because of recent partner violence [54]. A total of 30% to 50% of female homicide victims are murdered by a former or current partner, and more than 40% of them sought medical attention in the year before their death [55,56]. The greater their risk factors and the poorer their perceived health, the more likely they were to have multiple encounters for medical or mental health care [57].

Documentation, intervention, and referral

Unfortunately, in many cases, although the symptoms and signs are well documented in a medical record, their etiology is not. Many IPV patients are diagnosed with "forearm contusion" or "anxiety disorder" without the further documentation of abuse that led to that diagnosis [58].

IPV encounters in the ED should be carefully documented because there is a high likelihood of being reviewed in legal proceedings. The better the documentation, the less the burden is on the physician to recall the event later. When obtaining a history, the patient's words should be used whenever possible, placing them in quotation marks, describing what happened, how, when, and by whom.

Whenever possible, photographic documentation of injuries should be included in the medical record. It is important for both the patient and health care provider to recognize that some injuries may not be visibly prominent for hours to days after the initial visit, and follow-up photographs (usually with law enforcement) may be indicated. It is important to look for and diagram or photograph patterned injuries, such as cigarette burns, ligature marks, and handprints. Incidents of forced nonconsensual intercourse should also be documented. If clothing or other evidence is obtained, it should be documented and processed according to departmental protocols; often the date, time of collection, and person collecting the evidence needs to be recorded, and "chain of evidence" procedures need to be observed [59].

The risk of lethal IPV reinforces the need not only to screen for IPV but also to assess the patient's safety and ability to follow-up on discharge (Boxes 2 and 3) [60]. A danger assessment tool asking about escalation of violence, threats, stalking, availability of weapons, and substance abuse is readily available to help determine if a patient's safety is compromised [61]. If patients recognize acute risks, they may be more likely to seek assistance from a local family violence agency or law enforcement. Leaving an abusive relationship is recognized as the most dangerous time, however,

---

Box 2. Basic IPV safety plan

1. Move to a room with more than one exit, avoiding rooms with potential weapons (eg, kitchen knives).
2. Know the quickest route out of your home.
3. Know the quickest route out of your workplace. Find out what resources they have to protect employees.
4. Pack a bag with essential clothes, valuables, and documents for you and each of your children. Keep it hidden but make it easy to grab quickly.
5. Tell your neighbors about your abuse and ask them to call the police when they hear a disturbance.
6. Have a code word to use with your kids, family, and friends when you need help.
7. Have a safe place selected in case you ever have to leave.
8. Use your instincts.
9. You have the right to protect yourself and your kids.

Box 3. Discharge review: have the following been provided?

1. Screening for possible abuse (see Box 1)
2. Treatment for acute medical problems
3. Assessment and addressing of acute psychiatric risk, and evaluation and referral for mental health needs
4. Assessment of pattern and impact of abuse
5. Appropriate documentation and evidence collection
6. Validating
7. Safety assessment and plan (see Box 2)
8. Information about domestic violence in verbal and written form
9. Options for shelter, legal assistance, and counseling
10. Appropriate follow-up care (or referral) for medical, psychologic, and advocacy needs
11. Assurance of confidentiality

Adapted from Warshaw C, Ganley AL. Improving the health care system's response to domestic violence: a resource manual for health care providers. San Francisco: Family Violence Prevention Fund; 1998; with permission.

---

so patients' fears about leaving or retribution against children, other family members, or pets must be taken seriously.

It is important for health care providers to be aware of any reporting requirements to social service or law enforcement agencies, particularly if this might increase the patient's risk of increased violence [62]. Knowing and collaborating with local family violence, sexual assault, child protection, law enforcement, and animal control agencies is extremely helpful, because it can be difficult to determine and contact the appropriate resources after-hours, when most cases occur. They can usually provide most of the subsequent services or know where they can be obtained.

Several EDs have developed programs in conjunction with local or on-site advocacy programs or case management for IPV. Increased use of counseling and shelter services has been noted at these sites, although there is no good evidence that there has been a decrease in IPV-related ED visits [63,64].

Summary

IPV is a significant health care problem with numerous effects on individual and public health and safety. It affects individuals of all ages and socio-economic groups and both genders, and has significant effects on health and quality of life for the general public. Assessments and interventions for victims and perpetrators need continued development, implementation, and evaluation to decrease the financial, health care, and security burdens on society that currently exist because of intimate partner and related forms of violence.

References

[1] National Center for Injury Prevention and Control. Costs of intimate partner violence against women in the United States. Atlanta: Centers for Disease Control and Prevention; 2003.

[2] Rennison C. Intimate partner violence, 1993–2001. Publication No. NCJ 197838. Washington: Bureau of Justice Statistics, US Department of Justice; 2003.

[3] Rennison C. Intimate partner violence. Publication No. NCJ 178247. Washington: Bureau of Justice Statistics, US Department of Justice; 2000.

[4] Birnbaum A, Calderon Y, Gennis P, et al. Domestic violence: diurnal mismatch between need and availability of services. Acad Emerg Med 1996;3:246–51.

[5] Rickert VI, Wiemann CM, Harrykissoon SD, et al. The relationship among demographics, reproductive characteristics, and intimate partner violence. Am J Obstet Gynecol 2002;187:1002–7.

[6] Kyriacou DN, Anglin D, Taliaferro E, et al. Risk factors for injury to women from domestic violence against women. N Engl J Med 1999;341:1892–8.

[7] Rudolph MN, Hughes DH. Emergency assessments of domestic violence, sexual dangerousness, and elder and child abuse. Psychiatric Services 2001;52:281–2, 306.

[8] John R, Johnson JK, Kukreja S, et al. Domestic violence: prevalence and association with gynaecological symptoms. BJOG 2004;111:1128–32.

[9] Campbell JC. Health consequences of intimate partner violence. Lancet 2002;359:1331–6.

[10] Halpern CT, Young ML, Waller MW, et al. Prevalence of partner violence in same-sex romantic and sexual relationships in a national sample of adolescents. J Adolesc Health 2004;35:124–31.

[11] Barnes PG. It's just a quarrel. Am Bar Assoc J 1998;84:24–5.

[12] Kleinschmidt KC. Elder abuse: a review. Ann Emerg Med 1997;30:463–72.

[13] Edleson JL. The overlap between child maltreatment and woman battering. Violence Against Women 1999;5:134–54.

[14] Zink T, Kamine D, Musk L, et al. What are providers' reporting requirements for children who witness domestic violence? Clin Pediatr (Phila) 2004;43:449–60.

[15] Wahl RA, Sisk DJ, Ball TM. Clinic based screening for DV use of a child safety questionnaire. BMC Med 2004;2:25.

[16] Osofsky JD. Prevalence of children's exposure to domestic violence and child maltreatment: implications for prevention and intervention. Clin Child Fam Psychol Rev 2003;6:161–70.

[17] Jaffe PG. Legal and policy responses to children exposed to domestic violence: the need to evaluate intended and unintended consequences. Clin Child Fam Psychol Rev 2003;6:205–13.

[18] Muscari M. Juvenile animal abuse: practice and policy implications for PNPs. J Pediatr Health Care 2004;18:15–21.

[19] Ascione F. Battered women's reports of their partners' and their children's cruelty to animals. J Emotional Abuse 1998;1:119–33.

[20] Humane Society of the United States. First Strike Campaign 2001: report of animal cruelty cases. Washington: Humane Society of the United States; 2002.

[21] Flynn CP. Animal abuse in childhood and later support for interpersonal violence in families. Soc Anim 1999;7:161–71.

[22] Ascione F. Animal abuse and youth violence. OJJDP Juvenile Justice Bulletin, NCJ 188677; 2001. Available at: www.ncjrs.org/html/ojjdp/jjbul2001_9_2/contents.html. Accessed March 2, 2005.

[23] US Department of Justice, National Institute of Justice. Full report of the prevalence, incidence, and consequences of violence against women. 2000. NCJ 183781.14–15. Available at: http://www.ncjrs.gov/. Accessed August 16, 2006.

[24] Tjaden P, Thoennes N. National Institute of Justice Centers for Disease Control and Prevention research brief: stalking in America: findings from the National Violence Against Women Survey. Washington: US Department of Justice, Office of Justice Programs, National Institute of Justice; 1998.

[25] Partnership for Prevention. Domestic violence and the workplace. Washington: Partnership for Prevention. Available at: www.prevent.org. Accessed March 9, 2006.

[26] US Department of Labor, Bureau of Labor Statistics. Census of fatal occupational injuries: Table 4. Fatal occupational injuries by worker characteristics and event or exposure, 2003. Washington; 2004.

[27] Baldry AC. Bullying in schools and exposure to domestic violence. Child Abuse Negl 2003; 27:713–32.

[28] Cohn F, Rudman WJ. Fixing broken bones and broken homes: domestic violence as a patient safety issue. Jt Comm J Qual Saf 2004;30:636–46.

[29] Elliott BA. Screening for family violence: overcoming the barriers. J Fam Pract 2000;49: 137–8.

[30] Chamberlain L, Perham-Hester KA. The impact of perceived barriers on primary care physicians' screening practices for female partner abuse. Women Health 2002;35:55–69.

[31] Feldhaus KM, Koziol-McLain J, Amsbury HL, et al. Accuracy of 3 brief screening questions for detecting partner violence in the emergency department. JAMA 1997;277:1357–61.

[32] Sherin KM, Sinacore JM, Li XQ, et al. HITS: a short domestic violence screening tool for use in a family practice setting. Fam Med 1998;30:508–12.

[33] Webster J, Holt V. Screening for partner violence: direct questioning or self-report? Obstet Gynecol 2004;103:299–303.

[34] Director TD, Linden JA. Domestic violence: an approach to identification and intervention. Emerg Med Clin North Am 2004;22:1117–32.

[35] Family Violence Prevention Fund. National consensus guidelines on identifying and responding to domestic violence victimization in health care settings. San Francisco: 2004.

[36] Nelson HD, Nygren P, McInerney Y, et al. Screening women and elderly adults for family and intimate partner violence: a review of the evidence for the US Preventive Services Task Force. Ann Intern Med 2004;140:387–96.

[37] Nygren P, Nelson HD, Klein J. Screening children for family violence: a review of the evidence for the US Preventive Services Task Force. Annals of Family Medicine 2004;2:161–9.

[38] Anglin D, Sachs C. Preventive care in the emergency department: screening for domestic violence in the emergency department. Acad Emerg Med 2003;10:1118–27.

[39] Rhodes KV, Levinson W. Interventions for intimate partner violence against women: clinical applications. JAMA 2003;289:601–5.

[40] Taket A, Nurse J, Smith K, et al. Routinely asking women about domestic violence in health settings. BMJ 2003;327:673–6.

[41] Siegel RM, Joseph EC, Routh SA, et al. Screening for domestic violence in the pediatric office: a multipractice experience. Clin Pediatr 2003;42:599–602.

[42] Abbott J. Injuries and illnesses of domestic violence. Ann Emerg Med 1997;29:781–5.

[43] Muelleman RL, Lenaghan PA, Pakieser RA. Nonbattering presentations to the ED of women in physically abusive relationships. Am J Emerg Med 1998;16:128–31.

[44] Crandall ML, Nathens AB, Rivara FP. Injury patterns among female trauma patients: recognizing intentional injury. Journal of Trauma-Injury Infection and Critical Care 2004;57: 42–5.

[45] Muelleman RL, Lenaghan PA, Pakieser RA. Battered women: injury locations and types. Ann Emerg Med 1996;28:486–92.

[46] Strack GB, McClane GE, Hawley D. A review of 300 attempted strangulation cases. Part I: criminal legal issues. J Emerg Med 2001;21:303–9.

[47] McClane GE, Strack GB, Hawley D. A review of 300 attempted strangulation cases Part II: clinical evaluation of the surviving victim. J Emerg Med 2001;21:311–5.

[48] Corrigan JD, Wolfe M, Mysiw WJ, et al. Early identification of mild traumatic brain injury in female victims of domestic violence. Am J Obstet Gynecol 2003;188(5 Suppl):S71–6.

[49] Campbell J, Jones AS, Dienemann J, et al. Intimate partner violence and physical health consequences. Arch Intern Med 2002;162:1157–63.

[50] Felitti VJ, Anda RF, Nordenberg D, et al. Relationship of childhood abuse and household dysfunction to many of the leading causes of death in adults. The Adverse Childhood Experiences (ACE) Study. Am J Prev Med 1998;14:245–58.

[51] Bensley L, Van Eenwyk J, Wynkoop Simmons K. Childhood family violence history and women's risk for intimate partner violence and poor health. Am J Prev Med 2003;25:38–44.

[52] Roy CA, Perry JC. Instruments for the assessment of childhood trauma in adults. J Nerv Ment Dis 2004;192:343–51.

[53] Green CR, Flowe-Valencia H, Rosenblum L, et al. The role of childhood and adulthood abuse among women presenting for chronic pain management. Clin J Pain 2001;17:359–64.

[54] Crandall ML, Nathens AB, Kernic MA, et al. Predicting future injury among women in abusive relationships. Journal of Trauma-Injury Infection and Critical Care 2004;56:906–12 [discussion: 912].

[55] Campbell JC, Webster D, Koziol-McLain J, et al. Risk factors for femicide in abusive relationships: results from a multisite case control study. Am J Public Health 2003;93:1089–97.

[56] Wadman MC, Muelleman RL. Domestic violence homicides: ED use before victimization. Am J Emerg Med 1999;17:689–91.

[57] Sharps PW, Koziol-McLain J, Campbell J, et al. Health care providers' missed opportunities for preventing femicide. Prev Med 2001;33:373–80.

[58] Houry D, Feldhaus KM, Nyquist SR, et al. Emergency department documentation in cases of intentional assault. Ann Emerg Med 1999;34:715–9.

[59] Isaac NE, Enos VP. Documenting domestic violence: how health care providers can help victims. US Department of Justice; 20013. Publication No. NCJ 188564. Available at: http://www.ncjrs.gov/pdffiles1/nij/188564.pdf. Accessed August 16, 2006.

[60] Warshaw C, Ganley AL. Improving the health care system's response to domestic violence: a resource manual for health care providers. San Francisco: Family Violence Prevention Fund; 1998.

[61] Campbell JC. Danger assessment 2004. Available at: www.dangerassessment.com. Accessed August 16, 2006.

[62] Houry D, Sachs CJ, Feldhaus KM, et al. Violence-inflicted injuries: reporting laws in the fifty states. Ann Emerg Med 2002;39:56–60.

[63] Zun LS, Downey LV, Rosen J. Violence prevention in the ED: linkage of the ED to a social service agency. Am J Emerg Med 2003;21:454–7.

[64] Muelleman RL, Feighny KM. Effects of an emergency department-based advocacy program for battered women on community resource utilization. Ann Emerg Med 1999;33:62–6.

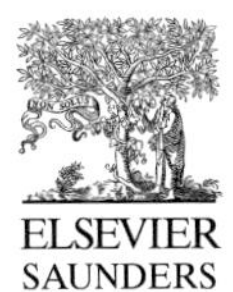

ELSEVIER
SAUNDERS

Emerg Med Clin N Am
24 (2006) 905–923

EMERGENCY
MEDICINE
CLINICS OF
NORTH AMERICA

Racial and Ethnic Disparities in the Emergency Department: A Public Health Perspective

Sheryl L. Heron, MD, MPH*,
Edward Stettner, MD,
Leon L. Haley, Jr, MD, MHSA

*Department of Emergency Medicine, Emory University School of Medicine,
69 Jesse Hill Jr Drive, Atlanta, GA 30303, USA*

The state of health care delivery seems to be filled with nothing but bad news, including continued concerns about rising health care costs, medical errors, patient safety, and the growing numbers of uninsured and underinsured Americans. To complicate matters further, the issue of racial and ethnic disparities in health care not only continues to exist in the delivery models, but also seemingly has worsened. In fact, according to the Centers for Disease Control and Prevention, despite years of attention to these disparities, the racial gap in American's health continues to widen [1].

Numerous studies, in both general medical literature and literature specific to emergency medicine, have previously documented racial and ethnic disparities showing differential use of cardiac angioplasty [2,3], coronary artery bypass surgery [4], mammography [5,6], influenza vaccine [7], pain management, and "gate keeping" activities [8–10]. African Americans die from nearly every major disease or cause at rates higher than whites, especially homicide (5.7 times higher) and HIV (8.7 times higher). The top three causes of death in the United States are the same for blacks and whites, but the rates of death for black people are strikingly higher: heart disease (30% higher), cancer (30% higher), and stroke (40% higher). African Americans also have higher rates of high blood pressure and many infectious diseases, especially those that are sexually transmitted [11]. To compound these concerns, minorities and non-English speakers have greater difficulties accessing health care services. Minorities are disproportionately more likely than the

---

* Corresponding author.
E-mail address: sheron@emory.edu (S.L. Heron).

emed.theclinics.com

general population to be uninsured, and are overrepresented among those in publicly funded health systems (ie, Medicaid [Fig. 1]) [12]. Even when individuals have the same health insurance and similar access to providers as nonminorities, research shows that racial and ethnic minorities tend to receive a lower quality of health care than white patients.

This article discusses these disparities from a public health perspective; specifically, why these racial and ethnic disparities threaten to impede efforts to improve the nation's health [13]. The authors (1) provide background information, including a review of the Institute of Medicine (IOM) report on health care disparities; (2) describe the racial and ethnic compositions of individuals in the emergency department (ED) setting from the perspective of both the patient and health care provider; (3) discuss the most prevalent disease presentations to the ED that are likely to have racial and ethnic disparities; and (4) give conclusions and general recommendations on how to address disparities in emergency health care.

What is the evidence: the Institute of Medicine report

In 1999, the IOM, a private, independent institute of the National Academy of Sciences, was charged by Congress with investigating whether racial and ethnic disparities in quality of care existed for those patients who enter the United States health care system. The specific charges of the committee were the following [13]:

1. Assess the extent of racial and ethnic differences in health care that are not otherwise attributable to known factors, such as access to care (ability to pay or insurance coverage, clinical needs, preferences, and appropriateness of the intervention)
2. Evaluate potential sources of racial and ethnic disparities in health care including the role of bias, discrimination, and stereotyping at the individual (provider and patient), institutional, and health system levels

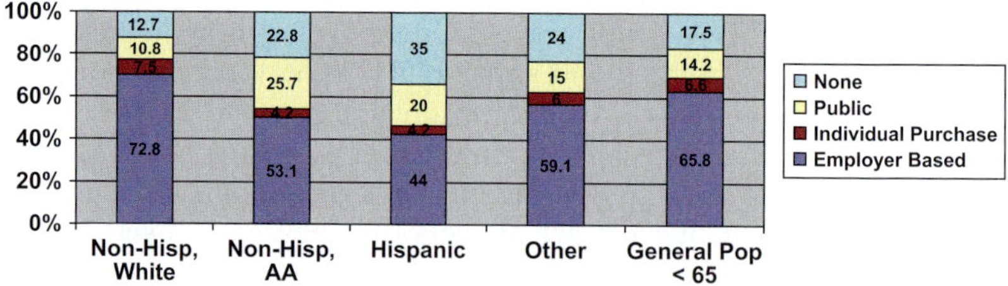

Fig. 1. Sources of health insurance for population under 65, by race and ethnicity, 1999. Numbers may not add to 100% secondary to additional sources of coverage and rounding. (*From* Fronstin P. Sources of health insurance and characteristics of the uninsured: analysis of the March 1999 Current Population Survey. EBRI Issue Brief 2000;217:1–26; with permission.)

3. Provide recommendations regarding interventions to eliminate health care disparities

It is also important to understand that the committee's charge was to focus on disparities in health care, not health outcomes. Many factors contribute to disparities in health outcome including access issues, insurance status, continuity of care, education, housing, employment, and other socioeconomic issues. To meet their charge, the IOM convened expert groups, reviewed over 600 papers on health disparities, and conducted public workshops and focus groups among several other activities. In addition to holding constant the variations in insurance status, patient income, and other access issues, many of the studies also controlled for other confounding factors, such as racial differences in the severity or stage of disease progression; the presence of comorbid illness; where the care was received (public or private hospitals); and other demographic data. Some studies that used more rigorous research designs followed patients prospectively, using data from clinical information abstracted from patient's charts, rather than administrative data used for insurance claims.

Most of the published literature indicates that minorities are less likely than whites to receive needed services, including clinically necessary procedures, even after correcting for access. In general, this research showed the following:

- African Americans and Hispanics tend to receive a lower quality of care across a range of disease areas, including cancer, cardiovascular disease, HIV-AIDS, diabetes, mental health, and other chronic and infectious diseases (Fig. 2) [13].
- African Americans are more likely than whites to receive less desirable services, such as amputation of all or part of a limb [13].
- Disparities are found even when clinical factors, such as stage of disease presentation, comorbidities, and disease severity, are taken into account [13].

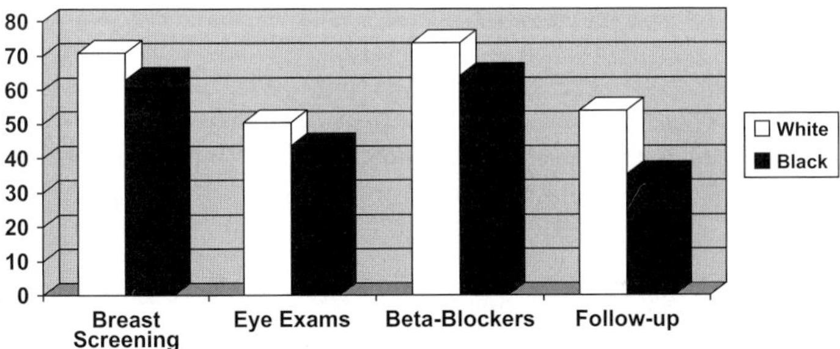

Fig. 2. Among Medicare beneficiaries enrolled in managed care plans, African Americans receive poorer quality of care. (*Data from* Schneider EC, Cleary PD, Zaslavsky AM, et al. Racial disparity in influenza vaccination: does managed care narrow the gap between African-Americans and whites? JAMA 2001;286:1455–60.)

- Disparities are found across a range of clinical settings including public and private hospitals, teaching and nonteaching hospitals [13].
- Disparities in care are associated with higher mortality among minorities who do not receive the same services as whites (eg, surgical treatment for small cell lung cancer) [14].
- Specific coverage of emergency medicine, as reported by Cone and coworkers [15], is minimal. There is brief discussion of the Emergency Medical Treatment and Active Labor Act in a chapter on patient and system-level factors that contribute to racial and ethnic disparities and discussion on the study by Lowe and coworkers [16] that found that after controlling for age, gender, time of day, type of managed care organization, and triage score, African Americans were approximately 1.5 times more likely than white patients to be denied authorization for their ED visit.

Potential sources of racial and ethnic disparities

The IOM report notes that many sources (including those related to characteristics of patients, health systems, and the clinical encounter) may contribute to racial and ethnic disparities in care (C. Gomes, T. McGuire, unpublished data, 2001). Some researchers speculate that there may be subtle differences in the way that members in different racial and ethnic groups respond to treatment, particularly with regard to some pharmaceutical interventions [17]. Others have speculated that minority patients may receive a lower quality of care because of differences in health-seeking behaviors. As such, they are more likely to refuse recommended services and delay seeking health care. These behaviors can develop as a result of a poor cultural match that in turn may lead to mistrust, misunderstanding of provider instructions, poor interactions with the health care system, and inadequate access. A small group of studies have found that African Americans are slightly more likely (approximately 3%–6%) to reject medical recommendations, but these small refusal rates do not explain the differences [13]. More research is needed to understand the reasons behind these refusals and, if explained, the different strategies for helping patients to make informed decisions.

As Fig. 3 depicts, the IOM study considered other causation factors that may be associated with disparities in health care. One of those additional factors is the operation of the health care system and the legal and regulatory climate in which it must operate. These include

Cultural or linguistic barriers (eg, the lack of interpretation services)
Fragmentation of the health care system
Factors related to minorities being disproportionately enrolled in lower-cost health plans where the demands on service use are controlled
Where minorities receive care (less likely to seek access in a private physician's office even when insured at the same level of whites)

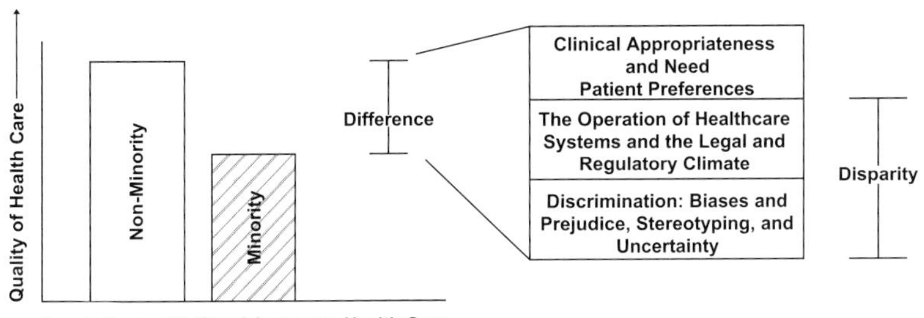

Fig. 3. Differences, disparities, and discrimination: populations with equal access to health care. (*From* Gomes C, McGuire T. Identifying the sources of racial and ethnic disparities in health care use. Unpublished manuscript; 2001, with permission.)

The other additional factor is related to the clinical encounter itself. According to the IOM, three mechanisms might be operative in health care disparities from the provider's side of the exchange:

Bias or prejudice against minorities
Greater clinical uncertainty when interacting with minority patients
Beliefs or stereotypes held by the provider about the behavior or health of minorities

Research on how patient race or ethnicity may influence physician decision-making and the quality of care for minorities is scant and still developing. As of yet, there is no direct evidence how prejudice, stereotypes, and bias influence care. It can be said that this creates a paradox: How can well-meaning and highly educated health care professions, working in their usual circumstances with diverse populations of patients, create a pattern of care that seems to be discriminatory? There is a large body of social psychology research that demonstrates that stereotyping is an almost universal human cognitive function. As such, stereotypes, conscious or not, endorse or guide the perception, interpretation, and retrieval of information [18].

Clearly, racial and ethnic disparities in health care exist and because they are associated with worse outcomes, these disparities are unacceptable. In addition, disparities occur in the context of a broader historical, contemporary social and economic inequity with evidence of persistent racial and ethnic discrimination in many sectors of American life.

In 1985, 15 years before the publication of the IOM report, the Department of Health and Human Service issued a report of the Secretary's Task Force on Black and Minority Health. The report was considered a landmark document at the time because it represented the first time Department of Health and Human Service had made a concerted effort to examine gaps in health care among ethnic groups. The task force observed that gross indicators of access and use of services, such as the number of annual visits to a physician, had narrowed as a result of the major insurance programs of Medicare and Medicaid [19]. The report also indicated that racial and ethnic groups continued to have poorer access to quality health care services and different patterns of use relative to white Americans, including a lower use of preventive services, a greater likelihood of not having a usual source of care, and a greater likelihood of being uninsured [19].

With these factors in mind, the role of the emergency medicine health care professional is significant as racial and ethnic communities seek health care in the ED. There is literature to suggest that an increase in the size of vulnerable populations served by EDs, such as ethnic minorities, the poor, and the working poor, is an important contributor to increases in ED visits [2,20–23]. Rather than be inclusive of the exhaustive literature on disparities in the health care arena, specific seminal and highlighted studies relevant to emergency medicine are the further focus of this article. Several articles in the emergency medicine literature have addressed racial disparities from an emergency medicine perspective [15,24–31]. Indeed, the Academic Emergency Medicine Consensus Conference in 2003 focused on disparities in emergency health care and was developed to examine current medical issues that impact the delivery of care to the emergency patient, specifically on health care disparities with attention to the ED setting [32].

This article also examines the literature on the racial and ethnic composition of individuals in the ED setting; reviews those systemic factors contributing to disparities in health care, and highlights medical conditions most likely to have disparate health presentations and outcomes in the ED. Lastly, the authors offer conclusions and future directions on how emergency medicine professionals can address these health care disparities.

The landmark report by the IOM highlights several strategies to address disparities in the United States health care delivery system [13]. This is a noteworthy discussion because the second overarching goal of the Healthy People 2010 initiative is to eliminate health disparities among segments of the population including but not limited to gender, race, or ethnicity and education [33].

The IOM report clearly notes patient, provider, and system level factors, beyond access-related issues, which may contribute to racial and ethnic health care disparities. This section of the report highlights ways in which health disparities can occur among various demographic groups in the United States, particularly as they relate to the aforementioned individual patient risk factors, such as lower socioeconomic status, environmental risks in minority communities, and health-related cultural beliefs of the patient and the health care provider [25]. The following section also examines the recommended strategy of workforce diversity, particularly as it relates to physician characteristics and related factors within the patient-physician dyad. The public health model of defining the problem, identifying the risk and protective factors, creating interventions, and evaluating the effect of these interventions is examined in the context of what the literature notes on health care disparities stated previously.

Individual factors

Lower socioeconomic factors

The impact of homelessness and poverty in the ED is discussed elsewhere in this issue. It is worthy to mention here, however, the question of disparities as it relates to socioeconomic status. Lillie-Blanton and colleagues [34] noted that minority patients were less likely than white patients to receive medical care from private physicians and less likely to have a primary care provider. In the Emergency Medicine Patients Access to Health Care Study, investigators noted that minority patients were more likely to access the ED for their general health care than white people, and reported financial reasons for seeking care in EDs [30]. This was also noted in a study of acute asthma among adults presenting to the ED, where ED management was similar for all racial groups but socioeconomic status accounted for most of the observed acute asthma differences [35]. Socioeconomic status is also linked to insurance status. Racial and ethnic minorities are less likely than white Americans to have health insurance, which is the most significant barrier to health care [36]. African Americans are less likely to have private or employment-based health insurance compared with white Americans and are more likely to have Medicaid or other publicly funded insurance. Native Americans, Alaska natives, Asian Americans, and Pacific Islanders also have a disproportionately high rate of uninsurance [36,37]. Lower socioeconomic status and lack of insurance in ethnically diverse communities is a significant barrier to health care access. As a result, many of these disadvantaged groups turn to the ED for health care. Despite these findings and the need for African Americans to seek care in the ED, Lowe and coworkers [16] noted that African American patients enrolled in managed care organizations were more likely than whites to be denied authorization for ED care.

Health-related beliefs of the health professional and the patient

Health care professionals are held to the highest professional standards and ethics, which ideally should prevent disparities in how health care is rendered in the physician-patient encounter. The work of van Ryn and Burke [38] supports the idea that physicians' perceptions of patients were influenced by patients' sociodemographic characteristics; specifically, physicians in her study tended to perceive African Americans and members of low socioeconomic status groups more negatively on a number of dimensions than they perceived whites or members of the middle and highest third of socioeconomic status. Clinical uncertainty, provider beliefs and stereotypes, and patient mistrust of the health care system are cited in the literature as important factors contributing to disparate treatment. The theory of uncertainty implies that a physician's vagueness in understanding and interpreting information from patients may contribute to disparities in care and can lead to minorities getting either more or less care than whites [13,39].

Workforce diversity

The physician-patient dyad has been based on the common belief of trusting one's doctor, yet physician bias may play a role in differences in the delivery of medical care. In a study by Schulman and coworkers [40], the race and sex of the patient influenced the recommendations of physicians independently of other factors. This may suggest bias on the part of the physicians. For example, African Americans were less likely to be referred for cardiac catheterization than whites. Of note, Burgess and coworkers [41] stated that stereotyping and bias is not simply a product of the individual provider but is caused by features of the health care setting that decrease cognitive capacity, such as fatigue, overload, and time pressure. Moreover, these conditions have been shown to be more prevalent in settings that predominantly treat minority patients. This is particularly noteworthy given the ED setting where fatigue, overload, and time pressure are natural parts of the work.

Indeed, as it is noted in the literature, this may speak to the need for workforce diversity and the role the minority physician plays in the care of minority patients [42,43]. For example, Cooper-Patrick and coworkers [44] noted that patients in race-concordant relationships with their physicians rated their visits as significantly more participatory than patients in race-discordant relationships. Other studies support concordance relationships [45,46]. In cases of language differences, this is even more evident. Language barriers and lack of interpreter services impede health care delivery in the ED setting. Bernstein and colleagues [47] noted that use of trained interpreters can increase clinic use, decrease 30-day total and ED return charges, and reduce disparities between English speaking patients and non-English noninterpreted patients in a number of services at the index ED visit.

What is the evidence: literature related to care in the emergency department

The IOM report was a landmark publication in that it was the first, large-scale government-sponsored examination of racial and ethnic disparity in health care. As mentioned previously, however, coverage of emergency medicine in this report is scant. Although this is caused in part by the relative paucity of academic research in this area, a number of studies have been published that merit consideration. Although a complete review of the breadth of literature on health care disparity is beyond the scope of this article, some of the most significant research in areas relevant to emergency medicine is addressed.

General medical care

The impetus to examine disparity in the ED stems from the overwhelming evidence on inequality in health care in general. A number of studies have examined racial disparities in the provision of general medical care without regard to specific diagnoses. A 1994 comparison of care provided to nearly 10,000 Medicare beneficiaries (including ordering of diagnostic studies, such as serum chemistries and chest radiographs, and the provision of therapies including diuretics and antibiotics) demonstrated significant deficiencies in the treatment of black patients [48]. An even larger study published in 1997 compared the provision of major therapeutic and diagnostic procedures in 77 disease categories among 1.7 million hospital encounters. African American patients were significantly less likely than whites to receive a major therapeutic procedure in nearly half of these categories [48]. Other researchers have demonstrated similar disparities with Hispanic patients. These studies provide a glimpse into the widespread and deeply ingrained problem of health care disparity.

Chest pain and acute coronary syndrome

The approach to chest pain and care of acute coronary syndrome (ACS) is perhaps the most comprehensively studied area of racial disparity. Although there is a paucity of ED-based literature on this topic, a number of studies have demonstrated significant race-related care discrepancies relevant to care provided in the ED. Almost universally, the data show that when diagnosed with acute myocardial infarction or unstable angina, African American patients are significantly less likely than whites to receive standard reperfusion therapies [2,3,49–51]. Similar disparities have been observed between Hispanic and white patients, although the difference is smaller [20]. More recent studies show that for those who do receive thrombolytics or percutaneous coronary intervention, door-to-therapy times are significantly longer for African American, Hispanic, and Asian patients [2]. Importantly, these studies all involved admitted patients with confirmed diagnoses of ACS, and represent a true disparity in provision of care, rather than a difference in access to care.

A number of investigators have attempted to identify the underlying causes of this inequality, with limited success. One study of cardiac care across a number of different hospitals found that the racial disparity could be partially attributed to care variation between participating hospitals, rather than within each of the individual sites. Even with multivariate analysis to factor out this effect, however, the study still reported that minority groups received substandard care [2]. An important message to recognize from this study is that the interhospital variability itself is an example of race-related disparity, because hospitals with poorer performance tended to treat a preponderance of African Americans, Hispanics, and Asians. Other studies have looked at whether the treatment gap can be explained by patient preference, socioeconomic factors, disease prevalence, differences in presentation, and regional variability; but no causative relationship has been found. In a review of the available literature, East and Peterson [21] rhetorically ask, "Have we elucidated the causes of racial inequality in care? No, but we have clarified what does not explain it."

One additional paper deserves close analysis: in 2003, a review of ED care of patients with suspected ACS was published. This study was unique in that it looked at chest pain care solely as it related to the ED; care after admission or discharge was not considered [50]. The results were striking: of patients diagnosed with acute myocardial infarction in the ED, 60% of white patients received cardiac catheterization, as opposed to only 39.6% of African Americans and 35.7% of all other non-whites. Additionally, in patients diagnosed with non–ST elevation myocardial infarction or unstable angina, white patients were more likely to undergo cardiac catheterization. Diagnostic work-up and medical therapy was similar for all groups with acute myocardial infarction or non–ST elevation myocardial infarction–unstable angina, with the exception of whites receiving glycoprotein IIb-IIIa inhibitors more often. Perhaps even more remarkable, however [50],

> Among patients with an ED diagnosis of non-ACS chest pain, African-Americans were less likely to undergo ECG acquisition within 10 minutes of ED presentation, laboratory evaluation, standard anti-ischemic medical treatment ... and invasive and noninvasive testing for CAD in comparison with whites ($P < .05$). Other nonwhites received less invasive testing and were admitted less often than whites with this diagnosis ($P < .01$).

Minority patients were significantly more likely to be diagnosed with "non-ACS chest pain" despite receiving fewer diagnostic tests, less medical therapy, and fewer hospitalizations then their white counterparts. This was the first study that demonstrated that not only is there unequal care in the immediate treatment of diagnosed ACS, but also in the work-up of patients with chest pain presenting to the ED.

Interestingly, there is evidence that this racial inequality can be overcome. An examination of nearly 1500 acute myocardial infarction patients within the equal-access, government-subsidized Department of Defense health care system demonstrated no race-based variability in the rate of immediate revascularization procedures [22]. The design of this health care system could help guide modifications to bridge the racial gap in cardiac care.

Trauma

As with cardiac care, there is a minimal amount of literature addressing disparities in ED care of the trauma patient. In the broader trauma literature, however, a number of examples are evident. From prehospital mortality rates to ED evaluation to postinjury recovery, trauma care is fraught with examples of the health care race gap.

Motor vehicle collisions are one of the leading causes of death in individuals younger than 34 years of age. Although in the past three decades there has been a steady decline in motor vehicle collision–related fatalities, Hispanics represent a disproportionate number of these deaths. A 1-year retrospective examination of motor vehicle collisions in rural North Carolina demonstrated a 0.037% mortality rate for whites as opposed to 4.4% for Hispanics. This equates to a death rate of 12.3 per 100,000 for whites as opposed to 166 per 100,000 for Hispanics [23]. In addition, Hispanic fatalities were more likely to have involved alcohol and be associated with lack of seat belt use. A larger study examining the fatality rates for African Americans and Hispanics and whites found similar disproportionate numbers, although by factoring in socioeconomic status they were able to account for some of the disparity [52]. These studies both provide examples of the disproportionate toll trauma takes on minority populations and propose educational strategies to bridge this gap.

Within the ED there is also evidence of disparate care. Although the literature is sparse, a few studies merit consideration. In an analysis of data from the National Trauma Data Bank, charts from nearly 7800 adolescent trauma victims were reviewed for frequency of alcohol and drug testing. The report found an increased rate of testing in both Hispanic and African American patients when compared with whites, but only the rates for Hispanic men and African American women reached statistical significance [53]. There was no relationship found between rates of testing and frequency of positive results among ethnic groups, indicating that the more frequent testing could not be clinically justified. Another study examined the treatment of mild traumatic brain injury in the ED and found significant disparities. African American patients were more likely to be treated by a resident and less likely to be referred to a primary care physician for follow-up. Hispanic patients were more likely to leave without being seen, to receive blood work including blood alcohol level testing, and to receive a nasogastric tube [27]. The authors of this study were unable to provide an explanation for some of these disparities, but believed they may be related to language barriers in the ED. Regardless, they recommended further study to elucidate the cause of these findings. Finally, another study reviewed the ED disposition for 1.5 million patients presenting with any traumatic injury and found that uninsured patients and African American women were less likely to be admitted than other demographic groups [54]. The provision of care for victims of trauma is unique to the ED environment, and the effect of race and ethnicity in this area remains poorly studied. It is likely that other areas of discrepancy may be found with further examination.

Cerebrovascular accident

The effect of stroke on the African American population is well documented. African Americans and Hispanics have a higher stroke frequency, higher mortality rate, and larger incidence of risk factors including diabetes and hypertension [55,56]. Literature examining this disparity, however, is scant.

One study examined the records of nearly 1200 ischemic stroke patients presenting to academic medical centers in 1999. The rates of administration of tissue-type plasminogen activator (tPA) were reviewed, and significant racial and ethnic differences were found in the use of this therapy. Although the most significant predictor of tPA use was stroke severity [57],

> Black tPA candidates were about one third as likely to receive tPA as those who were white (8.3% versus 24.6%; $P=0.04$). The magnitude of the difference was similar after adjustment for age, gender, insurance status, and stroke severity.

The study authors did note a trend toward more frequent contraindications to tPA among African Americans, including delayed presentation, but this did not account for the observed difference in treatment. Additionally, a significant gap was seen when considering only those patients who met inclusion criteria for administration of tPA. Although there continues to be some controversy regarding the role of tPA in acute stroke, this study makes clear that its use is not equal across all ethnic groups.

Asthma

It is well established that not only do African Americans and Hispanics have a greater incidence of asthma, but they also have more severe symptoms, are more frequently hospitalized, and often receive substandard outpatient care [31,58,59]. Recent investigations have sought to establish whether these disparities exist within the ED.

A review of more than 1800 adult patients enrolled in the Multicenter Airway Research Collaboration study examined whether racial or ethnic differences existed in the presentation and management of patients in the ED. The results were mixed. The investigators found that whereas African American and Hispanic patients presented with more severe respiratory symptoms and a history of more severe disease than did whites, the ED treatment they received was similar, and discharge rates were not statistically different. The disparity in asthma severity was largely eliminated through multivariate analysis for socioeconomic status. Interestingly, the study demonstrated more intense therapy for minorities in certain areas of care, such as amount of β-agonist administered and prescription of inhaled corticosteroids [31].

The same investigators conducted a similar study examining the presentation and treatment of children with asthma, and found similar results. With pediatric patients, minorities again had a history of more severe disease with more frequent hospitalizations, but intensity of ED therapy and rate of discharge was found to be equivalent. Interestingly, the investigators found that unlike in adults, all pediatric patients were equally likely to receive inhaled corticosteroids [60]. The authors expressed concern that given the more severe disease patterns and higher historical admission rates among African American and Hispanic children that they likely should have greater rates of corticosteroid prescription than whites.

Pain control

Some of the very first literature on health care disparity in the ED focused on management of acute pain and found some disturbing trends. In 1993, a retrospective cohort study compared analgesic use in Hispanic and non-Hispanic whites with isolated long bone fractures. After analyzing for multiple variables including injury severity, the investigators found that Hispanics were twice as likely as non-Hispanic whites to receive no analgesic in the ED [10]. The same investigators conducted a follow-up study to try to discover the reason for this striking discrepancy. Using a similar demographic population, Hispanic and non-Hispanic white patients with isolated extremity trauma, they asked both physicians and patients to estimate the severity of pain on a visual analog scale. They found no significant difference in either patient or physician estimates of pain severity between groups, and the degree of disparity between patient and physician estimates were similar for whites and Hispanics [61]. The authors concluded that physician capacity for assessing pain severity was similar for each ethnic group, and could not account for their early finding of disparate analgesic use.

A more recent study examined rate of analgesic use for African American and white patients with extremity fractures, and found that African Americans were much less likely to receive analgesia in the ED [9]. Again, none of the study's covariates could account for this discrepancy.

Two other studies merit consideration, because they analyzed analgesic prescription for a variety of conditions, including long-bone fractures, acute nontraumatic back pain, and migraine headache. The first presented volunteer physicians with a variety of scripted clinical vignettes using African American, Hispanic, or white patients presenting with migraine headache, back pain, or ankle fracture. The authors report no race or ethnicity-related difference in frequency of opioid prescription, but did find that patients with "socially desirable" characteristics (ie, a high prestige occupation and a strong relationship with a primary care provider) did increase rates of narcotic use [62]. The authors admit, however, that because their study was conducted on volunteer physicians in a nonmedical setting, their results may not translate into clinical practice. A study published that same year examined analgesic prescription rates among Hispanic, African American, and white patients with migraine headache, back pain, and isolated long bone fractures. Although rates of analgesia were similar for all three groups with extremity fractures, whites were more likely than both African Americans and Hispanics to receive pain control for headache and back pain [8]. Perhaps the similar results in pain control for long-bone fractures indicate heightened awareness of the need for analgesia in the ED, but there clearly remain areas of racial disparity.

Other studies and future directions

A few other studies have been published indicating disparity in other areas of ED care. An observational analysis of a full-year sample of pediatric appendicitis cases in California and New York demonstrated significantly increased rupture rates in Hispanic, Asian, and African American children, with some geographic variability [20]. A chart review of 1.2 million adolescent ED visits for sexually transmitted diseases demonstrated that not only are men more likely to be treated than women, but that Hispanic patients were particularly at risk for undertreatment [63].

These studies clearly demonstrate that racial and ethnic health care disparity exists within the ED. Many of these areas remain inadequately studied and there are other areas the literature has yet to address. Further examination of these and other disease presentations is needed to explore further areas of ethnic and racial inequality in ED care.

General recommendations

There is a need to increase awareness of racial and ethnic disparities in health care among the general public and key stakeholders, and to increase health care providers' awareness of disparities. Despite emergency medicine's philosophic, historical, and legislative mandate to care for all who present to the ED regardless of racial or ethnic background, clinicians are not immune to these problems.

Legal, regulatory, and policy recommendations

There are a number of important public policy steps that should be taken to eliminate racial and ethnic disparities. Among these steps there is a need to (1) avoid fragmentation of health plans along socioeconomic lines, and take measures to strengthen the stability of patient-provider relationships in publicly funded health plans; (2) increase the proportion of underrepresented United States racial and ethnic minorities among health professionals; (3) apply the same managed care protections to publicly funded HMO enrollees that apply to private HMO enrollees; and (4) provide greater resources to the US Department of Health and Human Services Office of Civil Rights to enforce civil rights laws [13].

Health system interventions

From a health systems perspective, there are a number of important potential interventions. These include (1) promoting the consistency and equity of care through the use of evidence-based guidelines; (2) structuring payment systems to ensure an adequate supply of services to minority patients, and limit provider incentives that may promote disparities; (3) enhancing patient-provider communication and trust by providing financial incentives for practices that reduce barriers and encourage evidence-based practice; and (4) promoting the use of interpretation services where community need exists. The use of community health workers and multidisciplinary treatment and preventive care teams should also be supported [13].

Education

Educational interventions are as important as health system and public policy interventions. There is a need to implement patient education programs to increase patients' knowledge of how best to access care and participate in treatment decisions. Emergency medicine literature also supports integrating cross-cultural education into the training of all current and future health professionals [64] and diversifying the medical and emergency medicine workforce [26,65].

As Jordan Cohen, President of the Association of American Medical Colleges, stated in the emergency medicine literature, "There must be a diverse medical student and faculty group in order for students to live and work and experience the diversity that is critical for developing the sensibilities that we call cultural competence. That is an important element in reducing disparities in health care over time" [66].

In emergency medicine, minorities are underrepresented in academic emergency medicine compared with other specialties and their status lags behind that of white academic emergency medicine physicians. Academic departments of emergency medicine must identify strategies to facilitate the recruitment, retention, and promotion of minority faculty [67]. As stated in the literature, efforts to recruit minorities and to eliminate disparities in health care require strong leadership [66].

Summary

Disparities in medical care in the emergency medical arena require continued attention and concerted efforts if there is to be a reduction in disparate health care outcomes of the patients we serve. Emergency medicine literature examining the issue is the first step toward finding solutions. The next step is in improved data collection, such as targeting methodologic issues (ie, study design that incorporates within-group comparisons of subgroups within the Hispanic or Asian population) and controlling for confounders. This methodology is a fundamental requirement for producing high-quality research on disparities [68]. Richards and Lowe [28] aptly note that emergency medicine has a different lens from other medical specialties in that ED professionals care for all comers and are more apt to respond uniformly given that reality. They also note that ED professionals must determine the extent of the problem within the specialty using rigorous databases and scientific research. Based on this scientific research, to the extent that disparities exist, the causal factors need to be identified and studied. This will lead to further action through the development of appropriate interventions and the tracking of outcome measures, and ultimately to progress toward eradicating racial disparities in health care [28].

References

[1] Keppel K, Pearcy J, Wagener D. Trends in racial and ethnic-specific rates for the health indicators: United States, 1990–98. Hyattsville: National Center for Health Statistics; 2002.

[2] Bradley E, Herrin J, Wang Y, et al. Racial and ethnic differences in time to acute reperfusion therapy for patients hospitalized with myocardial infarction. JAMA 2004;292:1563–72.

[3] Chen J, Rathore SS, Radford MJ, et al. Racial differences in the use of cardiac catheterization after acute myocardial infarction [see comment]. N Engl J Med 2001;344:1443–9.

[4] Johnson P, Lee T, Cook E, et al. Effect of race on the presentation and management of patients with acute chest pain. Ann Intern Med 1993;118:593–601.

[5] Gornick ME, Eggers PW, Reilly TW, et al. Effects of race and income on mortality and use of services among Medicare beneficiaries. N Engl J Med 1996;335:791–9.

[6] Jazieh AR, Buncher C. Racial and age-related disparities in obtaining screening mammography: results of a statewide database. South Med J 2002;95:1145–8.

[7] Schneider EC, Cleary PD, Zaslavsky AM, et al. Racial disparity in influenza vaccination: does managed care narrow the gap between African-Americans and whites? JAMA 2001;286:1455–60.

[8] Tamayo-Sarver J, Hinze S, Cydulka R, et al. Racial and ethnic disparities in emergency department analgesic prescription. Am J Public Health 2003;93:2067–73.

[9] Todd K, Deaton C, D'Adamo A, et al. Ethnicity and analgesic practice. Ann Emerg Med 2000;35:11.

[10] Todd K, Samaroo N, Hoffman J. Ethnicity as a risk factor for inadequate emergency department analgesia. JAMA 1993;269:1537–9.

[11] US Department of Health and Human Services. Health disparities experienced by black or African-Americans–United States. MMWR Morb Mortal Wkly Rep 2005;54:1–3.

[12] Fronstin P. Sources of health insurance and characteristics of the uninsured: analysis of the March 1999 Current Population Survey. EBRI Issue Brief 2000;217:1–26.

[13] Unequal treatment: confronting racial and ethnic disparities in health care. In: Brian D, Smedley AYS, Nelson AR, editors. Washington: Institute of Medicine; 2002.

[14] Bach PB, Cramer LD, Warren JL, et al. Racial differences in the treatment of early-stage lung cancer. N Engl J Med 1999;341:1198–205.

[15] Cone D, Richardson L, Todd K, et al. Health care disparities in emergency medicine. Acad Emerg Med 2003;10:1176–83.

[16] Lowe RA, Chhaya S, Nasci K, et al. Effect of ethnicity on denial of authorization for emergency department care by managed care gatekeepers. Acad Emerg Med 2001;8:259–66.

[17] Khandker R, Simoni-Wastila L. Differences in prescription drug utilization and expenditures between blacks and whites in the Georgia Medicaid population. Inquiry 1998;35:78–87.

[18] Mackie D, Hamilton D, Susskind J, et al. Social psychological foundations of stereotype formation. In: Macrae N, Stangor C, Hewstone M, editors. Stereotypes and stereotyping. New York: Guilford Press; 1996. p. 41–78.

[19] US Department of Health and Human Services. Report of the Secretary's Task Force on Black & Minority Health. Washington: US Department of Health and Human Services; 1985.

[20] Bertoni A, Goonan K, Bonds D, et al. Racial and ethnic disparities in cardiac catheterization for acute myocardial infarction in the United States, 1995–2001. J Natl Med Assoc 2005;97: 317–23.

[21] East M, Peterson E. Understanding racial differences in cardiovascular care and outcomes: issues for the new millennium. Am Heart J 2000;139.

[22] Taylor A, Meyer G, Morse R, et al. Can characteristics of a health care system mitigate ethnic bias in access to cardiovascular procedures? Experience from the Military Health Services System. J Am Coll Cardiol 1997;30:901–7.

[23] March JA, Evans M, Ward B, et al. Motor vehicle crash fatalities among Hispanics in rural North Carolina. Acad Emerg Med 2003;10:1249–52.

[24] Guagliardo MF, Teach SJ, Huang ZJ, et al. Racial and ethnic disparities in pediatric appendicitis rupture rate. Acad Emerg Med 2003;10:1218–27.

[25] Blanchard JC, Haywood YC, Scott C. Racial and ethnic disparities in health: an emergency medicine perspective. Acad Emerg Med 2003;10:1289–93.

[26] Hamilton G, Marco CA. Emergency medicine education and health care disparities. Acad Emerg Med 2003;10:1189–92.

[27] O'Connor RE, Haley L. Disparities in emergency department health care: systems and administration. Acad Emerg Med 2003;10:1193–8.

[28] Richards CF, Lowe RA. Researching racial and ethnic disparities in emergency medicine. Acad Emerg Med 2003;10:1169–75.

[29] Richardson L, Babcock Irvin C, Tamayo-Sarver J. Racial and ethnic disparities in the clinical practice of emergency medicine. Acad Emerg Med 2003;10(11):1184–8.

[30] Richardson L, Ragin D, Hwang U, et al. Emergency medicine patient's access to health care (EMPATH) study: racial/ethnic, gender and age related differences in emergency department use [abstract]. Acad Emerg Med 2003;10:524.

[31] Bazarian JJ, Pope C, McClung J, et al. Ethnic and racial disparities in emergency department care for mild traumatic brain injury. Acad Emerg Med 2003;10:1209–17.

[32] Biros MH, Adams JG, Cone DC. Executive summary: disparities in emergency health care. Acad Emerg Med 2003;10:1153–4.

[33] US Department of Health and Human Services. Healthy people 2010. Washington: Department of Health and Human Services; 2000.

[34] Lillie-Blanton M, Brodie M, Rowland D, et al. Race, ethnicity, and the health care system: public perceptions and experiences. Med Care Res Rev 2000;57(Suppl 1).218 35.

[35] Boudreaux ED, Emond SD, Clark S, et al. Acute asthma among adults presenting to the emergency department: the role of race/ethnicity and socioeconomic status. Chest 2003; 124:803–12.

[36] Hoffman C, Pohl M. Health insurance coverage in America: 1999 data update. Washington: The Kaiser Commission on Medicaid and the Uninsured; 2000.

[37] Brown R, Ojeda V, Wyn R. Racial and ethnic disparities in access to health insurance and health care. Los Angeles: UCLA Center for Health Policy Research; 2000.

[38] van Ryn M, Burke J. The effect of patient race and socio-economic status on physicians' perceptions of patients. Soc Sci Med 2000;50:813.

[39] Balsa A, McGuire T. Prejudice, uncertainty and stereotypes as sources of health care disparities. Boston: Boston University; 2001.

[40] Schulman K, Berlin J, Harless W, et al. The effect of race and sex on physicians' recommendations for cardiac catheterization [see comment]. N Engl J Med 1999;340:618–26 [erratum: N Engl J Med 1999;340:1130].

[41] Burgess D, Fu S, van Ryn M. Why do providers contribute to disparities and what can be done about it? J Gen Intern Med 2004;19:1154–69.

[42] Komaromy M, Grumbach K, Drake M, et al. The role of black and Hispanic physicians in providing health care of underserved populations. N Engl J Med 1996;334:1305–10.

[43] Moy E, Bartman B. Physician race and care of minority and medically indigent patients. JAMA 1995;273:1515–20.

[44] Cooper-Patrick L, Gallo JJ, Gonzales JJ, et al. Race, gender, and partnership in the patient-physician relationship. JAMA 1999;282:583–9.

[45] Saha S, Arbelaez JJ, Cooper LA. Patient-physician relationships and racial disparities in the quality of health care. Am J Public Health 2003;93:1713–9.

[46] Saha S, Komaromy M, Koepsell TD, et al. Patient-physician racial concordance and the perceived quality and use of health care. Arch Intern Med 1999;159:997–1004.

[47] Bernstein J, Bernstein E, Dave A, et al. Does the use of trained medical interpreters affect ED services, reduce subsequent charges, and improve follow-up? Acad Emerg Med 2000;7:523.

[48] Geiger HJ. Racial and ethnic disparities in diagnosis and treatment: a review of the evidence and a consideration of causes. In: Brian D, Smedley AYS, Nelson AR, editors. Unequal treatment: confronting racial and ethnic disparities in health care. Washington: The National Academic Press; 2003.

[49] Maynard C, Fisher L, Passamani E, et al. Blacks in the coronary artery surgery study (CASS): race and clinical decision making. Am J Public Health 1986;76:1446–8.

[50] Venkat A, Hoekstra J, Lindsell C, et al. The impact of race on the acute management of chest pain. Acad Emerg Med 2003;10:1199–208.

[51] Syed M, Khaja F, Rybicki B, et al. Effect of delay on racial differences in thrombolysis for acute myocardial infarction. Am Heart J 2000;140:643–50.

[52] Braver ER. Race, Hispanic origin, and socioeconomic status in relation to motor vehicle occupant death rates and risk factors among adults. Accid Anal Prev 2003;35:295–309.

[53] Marcin J, Pretzlaff R, Whittaker H, et al. Evaluation of race and ethnicity on alcohol and drug testing of adolescents admitted with trauma. Acad Emerg Med 2003;10:1253–9.

[54] Selassie A, McCarthy M, Pickelsimer E. The influence of insurance, race, and gender on emergency department disposition. Acad Emerg Med 2003;10:1260–70.

[55] Sacco RL. Preventing stroke among blacks: the challenges continue. JAMA 2003;289:3005–7.

[56] Sacco RL, Boden-Albala B, Abel G, et al. Race-ethnic disparities in the impact of stroke risk factors: The Northern Manhattan stroke study. Stroke 2001;32:1725–31.

[57] Johnston SC, Fung LH, Gillum LA, et al. Utilization of intravenous tissue-type plasminogen activator for ischemic stroke at academic medical centers: the influence of ethnicity. Stroke 2001;32:1061–8.

[58] Krishnan JA, Diette GB, Skinner EA, et al. Race and sex differences in consistency of care with national asthma guidelines in managed care organizations. Arch Intern Med 2001;161:1660–8.

[59] Simon PA, Zeng Z, Wold CM, et al. Prevalence of childhood asthma and associated morbidity in Los Angeles County: impacts of race/ethnicity and income. J Asthma 2003;40:535–43.

[60] Boudreaux ED, Emond SD, Clark S, et al. Race/ethnicity and asthma among children presenting to the emergency department: difference in disease severity and management. Pediatrics 2003;111.

[61] Todd KH, Lee T, Hofman JR. The effect of ethnicity on physician estimates of pain severity in patients with isolated extremity trauma. JAMA 1994;271:925–8.

[62] Tamayo-Sarver JH, Dawson NV, Hinze SW, et al. The effect of race/ethnicity and desirable social characteristics on physicians' decisions to prescribe opioid analgesics. Acad Emerg Med 2003;10.

[63] Beckmann KR, Melzer-Lange MD, Gorelick MH. Emergency department management of sexually transmitted infections in US adolescents: results from the national hospital ambulatory medical care survey. Ann Emerg Med 2004;43.

[64] Scott CJ, Martin M, Hamilton G. Training of medical professionals and the delivery of health care as related to cultural identity groups. Acad Emerg Med 2003;10:1149–52.

[65] Powe M, Neil R, Cooper LA. Diversifying the racial and ethnic composition of the physician workforce. Ann Intern Med 2004;141:223–4.

[66] Cohen JJ. Disparities in health care: an overview. Acad Emerg Med 2003;10:1155–60.
[67] Richardson LD, Wilets IF, Cydulka RK. Minority faculty in academic emergency medicine. Acad Emerg Med 2001;8:474.
[68] Weinick RM. Researching disparities: strategies for primary data collection. Acad Emerg Med 2003;10:1161–8.

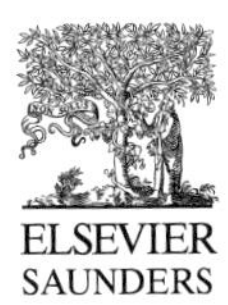

ELSEVIER
SAUNDERS

Emerg Med Clin N Am
24 (2006) 925–967

EMERGENCY
MEDICINE
CLINICS OF
NORTH AMERICA

The Impact of Alcohol, Tobacco, and Other Drug Use and Abuse in the Emergency Department

Gail D'Onofrio, MD, MS[a],*, Bruce Becker, MD[b], Robert H. Woolard, MD[b]

[a]Section of Emergency Medicine, Yale School of Medicine, 464 Congress Avenue, Suite 260, New Haven, CT 06519, USA
[b]Department of Emergency Medicine, Brown Medical School, Box G-A, Providence RI 02912, USA

Substance abuse is a major preventable public health problem affecting all racial, cultural, and socioeconomic groups with the total annual economic costs to the United States currently estimated at over $414 billion [1]. Over 500,000 deaths annually are attributable to alcohol, tobacco, or illicit drug use: 107,000 related to alcohol [2], 25,000 to illicit drugs [2], and 435,000 to tobacco [3]. Substance abuse is a risk factor for multiple diseases and a major risk factor for injury [4]. Tobacco use, especially cigarette smoking, is the leading cause of preventable disease and a major risk factor for heart disease, stroke, lung cancer, and chronic lung diseases [5]. It is responsible for more than 30% of all cancer deaths each year [6]. An estimated 18 million people have alcohol abuse problems, whereas an additional 5 million abuse other drugs [7]. Less than 3% of people with alcohol problems and fewer than 10% with drug problems receive treatment, despite the fact that substance abuse treatment has been demonstrated to be effective in reducing use and costs associated with substance abuse [8]. The consequences of substance abuse affect not only individuals, but also families, workplaces, and communities.

Alcohol use and abuse: prevalence and impact in the emergency department population

Alcohol problems are prevalent in the emergency department (ED) population and cover a wide spectrum of misuse, ranging from at-risk drinking

* Corresponding author.
E-mail address: gail.donofrio@yale.edu (G. D'Onofrio).

patterns to dependence (Fig. 1) [9]. Hazardous, also known as "at-risk," drinking levels are defined as those exceeding the National Institute of Alcohol Abuse and Alcoholism guidelines for low-risk drinking identified by the three recommended quantity and frequency screening questions outlined in the Appendix [10].

By definition these drinkers are at-risk for future medical, social, or legal consequences. Harmful drinkers are those patients who present with a negative consequence related to alcohol. It is estimated that approximately 20% of the population in the United States over the age of 12 are hazardous and harmful drinkers [11] and that they represent approximately 17% of patients seen in primary care practices [12], and a significant proportion of ED patients [13–15].

Emergency providers (EPs) routinely care for patients with hazardous and harmful drinking. There are an estimated 110 million ED visits each year, and between 10% and 46% of these visits are known to be associated with alcohol [16,17]. Cherpitel [13] screened all patients presenting to an ED and found that 17% were positive for harmful drinking. Patients presenting to the ED are more likely to have alcohol-related problems than those presenting to primary care. Cherpitel [18] recently compared patients presenting to an ED with those presenting to a primary care setting in the same metropolitan area. She found that ED patients were 1.5 to 3 times more likely to report heavy drinking, consequences of drinking, or ever having treatment for an alcohol problem than patients presenting to a primary care clinic. O'Brien and coworkers [19] found a higher likelihood of self-reported alcohol and drug use among patients who identified the ED as their regular source of care. A single alcohol-related ED visit has been shown to be an important predictor of continued problem drinking, alcohol-impaired driving, and possible premature death [20]. Problem drinkers average almost twice as many injury-related events per year as nonproblem drinkers and four times as many hospitalizations for injury [21]. In addition, it has

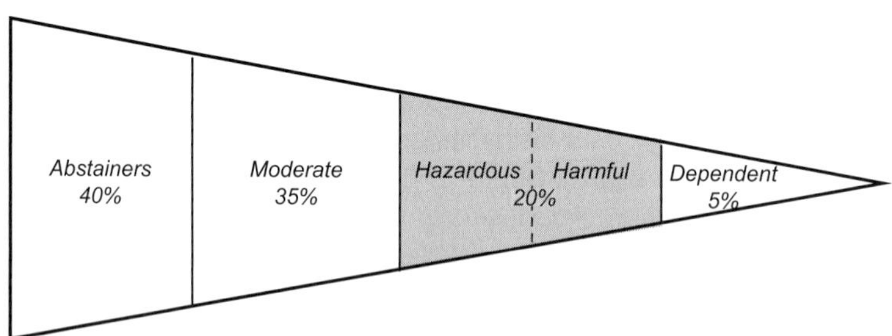

Fig. 1. The spectrum of alcohol use. (*From* D'Onofrio G, Pantalon MV, Degutis LC, et al. Development and implementation of an emergency practitioner-performed brief intervention for hazardous and harmful drinkers in the emergency department. Acad Emerg Med 2005;12:250; with permission from the Society for Academic Emergency Medicine.)

been shown that rates of heavy drinkers and alcohol-related problems among both injured and noninjured ED patients are higher than in the general population [14]. Hazardous and harmful drinkers who present to the ED have also been found to have a higher rate of ED use than patients who do not have alcohol problems [22].

Related issues regarding illness and injury

Alcohol is a major risk factor for virtually all categories of injury [23]. It has been demonstrated that alcohol is a factor in 60% to 70% of homicides, 40% of suicides, 40% to 50% of fatal motor vehicle crashes, 60% of fatal burn injuries, 60% of drownings, and 40% of fatal falls [24–28]. Nearly 50% of severely injured trauma patients are injured while under the influence of alcohol [29]. Alcohol is a risk factor in a variety of diseases including hypertension, stroke, diabetes, liver, and other gastrointestinal diseases, and breast and esophageal cancers [30]. The World Health Organization ranks disease burden by illness by region and country: in 2000, alcohol-use disorders were ranked second for 15 to 44 year olds at approximately 14%, in the United States, Canada, and Western Europe [31].

High-risk populations

A great proportion of patients who exceed the low-risk limits for drinking do not have contact with either alcohol treatment specialists or visit primary care medical practitioners. The ED may be their only contact with the health care system. Studies have shown that most patients without a chronic medical problem referred to primary care particularly in the uninsured population do not keep their visits or decrease their ED visits [32]. Young adults have the highest prevalence of binge and hazardous drinking in the United States. Excessive alcohol consumption is a continuing problem in the young adult age group. Data from the 2001 Behavioral Risk Factor Surveillance Survey demonstrate that 51.6% of respondents between the ages of 18 and 24 reported having three or more drinks on average per occasion [33]. Additionally, the consequences of excessive and underage drinking on college campuses are well documented [34]. Approximately 500,000 students between the ages of 18 and 24 are unintentionally injured under the influence of alcohol, and 1400 die each year from alcohol-related injuries. More than 600,000 students are assaulted by another student who has been drinking, 70,000 are victims of alcohol-related sexual assault, 400,000 have unprotected sex, and 2.1 million drive under the influence.

A missed opportunity for intervention and referral

EPs are often faced with a busy ED, conflicting demands, and ever-increasing responsibilities. Screening and intervention strategies must be brief and effective. Evidence suggests that an acute subcritical injury may be an important motivator to reduce drinking, and the time of the ED visit may be a valuable teachable moment [35]. The identification and initiation of treatment for individuals who are drinking at hazardous or harmful levels is beneficial in broadening the base of alcohol treatment. Unfortunately, despite high rates of heavy drinking among both injured and noninjured ED patients, routine screening and brief interventions are rarely performed in the ED. Because of this, an important opportunity to address alcohol-related problems is missed [36].

Treatment

Early identification of alcohol problems and referral to treatment are beneficial to individuals' health status and saves health care dollars. A recent study in Tennessee [37] demonstrated that less than 1% of patients with alcohol and other drug problems were identified and referred. ED patients with unmet substance abuse treatment need generated much higher hospital and ED charges than patients without such need. They were 81% more likely to be admitted to the hospital during their current ED visit (odds ratio [OR] 1.81; 95% confidence interval [CI], 1.27–2.64), and 46% more likely to have reported making at least one ED visit in the previous 12 months (OR 1.46; 95% CI, 1.12–1.84). Their use pattern was estimated at $777.2 million in extra hospital charges for Tennessee in 2000, an addition $1568 per ED patient with unmet substance abuse treatment need [38].

Brief interventions, which are described in detail later in this article, have been shown to be effective in multiple randomized, controlled trials [39]. The goal for at-risk or harmful drinkers is to reduce consumption into moderate range and to mitigate negative consequences. The goal for dependent drinkers is to negotiate referral to specialized treatment centers or acceptance of referral to self-help groups.

There is ample evidence that referral of patients with alcohol dependence is effective [40]. A review of observational and clinical trials reveals that two thirds of patients receiving treatment, either behavioral or pharmacologic, demonstrate a reduction in consumption by 50% at 1 year or a reduction in negative consequences, such as injury or loss of employment. One third of patients are either abstinent or drinking moderately without consequences [41]. A large-scale study on counseling for alcohol dependence showed that cognitive behavioral therapy, 12-step facilitation, and motivational-enhancement therapy were all effective treatments with similar efficacy. At 3 years, two thirds of the patients were abstinent.

Another opportunity for treatment is referral of patients to Alcoholics Anonymous. Alcoholics Anonymous is a free fellowship located in most communities. Participation, which includes attendance at meetings and having a sponsor, has been shown to be effective in promoting abstinence [42].

Screening for alcohol use and abuse

Screening includes diagnostic blood tests to determine blood alcohol concentrations either with blood samples or estimates using breathalyzers or saliva testing, or organ damage, such as liver function tests. Screening can also include structured questionnaires.

Structured questionnaires are very useful for detection and brief assessment of problem drinkers. A variety of instruments are available. Their effectiveness varies according to their availability, ease of administration, and test characteristics. Although structured interviews that can classify individuals into *Diagnostic and Statistical Manual of Mental Disorders-IV* categories may be best (eg, the Diagnostic Interview schedule [43], the Structured Clinical Interview for Diagnostic and Statistical Manual of Mental Disorders-III-R) [44], these are lengthy, time consuming, and not practical in the ED. Cherpitel [13] reported the sensitivities and specificities of several questionnaires in the ED setting. The CAGE [45] questionnaire was found to be 76% sensitive and 90% specific for dependence. Given the ease of administration and these results, the CAGE is an ideal instrument for the ED. It is not ideal, however, for at-risk and hazardous drinkers. The Alcohol Use Disorders Identification Test [46] was originally designed for harmful and hazardous drinkers; however, it is lengthy, including 10 questions, and needs to be scored.

Suggested options for use in the emergency department

The American College of Emergency Physicians has adopted the quantity and frequency questions suggested by the National Institute of Alcohol Abuse and Alcoholism to identify individuals drinking above recommended levels, followed by the CAGE questionnaire as part of their toolkit for screening and intervention [47]. The EP can then identify patients at risk by the first three quantity and frequency questions, and then proceed to the CAGE questions if patients are over the limits. Those with two or more positive answers should always be referred to specialized treatment. Those with one positive may be referred for further assessment or follow-up with their primary care provider. This algorithm can be completed in a step-wise fashion that takes the EP 5 to 45 seconds. To begin, one may ask, "Do you drink any beer, wine, or liquor"? This eliminates up to 40% of the general population who do not drink, and as many as 60% of ED populations. The following three quantity and frequency questions eliminate another substantial group that are moderate drinkers. The remaining patients who drink over low-risk limits are then asked the CAGE questions.

Interventions and referral for alcohol problems

Review of the literature in terms of efficacy in the emergency department

Brief interventions are short counseling sessions, ranging from 5 to 60 minutes, which incorporate feedback, advice, and motivational enhancement techniques to assist patients in reducing their alcohol consumption to low-risk guidelines, thereby reducing their risk of illness or injury. Brief intervention was first developed in 1994 in consultation with Dr. Stephan Rollnick for Project ASSERT in the ED [48,49]. There is compelling evidence in the literature that brief interventions for alcohol problems are effective in a variety of settings including the ED [48,50,51], primary care [52], and inpatient trauma settings [53]. There is some evidence that moderate drinkers may receive the greatest benefit from brief interventions [53].

Monti and colleagues [50] compared the effectiveness of standard care with that of a brief motivational interview (BMI) in reducing alcohol-related consequences and alcohol use among 94 adolescent patients ages 18 and 19 who presented to an ED with a positive blood alcohol concentration (BAC) or alcohol-related injury. At 6 months, both groups decreased their alcohol consumption, but those patients with BMI significantly reduced negative consequences regarding (1) drinking and driving (62% versus 86%); (2) being cited for a moving violation (3% versus 23%); (3) sustaining an alcohol-related injury (21% versus 50%); or (4) reporting fewer problems including problems with dates, friends, police, parents, and school.

Longabaugh and coworkers [51] evaluated the effectiveness of BMI in injured drinkers aged 18 and older who presented to an ED. Patients were eligible if they screened positive using testing methods for BAC, reported having ingested alcohol in the 6 hours before the injury, or scored positive on the Alcohol Use Disorders Identification Test screening questionnaire. Patients were randomized to standard care, brief intervention, or brief interventions with a booster that entailed a scheduled return visit 7 to 10 days after the initial brief interventions. At 1-year follow-up, participants in all three groups reported having reduced their days of heavy drinking, similar to the findings of Monti and coworkers [50]. Moreover, the brief interventions with a booster group reported significantly fewer alcohol-related negative consequences, such as injuries, and those items measured on the Drinking Inventory of Consequences, such as hangovers and lost work.

Other cohort studies provide evidence that identification of patients with alcohol problems and direct, timely linkage to specialized treatment centers enhances enrollment [49,54].

Drug use and abuse: overview

Drug users in the United States remain predominantly polysubstance abusers. Alcohol use with another drug remains the predominant pattern. Drugs are commonly used by youth in the United States. Marijuana use is most common, with 34% of youth reporting use (Fig. 2 and Table 1). Drug use mirrors the availability of different types and forms of drugs. In recent years, club drug use including 3,4-methylenedioxymethamphetamine ([MDMA] ecstasy), the most frequently abused club drug, has captured media attention. Use of prescription and opiates has increased in most areas, especially hydrocodone and oxycodone. Methamphetamine abuse has spread eastward from the west coast. Heroin use has remained at high levels where high-purity heroin powder is available. Cocaine, especially crack cocaine, continues to be widely available and a major problem in most urban areas. Benzodiazepines are widely abused and are used by drug abusers to enhance or control the effects of other drugs. Phencyclidine use also has increased in many areas (Fig. 3).

There are many consequences of drug use: motor vehicle crashes, injuries, HIV and STD infections, increased health care needs, crime, unemployment, and poor academic performance. Perhaps the largest immediate risk is posed by driving under the influence of substances. Whereas driving under the influence of alcohol is the most important factor associated with motor vehicle crashes and injury, public health and safety are also threatened by driving under the influence of other drugs, usually in combination with alcohol. An average of 4.2 million persons aged 16 to 20 reported driving under the influence of alcohol or illegal drugs during the past year. Of these, only 4% reported that they had been arrested [55].

Estimating the total cost of drug-related events, such as motor vehicle crashes, is difficult. There are few studies of the prevalence of other drug use (eg, opiates, cocaine, cannabinoids, and amphetamines) among drivers injured in road accidents. In one ED study 296 injured drivers aged 18 to 35 were compared with 278 noninjured patients. All were screened for drugs

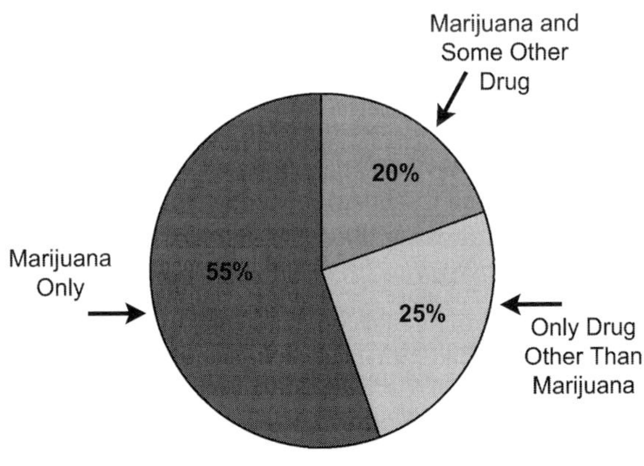

Fig. 2. Drug abuse-related ED visits involving narcotic analgesics, 1995 to 2002. (*From* Office of Applied Studies, SAMHSA, Drug Abuse Warning Network; 2002; with permission.)

Table 1
Reported drug and alcohol use by high school seniors, 2004

Drugs	% Used within the last	
	12 months	30 days
Alcohol	70.6	48
Marijuana	34.3	19.9
Stimulants	10	4.6
Other opiates	9.5	4.3
Tranquilizers	7.3	3.1
Sedatives	6.5	2.9
Hallucinogens	6.2	1.9
Cocaine	5.3	2.3
Inhalants	4.2	1.5
Steroids	2.5	1.6
Heroin	0.9	0.5

Data from Press release: Overall teen drug use continues gradual decline; but use of inhalants rises. University of Michigan News and Information Services, December 21, 2004.

in the ED. Only cannabinoids were found to be significantly present more often among drivers (14% of injured drivers versus 7.5% of uninjured). Cocaine and amphetamines were equally present at low levels among injured drivers and uninjured patients [56]. The presence of cannabis use among injured drivers is a grave concern. Alcohol use with cannabis has been associated with injury [57,58]. Driving under the influence of alcohol and marijuana is a growing concern and the focus of active intervention in some EDs [59].

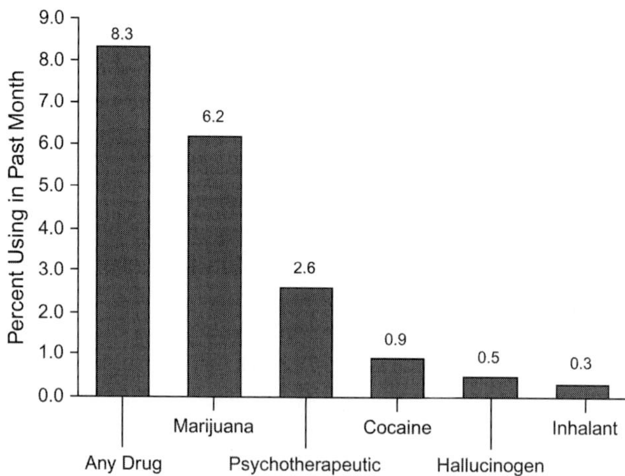

Fig. 3. Types of drugs used by past month illicit drug users aged 12 or older: 2002. (*From* Substance Abuse and Mental Health Services Administration. Results from the 2002 National Survey on Drug Use and Health: National Findings. Rockville (MD): Office of Applied Studies, NHSDA Series H-22, DHHS Publication No. SMA 03–3836; 2003.)

The relationship between illicit drug use and crime is significant. A higher prevalence and higher rates of crime are associated with more frequent use of heroin or cocaine. Addicts vary with regard to the type, amount, and severity of the crime committed. Drug use, especially cocaine use, among prisoners, parolees, probationers, and arrestees is high compared with the general population [60]. Ongoing drug use, especially cocaine use, reduces adherence and viral suppression among HIV-positive drug users [61].

There are many other problems faced differentially by drug abusers. They are more likely to be hospitalized and 2.3 times more likely to use an emergency room than nonabusers [62]. Teenagers that use alcohol or drugs are more likely to have sex than those who do not [63–66]. Those youths who engage in risk behaviors tend to take part in more than one risk behavior, including sexual experience. For teenagers and adults aged 18 to 30, having multiple sexual partners has been associated with use of alcohol or other substances [67]. Youth drug users remaining in school report a reduction in grades [68]. The employment of self-reporting drug users is also considerably less than nonusers in the United States and elsewhere [69]. There is also a problem with substance abuse in the workplace, especially among construction workers associated with injury and chronic pain [70].

Drug use and abuse: prevalence and impact in the emergency department population

Patients using drugs are encountered in most EDs on a routine basis. The specific drugs encountered reflect both national and local trends for use, with regional and city variation as drug crazes sweep through subcultures. Subcultures grow around the use of specific agents. Such drugs as marijuana, cocaine, amphetamines, ecstasy, prescription opiates, heroin, hallucinogens, or inhalants may predominate in any region at any time. Local drug use trends vary. For example, overall United States data indicate that cocaine abuse decreased between 1992 and 2002 [71]. Although cocaine abuse decreased by 60% or more in five states, it increased 100% or more in four other states.

EPs should recognize and screen for use of drugs when treating patients with an injury, change in mental status, respiratory distress, infection, depression, physical abuse, or loss of social support. A considerable part of emergency care is occupied with treating medical consequences of substance use. The abuse of drugs is often not addressed in the ED [72]. This unwillingness to identify drug abusers may relate to the fact that physicians, particularly EPs, use illicit drugs as often as the general population [73].

In 2000 there were 601,776 drug abuse–related ED visits. Most were alcohol in combination with other drugs (204,524), followed by cocaine (174,896), heroin or other opiates (97,287), and marijuana (96,446). From the prior year, ED visits involving heroin increased 15% and club drug ecstasy increased 58%. ED visits for prescription drugs containing oxycodone and hydrocodone have also dramatically increased over the past 2 years (Fig. 4) [74].

Polysubstance use leading to overdose, change in mental status, or incapacitation is the usual drug-related ED visit. Deaths are unusual, but near-death overdoses are often brought to EDs. Because management of these cases can be lifesaving and time consuming, EPs should be prepared to treat drug overdose and staffing should be planned to anticipate early evening cases in urban EDs [74]. Most ED deaths from drugs involve abuse of two or more drugs, often a drug and alcohol. Data from 2002 show that in most metropolitan areas drug-related deaths involve heroin or cocaine [75].

Marijuana (cannabis) is the most commonly used illicit drug in the United States, but leads to less ED visits than other drugs. There were an estimated 2.6 million new marijuana users in 2001. Over 14 million Americans aged 12 and older use marijuana at least once a month, and 3.1 million use marijuana daily [76]. Next to alcohol and tobacco, marijuana is the recreational drug of choice for American teenagers. Today's marijuana is more potent than that of the 1970s and 1980s, and may impact some ED visits among youth [77]. In 2002, marijuana was the third most common drug mentioned in ED visits in the United States. Marijuana mentions increased significantly (24%) from 2000 to 2002 [76].

A significant increase in the use of cocaine (other than crack) was seen among tenth-graders, from 1.1% in 2003 to 1.5% in 2004. Heroin, crack cocaine, hallucinogens other than lysergic acid diethylamide, phencyclidine, amphetamines, tranquilizers, sedatives, and methaqualone use, however, remained stable among youth from 2003 to 2004 [78]. Heroin use continues as a serious problem in America. A shift from injecting heroin to snorting or smoking has occurred. Heroin abuse is associated with fatal overdose; spontaneous abortion; and in users who inject the drug, infectious diseases,

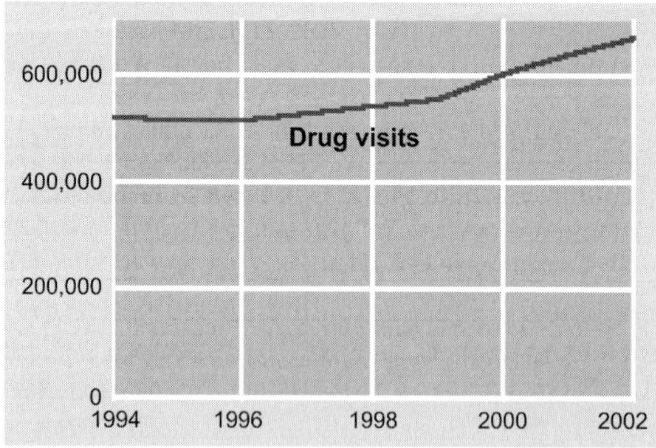

Fig. 4. Past month use of selected illicit drugs among persons aged 12 or older: 2002. (*From* Substance Abuse and Mental Health Services Administration. Results from the 2002 National Survey on Drug Use and Health: National Findings. Rockville (MD): Office of Applied Studies, NHSDA Series H-22, DHHS Publication No. SMA 03–3836; 2003.)

including HIV-AIDS and hepatitis. Opiate abuse increased from 2002 to 2003. Although the prevalence of lifetime nonmedical use of oxycodone increased significantly from 2002 to 2003, the prevalence of lifetime heroin use remained stable [79]. The means of drug use also changed. Between 1992 and 2002, inhalation as the route of administration increased from 20% to 33% among heroin abusers, whereas injection decreased from 77% to 62%. Many users who begin using heroin by inhaling, however, may switch to injecting later [80].

ED visits involving narcotic analgesics increased 153% from 1995 to 2002. More than one drug was involved in 75% of these drug abuse–related ED visits, and dependence was the motive underlying these ED visits [81]. Abuse of prescription medications has increased in all segments of the population. The Substance Abuse and Mental Health Services Administration estimates that in 2003, 6.3 million Americans abused prescription drugs. Most abused pain relievers (4.7 million); others abused tranquilizers (1.8 million), stimulants (1.2 million), and sedatives (0.3 million). Nonmedical use of oxycodone increased from 11.8 million users in 2002 to 13.7 million users in 2003. Most of these represent a group of opiate users distinct from heroin abusers. These users have a higher economic status [79]. Use of hydrocodone and oxycodone remains high; hydrocodone was at 2.5% for eighth graders, 6.2% for tenth graders, and 9.3% for twelfth graders. Oxycodone was at 1.7% for eighth graders, 3.5% for tenth graders, and 5% for twelfth graders. In 2003, about 4% and 4.5% of high school seniors reported nonmedical use of oxycodone (Fig. 5) [82].

Although heroin, cocaine, and marijuana remain the most frequently abused drugs leading to ED visits, new drugs also are being used by patients. Ecstasy, amphetamine-like drugs, γ-hydroxybutyrate (GHB), ketamine, amyl nitrite, and nitrous oxide use although increasing, may be less familiar to ED staff [83]. In 2002, there were 676,000 ecstasy users. Club drugs are favored over marijuana, lysergic acid diethylamide, methamphetamine, and opiates because they are believed to enhance social interaction [84,85]. The most widely used club drugs are ecstasy, GHB, flunitrazepam, and ketamine. These drugs are low cost and available in pills, powders, or liquids. Club drugs are taken orally, frequently in combination with each other and alcohol (Table 2).

Stimulants remain an abused group of drugs. Most frequently used are methamphetamines, diet pills, methylphenidate, and dextroamphetamine. Stimulant abuse is significantly higher in the West where methamphetamine use is most common [86]. Smoking methamphetamines or amphetamines has increased over other routes. For stimulant addicts, 50% smoked in 2002 compared with 12% in 1992. In 2003, an estimated 378,000 persons in the United States met the diagnostic criteria for stimulant dependence or abuse [87].

A trend that continues to influence drug culture is the Internet marketing of drugs. During a 1-week analysis, 495 web sites were identified advertising controlled prescription drugs. Drugs marketed included painkillers (oxycodone, oxycodone-acetaminophen, propoxyphene, and hydrocodone

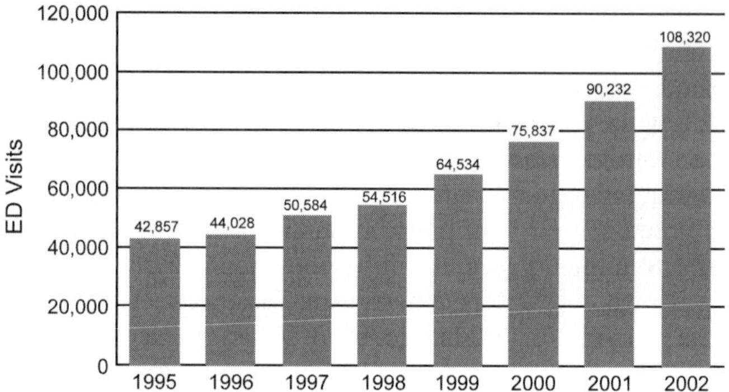

Fig. 5. Total number of ED drug visits, 1994 to 2002. (*From* US Department of Health and Human Services, SAMHSA, Office of Applied Studies, Emergency department trends from the Drug Abuse Warning Network: final estimates 1995–2002; 2003.)

bitartrate–acetaminophen); stimulants (dextroamphetamine, methylpheni-date, and amphetamine-dextroamphetamine); and sedatives (diazepam and alprazolam). Other sites advertise ecstasy-like or other club-type drugs, made in home laboratories. New sites and drugs become available daily [88].

EPs should have some understanding of drug culture and phenomena. Rave attendance may have been a modern rite of passage for many youth and will be replaced by another soon. An intoxicated or incapacitated youth should be considered a polydrug user, using unknown agents. Fortunately, the patient or companions usually reveal the drugs used.

Related issues regarding illness and injury

Drugs produce many clinical syndromes, such as anxiety, hallucination, respiratory depression, or drug-seeking behavior, in the ED. Each drug

Table 2
Street names for club drugs

Drug	Street name
MDMA	Ecstasy, X, M, E, XTC, rolls, beans, Clarity, Adam, lover's speed, hug drug
GHB	G, liquid ecstasy, Grievous Bodily Harm, gib, soap, scoop, nitro
GBL	Blue Nitro, GH Revitalizer, Gamma G
BD	Weight Belt Cleaner, Serenity, Thunder Nectar, Revitalize Plus
Flunitrazepam	Mexican valium, circles, roofies, la rocha, roche, rophies, R2, rope, forget-me pill
Ketamine (ketalar)	K, special K, super K, vitamin K, kit-kat, keets, super acid, jet, cat valiums

Data from Gahlinger PM. Illegal drugs: a complete guide to their history, chemistry, use and abuse. New York: Plume; 2004. p. 169–172.

has an associated group of presentations in the ED. Syndromes of recreational use, overdose, withdrawal, and medical complications can be unique to the drug, mode of delivery, and dose. Although recreational drug overdose can be fatal, the most commonly identified drugs taken in fatal overdose are not recreational drugs but are acetaminophen, benzodiazepines, and antidepressants. Only one is a class of abused drugs. Recreational overdose is an unusual cause of death or hospital admission [89].

ED staff should become familiar not only with common drugs but also with new drugs of abuse. Examples of a relatively new group of abused drugs are club drugs, which are consumed during raves and at late night dance clubs. Overdose should be considered polydrug with the actual substance unknown. Management is supportive with control of central nervous system stimulation or depression. There are no specific antidotes for club drugs except for flunitrazepam, a benzodiazepine that responds to flumazenil. Most club drug overdoses resolve with full recovery within 7 hours without critical care interventions [90]. MDMA, the usual rave drug, causes both amphetamine and hallucinogenic drug effects [91]. Users of ecstasy report heightened sensations, feelings of empathy, and well-being. Common effects of ecstasy are sweating, tachycardia, fatigue, and muscle spasms [92]. Raves occasionally result in severe dehydration, respiratory collapse, violent agitation, or death. Ravers seek euphoria through a marathon of trance dancing, club drug use, and music. Ecstasy use can cause a sharp increase in body temperature, which can lead to liver, kidney, and cardiovascular failure. It also increases heart rate and blood pressure and causes other symptoms, such as teeth clenching, nausea, blurred vision, faintness, and sweating [93]. With ecstasy, alcohol use is unusual, although cannabis is also popular among ravers [94]. There are now many reports of ecstasy toxicity and deaths [89]. In severe and fatal cases hyperthermia, disseminated intravascular coagulation, rhabdomyolysis, renal failure, cardiac arrhythmias, and seizures have been observed [89,90,95]. Management of toxic ecstasy ingestion includes active cooling, muscle relaxants, anticonvulsants, and benzodiazepines [95].

Methamphetamine, GHB, and ketamine are often available at clubs and rave scenes [96]. GHB use is not as common as it was 1 or 2 years ago. GHB has an onset within 15 to 30 minutes and duration of 3 hours. GHB causes behavioral changes, aggression, impaired judgment, nystagmus, and ataxia. Apnea or violent combativeness have brought some patients to EDs. Even low doses of GHB can produce profound central nervous system depression synergistic with alcohol [97]. At lower doses amnesia and hypotonia occur, whereas higher doses cause anesthesia, coma, seizures, and respiratory depression. GHB causes random clonic movements of the face and extremities. GHB overdose presents with profoundly decreased level of consciousness and respiratory depression. Management is primarily supportive. GHB respiratory depression and apnea can be followed by violent combativeness. Patients generally recover rapidly. Studies have suggested that intubation is not necessary in pure GHB coma [98,99], and most recover after simple supportive measures. Prolonged use of GHB results in dependence. Withdrawal occurs 1 to 6 hours after cessation, and can cause insomnia, anxiety, hallucinations, and tremor that may progress to delirium with autonomic instability. Treatment of GHB withdrawal has been successfully accomplished with the use of benzodiazepines, often at high doses [100–102].

Ketamine use has become more popular. It is a rapid-acting hypnotic, analgesic, and amnesic without respiratory depression. Ketamine produces "out of body" experiences and vivid dreams. Ketamine-induced hallucinations may lead to an ED visit [103]. At higher doses, respiratory depression can occur. Common complaints are anxiety, chest pain, and palpitations. Tachycardia and hypertension are seen [104]. Adverse events associated with ketamine are less frequent, but include stridor, laryngospasm, emesis, and aspiration. Protecting the airway may be the priority in a ketamine emergency [105].

Fortunately most ravers, whatever drug they use, survive unharmed, never needing medical attention. The average club drug user's participation is limited to about 2 years of drug use. Treatment of chronic abuse is usually not required [92]. Club drug use is but one example of drug culture with which the EP should be familiar.

Another drug becoming more commonly abused is methylphenidate and similar prescription drugs that might become the next youth drugs. Methylphenidate is prescribed for attention-deficit/hyperactivity disorder. It is similar to other amphetamines. Abuse of the drug leads to serious signs of toxicity; tolerance and dependence develop. EPs may need to treat complications and offer advice to reduce the potential of harm. Overdose presents as a sympathomimetic toxidrome with tachycardia, hypertension, dysrhythmias, flushing, angina, acute myocardial infarction, congestive heart failure, diaphoresis, headache, altered mental status, seizures, intracranial hemorrhage, mydriasis, muscle spasms, jaw clenching, or severe fatigue. Serious effects include hyperthermia; fluid and electrolyte imbalance, such as hyponatremia; cardiac arrhythmia; disseminated intravascular coagulation; rhabdomyolysis; acute renal failure; and hepatic toxicity. Supportive care and benzodiazepines should be given for agitation and seizures.

Cocaine is a strong central nervous system stimulant. Cocaine users can experience acute myocardial infarction or stroke and sudden death, and cocaine-related deaths are usually the result of cardiac arrest or seizure. Euphoria is commonly reported by cocaine abusers. Physical effects include constricted blood vessels; dilated pupils; and increased temperature, heart rate, and blood pressure. The effect of snorting lasts 15 to 20 minutes, whereas the effects from smoking may last 5 to 10 minutes. Use of cocaine occurs in a binge pattern, during which the drug is repeatedly taken at high doses. Complications associated with cocaine use include paranoia, psychosis, arrhythmias, and chest pain. When people mix cocaine and alcohol consumption they produce cocaethylene, which intensifies cocaine's euphoric effects and increases the risk of sudden death.

Inhalants are chemical vapors that produce mind-altering effects and are common home products, such as spray-paints, glues, and cleaning fluids. Adolescents can easily obtain them. Inhalants produce short-term effects similar to anesthetics. Highly concentrated amounts of chemicals (butane, propane, and other aerosols) can directly induce heart failure and death, referred to as "sudden sniffing death" [106].

Hallucinogens are less commonly used. The effects of lysergic acid diethylamide are unpredictable depending on amount, personality, mood, and surroundings. The effects of the drug, occurring after 30 to 90 minutes, include dilated pupils, higher body temperature, increased heart rate and blood pressure, sweating, loss of appetite, sleeplessness, dry mouth, and tremors. Sensations and feelings change dramatically. In large doses, delusions, visual hallucinations, and panic occur. Most users of lysergic acid diethylamide voluntarily decrease or stop its use over time. Lysergic acid diethylamide is not considered addictive [107].

After injection of heroin, euphoria (rush), flushing of the skin, and dry mouth occur. A wakeful or drowsy state ensues with clouded mental functioning. Heroin abuse during pregnancy and its many associated environmental factors (eg, lack of prenatal care) have been associated with adverse consequences including low birth weight, an important risk factor for later developmental delay. Tolerance develops so the abuser must use more to achieve the same effect. Withdrawal may occur a few hours after the last dose with drug craving, restlessness, muscle and bone pain, insomnia, diarrhea and vomiting, cold flashes with goose bumps, and kicking, which peak between 48 and 72 hours. Patients present to EDs with opioid overdose or withdrawal syndrome. Opioid overdose causes respiratory depression easily reversed by naloxone, although high doses may be needed. The onset, severity, and duration of withdrawal symptoms depend on the opioid abused and the extent of dependence. The shorter is the half-life of the opioid, the shorter to onset of symptoms, and the greater the intensity of withdrawal. Opioid withdrawal is managed by supportive care. A long-acting, cross-tolerant opioid, such as methadone, is very effective for treatment of withdrawal. ED staff must maintain a high index of suspicion for serious coexisting illness especially with injection drug users.

High-risk populations

Although anyone may use drugs, youths in general are at higher risk for drug experimentation. The lower the income, the more likely that youths use drugs. Youth drug use is common, but the drugs used vary. For example, youths in families with annual incomes of $75,000 or more are less likely to use most drugs, but as likely to use alcohol or inhalants as those with incomes of less than $20,000 [108].

Events and availability of drugs rather than patient demographics may better define risk for specific type of drug use. For example, among

253,286 spectators at rock concerts, about half of first aid visits involved drug or alcohol use. First aid station use was 1.2 per 1000 spectators. The most common diagnoses were minor trauma (42%) and ethanol or illicit drug intoxication (32%). Physicians working near rock concerts should be aware of the current drug use patterns and should be prepared to treat drug use [109].

A missed opportunity for intervention and referral

EPs should identify and refer substance users to drug treatment programs. Although studies have shown the efficacy of alcohol identification and referral in the ED, the effectiveness of drug referral remains explicitly to be demonstrated. The benefit of treatment is proved. Referring heroin users to needle exchange programs has reduced ED use. Future studies should demonstrate other concrete benefits of other ED referrals of drug users [110,111].

Treatment

In 2002, according to the Substance Abuse and Mental Health Services Administration, 7.1 million Americans (3.2%) ages 12 or older had drug abuse or dependence. Almost half of these abused both alcohol and drugs. It is important for the EP to recognize drug addiction as a treatable disorder like diabetes or heart disease. Many types of treatment have proved effective including counseling, psychotherapy, support groups, and family therapy. Medications that suppress withdrawal, craving, or the effects of drugs are beneficial and represent an area of active research [112]. Five substances accounted for 95% of all treatments: (1) alcohol (43%); (2) opiates (18%; primarily heroin); (3) marijuana or hashish (15%); (4) cocaine (13%); and (5) stimulants (7%) [113].

Heroin and opiates

Treatment for heroin abuse increased from 11% of all admissions in 1992 to 15% in 2002. Sixty-two percent of primary heroin admissions reported injection as the route of administration, 33% reported inhalation, and 3% reported smoking. Treatment for opiates other than heroin increased from less than 1% of all admissions in 1992 to 2% in 2002. Three-quarters (75%) of primary nonheroin opiate admissions reported oral as the route of administration. For heroin addiction, studies show that treatment using methadone with behavioral therapy reduces death and health problems, cost of treatment, crime, and unemployment. Medically assisted withdrawal minimizes discomfort but does not (without further treatment), however, improve outcome. Maintenance treatment for heroin addicts involves daily oral synthetic opiate, usually methadone. Buprenorphine is a medication now available for treating addiction to opiates. There is less risk of addiction to buprenorphine than methadone. Some opiate abusers do not require maintenance therapy, particularly if there is only a brief history of drug dependence. Several other medications for use in heroin treatment programs are also under study. Counseling for heroin addiction is usually part of a medical treatment program and often continues when medications are stopped. Counseling includes contingency management and cognitive-behavioral interventions designed to modify expectancies and increase life skills [114]. It is estimated that it costs approximately $3600 per month for a drug abuser untreated in the community. Incarceration costs approximately $3300 per month and methadone maintenance about $290 per month. Of note, these costs are similar to treatment for other chronic illnesses [115].

Cocaine

The proportion of admissions for primary cocaine abuse declined from 18% in 1992 to 13% in 2002. Smoked cocaine (crack) represented 73% of all primary cocaine admissions in 2002. Cognitive behavioral therapies can be effective in decreasing cocaine use. Drugs to treat cocaine addiction are under development [116].

Marijuana

In a survey, teenagers in treatment for marijuana dependence and abuse increased 142% since 1992. Teenagers are three times more likely to be treated for marijuana than for alcohol, and six times more likely to be in treatment for marijuana than for all other drugs combined. The proportion of admissions for primary marijuana abuse increased from 6% in 1992 to 15% in 2002. One study found comparable benefits from a 14-session cognitive-behavioral group treatment and a two-session individual treatment that included motivational interviewing and advice for men in their early thirties who had smoked marijuana daily for more than 10 years. These results suggest that if brief interventions are initiated in the ED, they may be effective [117]. No medications are currently available for treating marijuana abuse. Recent discoveries about the working of the tetrahydrocannabinol receptors have raised the possibility of developing a medication that blocks the intoxicating effects of tetrahydrocannabinol [76].

Stimulants

The proportion of admissions for abuse of stimulants increased from 1% to 7% between 1992 and 2002. Treatment is similar to cocaine.

Screening for drug use and abuse

Screening tools

In the ED the routine history often includes a single generic question about drug use. The EP is trained to ask this question when use is suspected, especially when the medical condition may be a complication of drug use. Screening using standard substance abuse screening questions for quantity and frequency in the last month or other questions to uncover drug problems is not routine. EPs are generally not familiar with drug screening tools. Screening questions have been embedded into health history surveys, however, and included in alcohol research projects by emergency researchers [49]. Bernstein and coworkers [49] have used, and reported on, the 10-item drug abuse severity test for clinical screening in a clinic population with frequent ED use. In this study, a drug problem was determined on the basis of current use of any drug and a drug abuse severity test score indicating moderate use severity [59,118–120]. Woolard is studying problematic alcohol and marijuana use in ED patients. The association of any injury with conjoint marijuana and alcohol use is considered problematic. His group has found that a simple screening question, "Have you used both alcohol and marijuana together in the last month or year?" identifies users of both substances who need referral for counseling. They have developed research instruments to screen for consequences of abuse. These are too long, however, for ED staff use [59].

Simple screening methods for other drugs need to be developed and validated in EDs. At the present time, however, common sense questions, such as "Do you use drugs?" and "Would you like to talk to someone about drug use?," can and should be more widely applied to screen most ED patients.

Interventions and referral for drug use and abuse

Review of the literature in terms of efficacy in the emergency department

BMI is one approach to modify drug use behavior. Its brevity makes it attractive in the ED. Drug abusers seeking treatment or currently in treatment have had contradictory results, however, from BMI (eg, enhanced treatment outcomes or no effect on outcomes) [121–125]. Counseling and medical treatment of drug use may require long-term therapy. Outpatient drug treatment often includes regular individual or group counseling. Early identification and advice to novice users at an early stage could be effective. It is difficult, however, to generalize BMI treatment results from individuals seeking or in treatment to ED patients who are not in treatment [72]. BMIs have been piloted with out-of-treatment drug users in medical settings outside the ED [126]. BMI has not yet been adequately tested for drug users [127].

Some positive effects of BMI have been reported. In ED settings, outreach workers screened 7118 patients for substance abuse and provided BMI and treatment referral to 1096. Among a subset of 245 patients followed for 3 months, there was a 45% reduction in drug abuse and a 50% increase in the rate of contact with substance abuse treatment providers. For opiates use, the difference (29% versus 25%) was not significant with or without BMI. For abstinence from both drugs, 17.4% of the BMI group were drug-free compared with 12.8% of the control group (adjusted OR 1.51; 95% CI, 0.98–2.26; $P = 0.052$). Among participants in the intervention group, 22.3% were abstinent from cocaine at 6 months postintervention compared with 16.9% of the controls (adjusted OR 1.51; 95% CI, 1.00–2.47; $P = .050$). For cocaine, there was greater improvement in the intervention group (29% reduction versus a 4% reduction for the control group). Further research may replicate these and other positive effects of BMI in the ED [72]. Studies have shown that enrolling patients undergoing detoxification from alcohol, heroin, or cocaine into a health evaluation link to primary care clinic was effective for alcohol and illicit drug problems [128].

Tobacco use: prevalence and impact in the emergency department population

Tobacco is the single greatest cause of disease and premature death in America today and is responsible for more than 430,000 deaths each year [129]. People who smoke are at increased risk of heart disease, cancer, and other smoking-related illnesses [130]. Nearly 25% of adult Americans currently smoke [131]. The societal costs of tobacco death and disease approach $100 billion. Americans spend an estimated $50 billion annually on direct medical care for smoking-related illnesses. Lost productivity and forfeited earnings caused by smoking-related disability account for another $47 billion per year [129].

It has been suggested that smoking should be the new vital sign wherever patient care is administered and strategies have been suggested by the US Public Health Service for implementation. In hospitals, specifically, there should be systems-based tobacco-user identification; provision of education, resources, and feedback to providers treating smokers; existence of dedicated staff to provide tobacco-dependence treatment; and policies for overall support [129]. Smoking cessation efforts may be the nexus for the fields of emergency medicine and public health. Smokers account for a disproportionate share of ED patients. Although about 25% of all American adults smoke, nearly 40% or more of adult ED patients smoke. Overall, 70% of United States adults who smoke want to quit [132]. In a multicentered study by Boudreaux and coworkers [133], ED patients at four Boston EDs were screened for smoking and queried regarding their interest in smoking cessation. Of 754 eligible patients, 530 (70%) were screened; 26% were current smokers, 31% former smokers, and 43% never smokers. This study found that 72% of current smokers had tried to quit in the past year, and 33% wanted an outpatient referral. Another study conducted by Lowenstein and coworkers [134] looked at the smoking habits, levels of addiction, readiness to quit, and access to primary care in ED patients at a university hospital. This study enrolled 336 (89%) eligible patients, finding 41% to be current smokers (95% CI, 0.36–0.46); with 68% stating that they wanted to quit, and 49% within the month; with 56% never having been told to quit smoking by any physician. When asked about primary care, 56% reported relying on the ED for most or all of their routine, primary health care; with 55% (95% CI, 0.46–0.64) of these patients being current smokers. Many adult ED patients are active smokers who use the ED as their regular source of care, and who want to quit; no one can afford to be unaware that incorporating smoking cessation counseling into standard ED care is warranted and necessary.

A missed opportunity for intervention and referral

In a study by Prochazka and coworkers, EPs were asked about training received for smoking cessation counseling, understanding of pharmacologic treatment techniques, current practice, and barriers to clinical application in an ED setting [134a]. A 26-item questionnaire was mailed to 256 members of the Colorado Chapter of the American College of Emergency Physicians. The responses, received from 77% of members, suggested that most EPs lack formal smoking cessation training (55%) and felt poorly prepared to counsel patients about smoking cessation (65%). Only 27% reported routinely asking patients to quit smoking; those with formal smoking cessation training were more likely to counsel and refer patients (34% versus 20%, $P =$ .03). The barriers cited were lack of time, perception of patient disinterest, inappropriateness of counseling in an ED setting, and a belief that counseling is ineffective [135]. In another study published in JAMA, only 21% of practicing physicians said that they received adequate training to help their patients stop smoking [135a]. According to a recent survey of United States medical school deans, most medical schools do not require clinical training in smoking cessation techniques [136].

Screening for tobacco use in the emergency department

Questions for screening for tobacco use are often limited to: "Do you currently smoke?" and "What are the average number of cigarettes smoked per day?" or "How many years have you been smoking." Nicotine can be both absorbed and inhaled, however, and the patient should ideally be queried about all types of tobacco use including cigarettes, cigars, pipe, smokeless chew, smokeless dry snuff, smokeless wet snuff, bidis, herbal cigarettes, omni cigarettes, and tobacco lozenges for the amount used each day and the number of years of use. The Comprehensive Tobacco Center in Jackson, Mississippi, has outlined all these forms (Table 3).

Interventions and referral for tobacco use

Review of the literature in terms of efficacy in the emergency department

Although intensive clinic-based behavioral treatments are effective, only a small percentage of highly motivated smokers seek out this kind of assistance [137–139]. The development of novel interventions and delivery systems that can reach, motivate, and treat the population of smokers is greatly needed [137,140,141].

One innovative approach has been proactively to reach out to and intervene with smokers in medical settings. Smoking cessation interventions delivered in medical settings have great potential to reach a wide range of smokers who otherwise might not present for smoking treatment and can be leveraged to take advantage of teachable moments. The term "teachable moment" has been used to describe naturally occurring life events that may motivate an individual to change his or her health behaviors [142]. Timing interventions to coincide with naturally occurring teachable moments may increase the efficacy of those interventions.

Although the medical setting may seem to be an ideal teachable moment for delivering smoking cessation interventions, it is likely that all teachable moments are not of equal value in prompting behavior change. Studies of these interventions delivered in medical settings have produced widely varying rates of success. For example, physician advice given to smokers during a routine visit produces cessation rates of about 3% to 10% [143–150], with higher cessation rates associated with sick visits as opposed to routine checkups [151–153].

Table 3
Tobacco products

Type tobacco product	Description
Cigarettes	First developed in 1800s using flue-cured tobacco leaf, making it easier to inhale. Extremely effective method to facilitate nicotine uptake. Rolled in flame-retardant paper; filter usually added.
Cigars	Tobacco rolled in tobacco leaf; engineered for mucosal absorption; can deliver as much nicotine as 5–20 cigarettes.
Pipe	Tobacco is chopped, flavored, and scented. Not intended for inhalation, but usually is. High level of nicotine delivery.
Smokeless chew	Plug or loose form; flavored; held in mouth; very high levels of nicotine.
Smokeless dry snuff	Scented fine powder; snorted into nose.
Smokeless wet snuff	Also called dip; finely chopped, moist, and flavorful; held in mouth.
Bidis	Considered cool by younger smokers, these are very strong, flavored cigarettes. They produce three times as much nicotine and five times as much tar as regular cigarettes.
Herbal cigarettes	Produce tars and CO, and often have tobacco mixed in.
Omni cigarettes	Very low-nicotine delivery, but produce comparable tar levels.
Ariva	Tobacco lozenges (not to be confused with the Commit nicotine lozenge); likely carries same risk as smokeless tobacco.

Adapted from Treating the tobacco user: a health care provider's guide. The ACT Center (A Comprehensive Tobacco Center). Available at: http://actcenter.umc.edu/. Accessed August 14, 2006.

In contrast, hospitalization for serious illness, such as myocardial infarction or cardiac bypass surgery, can be a highly motivating experience and has been associated with quit rates above 50% even without additional intervention for smoking cessation [154–156]. For example, Rigotti and colleagues [157] found that 51% of smokers who had undergone coronary bypass surgery had quit from smoking 1 year postdischarge. Although the experience of hospitalization for cardiac illness seems to motivate many smokers to quit, the effect of a brief hospitalization on motivation to quit smoking and cessation rates is not known.

One small controlled trial has examined smoking interventions for adult ED patients. Richman and colleagues [158] randomized 152 patients into an intervention group or a standard care group. The intervention group received an educational brochure, brief standardized physician counseling, and a referral to an outpatient smoking treatment program, whereas the control group received only the educational brochure. At 3-month follow-up, cessation rates between the intervention and control groups were equivalent, at about 11%. The study suffered from significant limitations, however, including a small sample size, a very minimal impact intervention, and a $200 fee associated with the outpatient smoking cessation program to which patients were referred. The authors emphasized that larger studies using more intensive, multimodal, or tailored interventions are needed.

Becker and associates at Brown University designed and implemented a large study focusing on one particular subgroup of ED patients: those admitted to an ED observation unit with chest pain. An estimated 5.6 million visits are made to EDs in the United States for chest pain at a cost of more than $5 billion each year [159]. Most of these patients are at low risk for myocardial infarction [160]. Between 85% and 90% of patients who present to the observation unit with chest pain are ruled out for myocardial infarction and other serious cardiac events [161–163].

The ED observation unit constitutes an intermediate care unit, a step down from intensive inpatient care, but more prolonged than the typical ED visit [164]. During most of the ED observation unit stay, the patient remains at rest with no entertainment or stimulation, and can be provided with interviews, counseling interventions, and other educational endeavors. Currently, no preventive health interventions are being delivered to patients in the ED observation unit.

The research team focused on patients who smoked who were admitted to an ED observation unit with chest pain. Patients were interested and motivated to receive counseling (only 10.4% of eligible patients refused participation in this study). Moreover, both measures of motivation, the Contemplation Ladder [165] and the single-item Readiness measure, indicated moderate levels of motivation to quit smoking. Smoking rates observed in this sample are similar to those seen in other studies of adult smokers [166,167]. Almost half of all participants lived with another smoker in their home.

The mean nicotine dependence score was moderate, indicating that these smokers are not likely to be especially resistant to treatment [168]. The wide range of observed dependence scores suggested, however, that nicotine-replacement therapy is necessary for those who are highly nicotine dependent.

Given its link to heart disease, smoking cessation may be a particularly salient intervention to deliver to ED observation unit patients who are experiencing chest pain and are likely to be concerned that they may be experiencing heart disease. The link between heart disease and chest pain is not apparent, however, to many patients. Thirty-nine percent of study participants said that they did not have any symptoms of a disease or illness that was caused or made worse by smoking; nevertheless, results indicated that readiness to quit smoking was significantly associated with perceived risk.

The investigators then launched an intervention study with these patients. The Chest Pain Smoking Study was a randomized, controlled clinical trial designed to examine the relative efficacy of a brief, motivationally tailored smoking cessation intervention compared with usual care on abstinence rates and motivation to quit smoking among patients presenting to the hospital ED observation unit with symptoms of chest pain. All participants who agreed to quit smoking were offered nicotine-replacement therapy in the form of patches.

Over half (58%) of participants had made at least one 24-hour quit attempt in the previous year. A total of 59%, however, had never before used nicotine-replacement therapy (gum or patch). Among the sample of study completers, at 1 month 16.8% of those given usual care and 27.3% of those given the tailored intervention had stopped smoking. At Month 3, the percentages quit were 19.2% and 28.7% in the usual care and tailored arms, respectively. At Month 6 the percentages quit were 18.8% and 21.7%, respectively. Most individuals who quit did so by Month 1. By Month 6, 25% of those who had quit at Month 1 were smoking. Approximately one third of those quit at each time point relapsed by the following assessment.

Results of this study demonstrate that admission to an ED observation unit for symptoms of chest pain provides a teachable moment during which patients can be helped to increase their motivation to quit smoking. Although the experience alone produced initial cessation rates of nearly 10% among usual care participants, the addition of a motivational counseling session significantly increased successful quit attempts by nearly 70%. Approximately 5.6 million individuals present to hospital EDs with chest pain each year [169]. Currently, over 22% of adults smoke [170], and over 25% of all ED visits annually are made by smokers [169]. Broad application of smoking interventions in this population could reach over 10 million smokers per year.

Although these results cannot be extrapolated to smokers receiving treatment for other problems in EDs, the investigators are currently completing a smoking cessation trial targeting adults being treated for acute respiratory illness in EDs. The initial results are promising. Treating the millions of smokers who present to EDs each year could have substantial impact on the public health of the nation.

Brief interventions for alcohol, tobacco, and other drug problems

Components of a brief intervention

Brief interventions, specifically known as the "Brief Negotiation Interview," were adapted to the ED setting with the help of Dr. Stephen Rollnick at Boston City Hospital, currently known as Boston Medical Center [48,49]. In a recently published paper, D'Onofrio and coworkers [171] describe the Brief Negotiation Interview steps and associated necessary provider training. Their intervention consists of four major components, which are outlined in the following steps: (1) raise the subject of alcohol consumption, (2) provide feedback on the patient's drinking levels and effects, (3) enhance motivation to reduce drinking, and (4) negotiate and advise a plan of action. Each step has specific objectives that can in most cases successfully be achieved if the EP adheres to the explicitly scripted procedures shown in Table 4. The EP should be nonconfrontational, nonstigmatizing, and the interview should always be conducted in a constructive manner.

Raise the subject

In this first step of the Brief Negotiation Interview, the EP addresses the issue of alcohol use and possible consequences by introducing himself or herself and asking permission to discuss the patient's drinking.

Provide feedback

The EP reviews the patient's drinking amounts and patterns and asks what if any connection exists between drinking and the ED visit or other health consequences. The ED visit offers a potential teachable moment because of the possible negative consequences associated with the event [172]. If the patient does not make the connection, the practitioner can provide this information. For example, even if a motor vehicle crash is not technically the patient's legal fault, one can state that reaction times are slowed after even one drink and certain cues that one relies on to drive defensively may be lost because of impaired judgment caused by the alcohol. Low-risk amounts of alcohol consumption appropriate for the patient's age and sex are reviewed.

Enhance motivation

The primary objective of this step is to elicit and reinforce the patient's motivational statements regarding change. Assessing motivation is addressed by asking, "On a scale from one to ten, how ready are you to change any aspect of your drinking?" where 1 is not ready and 10 is very ready (Fig. 6). Once a number along the continuum is chosen by the patient, the

Table 4
BNI steps

Raise subject	Hello, I am _______. Would you mind taking a few minutes to talk with me about your alcohol use? < <PAUSE> >
Provide feedback	
Review screen	From what I understand you are drinking [insert screening data]... We know that drinking above certain levels can cause problems, such as [insert facts]... I am concerned about your drinking.
Make connection	What connection (if any) do you see between your drinking and this ED visit? If patient sees connection: reiterate what patient has said If patient does not see connection: make one using facts
Show NIAAA Guidelines and norms	These are what we consider the upper limits of low risk drinking for your age and sex. By low risk we mean that you would be less likely to experience illness or injury if you stayed within these guidelines.
Enhance motivation	
Readiness to change	[Show readiness ruler] On a scale from 1–10, how ready are you to change any aspect of your drinking?
Develop discrepancy	If patient says: ≥ 2 ask Why did you choose that number and not a lower one?; ≤ 1 or unwilling, ask What would make this a problem for you?...How important would it be for you to prevent that from happening?...Have you ever done anything you wish you hadn't while drinking? Discuss pros and cons.
Negotiate and advise	
Negotiate goal	Reiterate what patient says in Step 3 and say, What's the next step?
Give advice	If you can stay within these limits you will be less likely to experience [further] illness or injury related to alcohol use.
Summarize	This is what I've heard you say...Here is a drinking agreement I would like you to fill out, reinforcing your new drinking goals. This is really an agreement between you and yourself.
Provide handouts	Provide: Drinking agreement [patient keeps 1 copy] Project ED Health Information Sheet
Suggest PC f/u	Suggest PC f/u to discuss drinking level or pattern
Thank patient	Thank patient for his or her time

From D'Onofrio G, Pantalon MV, Degutis LC, et al. Development and implementation of an emergency practitioner-performed brief intervention for hazardous and harmful drinkers in the emergency department. Acad Emerg Med 2005;12:249–56; with permission from the Society for Academic Emergency Medicine.

EP should then ask, "why not less?." So, if the patient chooses a five, the EP responds positively, "That's great, you are 50% ready for change. Tell me why you did not choose a three or a four? In other words, what are some of the reasons you are ready to make a change?" This generates motivational statements that can then be repeated or reflected back to the patient, thereby reinforcing their own incentives for change [173]. Patients are often ambivalent about change, developing discrepancies between the patient's present drinking patterns and his or her own expressed concerns may tip the scales toward readiness to change. To strengthen or reinforce these motivational statements (eg, patient listing reasons why he or she should reduce their use of alcohol), the technique of reflective listening is useful. Here the EP reiterates or reflects back to the patient what he or she said, and may have the patient elaborate on it briefly. This technique is based on an effective method used with a wide range of substance-using individuals to promote change [174]. Patients most often choose a number between 2 and 10. Infrequently, a patient may choose a one or be unwilling to self identify a number along the ruler. Most often these are young adults. Strategies for continuing the discussion may be asking the patient "Have you ever done anything you wished you had not while drinking?" or asking "What would make this a problem for you?" (encouraging the patient to think about the future). If the patient gives an appropriate response to the second question, then ask, "How ready are you to work toward preventing this?" Other strategies include a discussion of the pros and cons of the patient's current level of drinking, encouraging patients to think about previous times they have cut back on their drinking, and praising their willingness to discuss such a sensitive topic and their willingness even to consider change.

Negotiate and advise

The goal here is to negotiate a realistic and constructive goal with regard to a patient's drinking amounts and patterns. The best approach is by asking the patient the open-ended question of, "Given what we have discussed, what is the next step with regard to your drinking or what, if anything, might you consider changing about your use of alcohol?" Reinforce that for a patient with a strong family history of alcohol dependence, the goal

Readiness to Change Ruler

Not ready   Very ready

| | | | | | | | | |
1   2   3   4   5   6   7   8   9   10

Fig. 6. Readiness to change ruler. (*From* D'Onofrio G, Pantalon MV, Degutis LC, et al. Development and implementation of an emergency practitioner-performed brief intervention for hazardous and harmful drinkers in the emergency department. Acad Emerg Med 2005;12:253; with permission from the Society for Academic Emergency Medicine.)

is to stay within the low-risk guidelines. If they cannot stay within these limits, however, abstinence may be necessary. If the goal exceeds the recommended guidelines the EP may tell the patient that, based on medical opinion, the best recommendation is to cut back to low-risk drinking limits, but that any step in that direction is a good start.

At the end of the negotiation, the patient's goal can be written on the discharge instruction sheet or a separate drinking agreement. Confronting or pressuring the patient only leads to an increase in resistance, resulting in the patient stopping the encounter altogether. The EP should summarize the agreement and provide follow-up to a primary care physician or specialized treatment facility and provide a handout with information similar to that provided in the Appendix. Finally, thanking the patient for his or her time is essential. The actual role play of a Brief Negotiation Interview is provided in Table 5. Sometimes additional motivational strategies are necessary to assist the patient in changing their drinking behavior. There are some hints to help the EP from falling into traps that may bolster the patient's resistance, outlined in Table 6. In addition, common problems encountered during the Brief Negotiation Interview and potential solutions are outlined in Table 7.

Barriers to screening for alcohol, tobacco, and other drug use and providing intervention and referral: a climate change

Real and perceived barriers

The failure of ED staff to detect, intervene, and refer patients for counseling is well documented [24,38]. The chaotic ED environment, lack of sufficient staff and resources, and practitioner characteristics, such as low levels of confidence in their skills and negative attitudes toward patients with drinking problems, are often cited as significant obstacles to such screening and intervention [24,175]. Graham and colleagues [175] surveyed 569 members of the Michigan College of Emergency Physicians about their attitudes toward using interventions with ED patients who have alcohol problems. Of the 257 members who responded (46% of those surveyed), 75% agreed that alcohol abuse and dependence are treatable illnesses, and only 15% stated they would not support ED interventions. Both supporters and nonsupporters thought that lack of time was a major obstacle to screening and intervention. Interventions used in previous alcohol studies were often lengthy, lasting 30 to 60 minutes, and were not performed by existing ED staff, but rather by non-ED staff, including a doctoral level psychologist [53] and social workers or graduate students [50,51]. The need for an effective intervention aimed at reducing the deleterious effects of alcohol, tobacco, and other drug use that is feasible for administration by ED staff is critical. For this to be translated into practice, however, the intervention needs to be acceptable to ED staff and feasible for EPs to provide in a real-world setting.

Table 5
Case example of BNI dialogue

Speaker	Dialogue	Procedure
Physician	Hello, I am Dr. Jones. Would you mind spending a few minutes talking about your use of alcohol?	Raise the subject
Patient	Ok, like what?	
Physician	From what I understand you were drinking tonight and were involved in a car crash. You told the nurse that you drink 2–3 days a week and usually have 6–8 beers per occasion. I am concerned because that level of drinking can put you at risk for illness or injuries, such as why you are here today. What connection do you see between your drinking and this ED visit?	Provide feedback Make connection
Patient	None really. I mean, I really had the right of way. I had a few beers. What is the problem with that? I can hold my alcohol well. He ran into me. You know that intersection between Grand and College Ave. I was going south on College and he just smacked right into me. I did not see him at all. I am in kind of a rush. I need to get out of here, but it was not my fault.	
Physician	I believe that is was not your fault. I know that busy intersection. We know, however, that drinking even small amounts, such as 1 or 2 drinks, can reduce your reaction time. As you know, we avoid crashes almost every day. Drivers run stop signs, backup without looking, etc. At that very intersection there are near- misses everyday. Do you think that you might have seen that other car approaching and avoided the crash if you had not been drinking? I do not know for sure, I was not there, but it is one thing I would like you to consider.	
Patient	Well, I said that I didn't see him at all. I didn't see him until the crash.	
Physician	So one thing, you might have seen him if you were not drinking any amount. It is clear that legally you had the right of way. I am also concerned about the amount you drink. Based on a large amount of research and national information we know that if you drink above certain levels it puts you at risk for injuries and illness. For your age and sex that means the upper limits of low-risk drinking are no more than 14 drinks per week, and no more than 4 drinks on any occasion. A standard drink is one 12-oz of beer, 5 oz of wine, or 1.5 oz of distilled spirits.	Show NIAAA guidelines
Patient	Yeah, I guess I am over that.	

Table 5 (*continued*)

Speaker	Dialogue	Procedure
Physician	Well now that we have discussed the risks of further injury when drinking over the recommended amounts, how ready are you to change any aspect of your drinking?	Enhance motivation Readiness to change
Patient	I do not know, maybe a 5	
Physician	OK, so that is good, you are halfway or 50% there. Why not less? In other words, why did you not pick a 1 or 2? What are some reasons why you think some changes need to be made?	Develop discrepancy
Patient	Well, I am here I guess, and I can tell that my neck and back are really going to hurt tomorrow. But I really do like to drink with my friends. Normally I do not drink and drive, but I needed to be somewhere after, so I drove myself.	
Physician	So you already know that drinking and driving is not a good idea and that was a rare event for you. But rare events can sometimes lead to consequences, like today. So I guess you are ready because you do not think that it is a good idea to drink and drive. On the other hand, you enjoy drinking with your friends. Any disadvantages to that?	Reflection
Patient	We normally go out on Friday and Saturdays. Sometimes on Thursdays and then I'm a little late to work on Friday. It takes the morning and lots of coffee to clear my head.	
Physician	So what I hear your saying is that there are two reasons why you are dissatisfied with your drinking. First is that you ended up in the ED and will probably have some muscles aches and pains for a few days, and second that sometimes you are slow at work. That could cause you trouble I suspect with your boss. In addition I have given you some information regarding the risks of drinking over the recommended limits. So, where does that leave you now? (or what is the next step?) What agreement could you make between you and yourself regarding your drinking levels?	Negotiate and Advise Summarize Negotiate goal
Patient	Well, I am definitely not going to drink and drive. That is a big deal because even though I thought I could, I probably cannot. I do not know about the limits. I can stay within 14 a week, but I do not know about the 4 at a time. I will try but it is often a long game we are watching.	
Physician	So no more drinking and driving, and you are going to try to keep it to 4 beers per occasion, knowing that it is tough at times but you are willing to try.	

Table 5 (*continued*)

Speaker	Dialogue	Procedure
Patient	OK	
Physician	Good luck. I would also recommend that you follow-up with your primary care doctor and discuss how you are doing with the agreement. Thanks for your time.	Follow-up Thank patient

From D'Onofrio G, Pantalon MV, Degutis LC, et al. Development and implementation of an emergency practitioner-performed brief intervention for hazardous and harmful drinkers in the emergency department. Acad Emerg Med 2005;12:249–56; with permission from the Society for Academic Emergency Medicine.

How to bring about change

Changing practitioner behavior regarding screening and intervention is difficult. There are documented strategies that may be helpful. These include the use of educational techniques that involve skills-based learning; eliciting opinion leaders in all practitioner groups; instituting system changes, such as prompts or screening questions on triage forms, computer-generated screening, and so forth; providing ongoing feedback to the practitioners; and providing incentives to the staff [176]. Improvement in screening and intervention for alcohol problems has been documented when emergency medicine residents received a skills-based structured educational intervention for alcohol problems [177]. Governmental agencies have become aware of the importance of screening for alcohol-related problems in ED patients. This is evidenced by the passage of Public Act 98-201 in the State of Connecticut [178]. This Act mandates substance abuse screening for injured patients who are admitted for treatment of injuries to any acute care hospital in the state. In addition, this act mandates the development of model continuing education standards related to alcohol and other drug screening for health care practitioners.

Creative models

Innovative approaches to screening and intervention in the emergency department

Several studies have reported innovative methods for screening and intervention in the ED. Rhodes and colleagues [179] described the use of a computer-based approach for screening a variety of health issues, including alcohol and other drug problems. In this study, 542 adult ED patients (89% of those approached) with nonurgent conditions were assigned either to the computer intervention (a self-administered computer survey generating individualized health information) or usual care (ie, no intervention). In the intervention group, 85% of participants reported one or more behavioral risk factors for alcohol and other drug problems, including problem drinking (19%), or driving within 4 hours of having two or more drinks (11%). Ninety-five percent of patients in the intervention group requested

Table 6
Motivational strategies for use during BNI

Motivational strategies	Patient response	Provider response
Refrain from directly countering resistance statements	"How can I have a drinking problem when I drink less than all my buddies?"	Reply without insisting that there is a problem, but an issue worthy of further assessment and discussion
Focus on the less resistant aspects of the statement	Patient may be wondering how much drinking causes a problem	Restate patient concern and ask about their level of drinking. Make the statement, "It sounds like you are confused about how you could have an issue with your drinking if you drink less than all your friends. I would like to tell you."
Restate positive or motivational statements	"You know, now that you mention it, I feel like I have been overdoing it with my drinking lately; I guess I might have to change my drinking"	"You do not need me to tell you you have been drinking a little too much lately, you have noticed yourself; It sounds like you have been thinking about changing because (insert patient reasons)."
Other helpful hints		Encourage patients to think about previous times they have cut back on their drinking. Praise patients for their willingness to discuss such a sensitive topic, and their willingness to even consider change. View the patient as an active participant in the intervention.

From D'Onofrio G, Pantalon MV, Degutis LC, et al. Development and implementation of an emergency practitioner-performed brief intervention for hazardous and harmful drinkers in the emergency department. Acad Emerg Med 2005;12:249–56; with permission from the Society for Academic Emergency Medicine.

further health information and 62% of the intervention group remembered receiving advice on what they could do to improve their health 1 week after the ED visit. The investigators concluded that computer technology may help physicians use the patients' waiting time for health promotion and targeting patients at risk for various health problems.

Gregor and colleagues [180] examined the feasibility of using an interactive computer program in the ED to prevent alcohol misuse among adolescents. They enrolled patients ages 14 to 18 who visited the ED within 24

Table 7
Problems sometimes encountered during the BNI

Problem	Overview and solution
Refusal to engage in discussion of their drinking	Most patients will agree to discuss drinking, but if someone outright refuses to discuss it at all, tell them that you will respect their wishes and give them 3 pieces of information: 1. Their drinking exceeds low-risk drinking limits (or is harmful) 2. Low-risk drinking limits recommended for their age and sex 3. You are concerned and that they should cut down to low-risk drinking limits to avoid future harm.
Refusal to self-identify along the readiness ruler	When this happens, it is usually a problem with understanding the numbers. There are several ways of dealing with this: 1. Anchor the numbers with descriptors, such as "1" means not ready at all or 0% ready and 10 means completely ready or 100% ready to change. 2. Ask "What would make this a problem for you?" Or, "How important is it for you to change any aspect of your drinking?" 3. Discussion of pros and cons (refer to list).
Unwilling to associate visit with alcohol use	Do not force the patient to make the connection, but be sure that he or she hears that in your medical opinion there is a connection. However, this connection may not be the thing that ultimately motivates the patient to change. If this happens try to find some other negative consequence of drinking that the patient can agree is related to alcohol and bothersome enough to consider drinking less.
Not ready to change drinking patterns to lower-risk	Tell the patient that the best recommendation is to cut back to low-risk drinking limits, but that any step in that direction is a good start.

From D'Onofrio G, Pantalon MV, Degutis LC, et al. Development and implementation of an emergency practitioner-performed brief intervention for hazardous and harmful drinkers in the emergency department. Acad Emerg Med 2005;12:249–56; with permission from the Society for Academic Emergency Medicine.

hours of an acute injury. Overall, 71% reported ever drinking alcohol and about 63% reported recent alcohol use. The program consisted of an interactive house party with audio. Each participant chose a "party pal" from a group of five teenaged cartoon characters and was exposed to various scenarios depicting important concepts regarding alcohol misuse. Of the recent drinkers participating in the study, 74% reported that the program made them rethink their alcohol use, 94% liked the program, and only about 5% required assistance with it. Outcomes recently published comparing the intervention with a control group did not show an effect in alcohol consumption at 12 months between conditions. A subgroup analysis suggested, however, that the intervention may have an effect among subjects with experience drinking and driving [181].

Another innovative model of screening and intervention approach, Project ASSERT, uses health promotion advocates or community outreach workers to screen, intervene, and refer patients with alcohol and other drug problems. The program, first described at Boston Medical Center [49], is also implemented at hospitals in New Haven, Connecticut (Yale–New Haven Hospital [182] and Hospital of Saint Raphael). Results from Boston were previously described. A 5-year evaluation at Yale–New Haven Hospital [54] demonstrated that nearly 24,000 patients were screened for alcohol, tobacco, or other drug use use. Approximately 75% of the 3249 patients who were referred to specialized treatment facilities were contacted at 1-month follow-up. Of these, 88% enrolled into a treatment program. These results suggest that this model of screening and direct linkage to treatment is feasible. Moreover, the program is cost-effective, because at both participating institutions, Project ASSERT is funded by health promotion advocates' consultation fees that are included in the hospitals' facility fees.

Best practices for alcohol screening, brief intervention, and referral to treatment include the following:

1. Development of a specific community-based resource list including alcohol, tobacco, or other drug use services, Alcohol Anonymous, AL-NON, needle exchange programs, and so forth.
2. Availability of information sheets, such as "How Much is Too Much to Drink" and safe sex, and offer advice on such subjects as avoiding substance use while driving.
3. Screening protocols for alcohol, tobacco, or other drug use that can be used by a variety of emergency practitioners, or kiosk or computer generated.
4. Educational programs for emergency practitioners (physicians, nurses, physician associates) to perform brief interventions for alcohol, tobacco, or other drug use problems.
5. Enlist opinion leaders from all practitioners to assist with system changes, education, and feedback.
6. Development of feedback mechanisms so that EPs become aware of successes, such as linkage to treatment, sobriety, and so forth and not always only relapses.
7. Development of a peer educator program so that patients can be linked directly with specialized treatment facilities and that partnerships with these centers can be developed and maintained.

Summary

Unhealthy alcohol, tobacco, and other drug use is prevalent in ED populations. Evidence suggests that screening, intervention, and referral can be effective in changing patterns of use and reducing negative consequences. ED practitioners can learn these skills. System changes are needed to incorporate best practices.

Appendix: NIAAA screening questions and guidelines for low-risk drinking

NIAA screening questions

Ask current drinkers:
- On average, how many days per week do you drink alcohol?
- On a typical day when you drink, how many drinks do you have?
- What's the maximum number of drinks you had on a given occasion (or day if age >65) in the last month?

If you drink more than this, you can put yourself at risk for illness and/or injury:

Men: >14 drinks per week or >4 drinks per occasion
Women: >7 drinks per week or >3 drinks per occasion
Age over 65: >7 drinks per week or >1 drink

WHAT IS A STANDARD DRINK?

1 shot of liquor (whiskey, vodka, gin, etc.) 1.5 oz.	1 regular beer 12 oz.	1 glass of wine 5 oz.

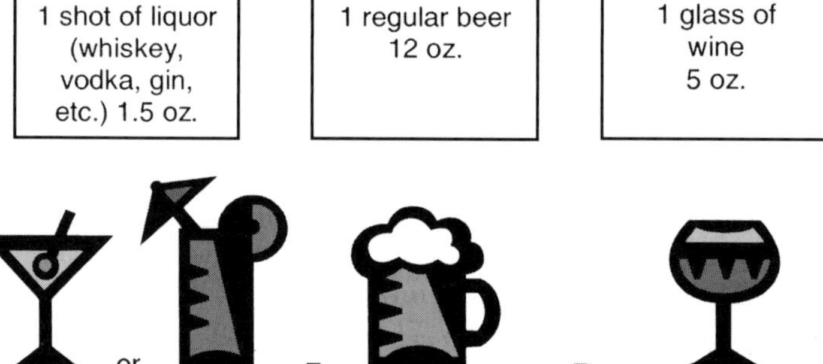

Each of these drinks has about ½ oz. of pure alcohol.

Adapted from US Department of Health and Human Services. National Institutes of Health. National Institute on Alcohol Abuse and Alcoholism. Helping patients with alcohol problems: a health practitioner's guide [NIH publication no. 04-3769]. Washington, DC: Government Printing Office; 2004.

References

[1] Schneider Institute for Health Policy. Substance abuse: the nation's number one health problem. Robert Wood Johnson Foundation, annual report; 2001.

[2] NIDA's economic costs of alcohol and drug abuse in the United States, 1992. Available at: http://www.nida.nih.gov/EconomicCosts/Chapter5.html#5.2. Accessed August 11, 2006.

[3] Reducing the health consequences of smoking: 25 years of progress. A report of the Surgeon General. Washington: Centers for Disease Control, National Center for Chronic Disease Prevention and Health Promotion, Office on Smoking and Health; 1989.

[4] Department of Health and Human Services. Ninth special report to Congress on alcohol and health. National Institute on Alcohol Abuse and Alcoholism. Rockville (MD): Department of Health and Human Services; 1997.

[5] Centers for Disease Control and Prevention. Chronic diseases and their risk factors: the nation's leading causes of death; 1999.

[6] Center for Disease Control and Prevention. Smoking-attributable mortality and years of potential life lost—United States, 1984. MMWR 1997;46:444–51.

[7] Institute of Medicine. Pathways of addiction: opportunities in drug abuse research. Washington: National Academy Press; 1996.

[8] Gerstein DR, Harwood HJ, Sutter N, et al. Evaluation recovery services: the California drug and alcohol treatment assessment. Sacramento (CA): State of California Department of Alcohol and Drug Programs; 1994.

[9] Broadening the base of treatment for alcohol problems. Report of a study by a committee of the Institute of Medicine. Washington: National Academy Press; 1990.

[10] US Department of Health and Human Services. National Institutes of Health. National Institute on Alcohol Abuse and Alcoholism. Helping patients with alcohol problems: a health practitioner's guide. NIH publication No. 04–3769. Washington: Government Printing Office; 2004.

[11] Secretary of Health and Human Services. Tenth special report to the US Congress on alcohol and health. NIH publication No. 00–1583. Washington: Government Printing Office; 2000.

[12] Manwell LB, Fleming MF, Johnson K, et al. Tobacco, alcohol, and drug use in a primary care sample: 90 day prevalence and associated factors. J Addict Dis 1998;17: 67–81.

[13] Cherpitel CJ. Screening for alcohol problems in the emergency department. Ann Emerg Med 1995;26:158–66

[14] Cherpitel CJ. Alcohol consumption among emergency room patients: comparison of county/community hospitals and an HMO. J Stud Alcohol 1993;54:432–40.

[15] Whiteman PJ, Hoffman RS, Goldfrank LR. Alcoholism in the emergency department: an epidemiologic study. Acad Emerg Med 2000;7:14–20.

[16] Cherpitel CJ. Breath analysis and self-report as measures of alcohol-related emergency room admissions. J Stud Alcohol 1989;50:155–61.

[17] Bernstein E, Tracey A, Bernstein J, et al. Emergency department detection and referral rates for patients with problem drinking. Subst Abus 1996;7:69–76.

[18] Cherpitel CJ. Drinking patterns and problems: a comparison of primary care with the emergency room. Subst Abus 1999;20:85–95.

[19] O'Brien GM, Stein MD, Zierler S, et al. Use of the ED as a regular source of care: associated factors beyond lack of health insurance. Ann Emerg Med 1997;30:286–91.

[20] Davidson P, Koziol-McLain J, Harrison L, et al. Intoxicated ED patients: a 5-year follow-up of morbidity and mortality. Ann Emerg Med 1997;30:593–7.

[21] National Highway Traffic Safety Administration. Current research in alcohol. Ann Emerg Med 1997;30:817–9.

[22] Degutis LC. Screening for alcohol problems in emergency department patients with minor injury: results and recommendations for practice and policy. Contemp Drug Prob 1998;25: 463–75.

[23] Freedland ES, McMicken DB, D'Onofrio G. Alcohol and trauma. Emerg Med Clin North Am 1993;3:225–39.

[24] Lowenstein SR, Weissberg M, Terry D. Alcohol intoxication, injuries, and dangerous behaviors-and the revolving emergency department door. J Trauma 1990;30:1252–7.

[25] Cherpitel CJ. Alcohol and violence-related injuries: an emergency room study. Addiction 1993;88:79–88.

[26] Cherpitel CJ. Alcohol and injuries: a review of international emergency room studies. Addiction 1993;88:651–65.

[27] Howland J, Hingson R. Alcohol as a risk factor for injuries of death due to fires and burns; review of the literature. Public Health Rep 1987;102:475–83.

[28] Hingston R, Howland J. Alcohol as a risk factor for injury or death resulting from accidental falls: a review of the literature. J Stud Alcohol 1987;48:212–9.

[29] Dunn CW, Donovan DM, Gentilello L. Practical guidelines for performing alcohol interventions in trauma center. J Trauma 1997;42:299–304.

[30] Lieber CS. Medical disorders of alcoholism. N Engl J Med 1995;333:1058–65.

[31] World Health Organization. Burden of disease statistics, 2000. Available at: www.who.org. Accessed August 14, 2006.

[32] McCarthy ML, Hirshon JM, Ruggles RL, et al. Referral of medically uninsured ED patients to primary care. Acad Emerg Med 2002;9:639–42.

[33] Behavioral Risk Factor Surveillance System. BRFSS prevalence data–age grouping. Available at: http://apps.nccd.cdc.gov/brfss. Accessed August 14, 2006.

[34] Hingston RW, Heeren T, Zakocs RC, et al. Magnitude of alcohol-related mortality and morbidity among US college students ages 18–24. J Stud Alcohol 2002;63:136–44.

[35] Becker BM, Woolard RH, Longabaugh R, et al. Alcohol use among subcritically injured emergency department patients and injury as a motivator to reduce drinking. Acad Emerg Med 1995;2:784–90.

[36] Soderstrom C, Crowley R. A National Alcohol and Trauma Center survey: missed opportunities, failures of responsibility. Arch Surg 1987;122:1067–71.

[37] Rockett IRH, Putnam SL, Jia H, et al. Unmet substance abuse treatment need, health services utilization and cost: a population-based emergency department study. Ann Emerg Med 2005;45:118–27.

[38] Rockett IRH, Putnam SL, Jia H, et al. Assessing substance abuse treatment need: a statewide hospital emergency department study. Ann Emerg Med 2003;41:802–13.

[39] D'Onofrio G, Degutis LC. Preventive care in the emergency department: screening and brief intervention for alcohol problems in the emergency department. A systematic review. Acad Emerg Med 2002;9:627–38.

[40] Saitz R. Unhealthy alcohol use. N Engl J Med 2005;352:596–607.

[41] Miller WR, Walters ST, Bennett ME. How effective is alcoholism treatment in the United States? J Stud Alcohol 2001;62:211–20.

[42] Montgomery HA, Miller WR, Tonigan JS. Does Alcoholics Anonymous involvement predict treatment outcome? J Subst Abuse Treat 1995;12:241–6.

[43] Robins LN, Helzer JE, Croughan J, et al. National Institute of Mental Health Diagnostic Interview Schedule. Arch Gen Psychiatry 1981;38:381–9.

[44] Spitzer RL, Williams JBW, Gibbon M, et al, editors. User's guide for the structured clinical interview for DSM-III-R. Washington: American Psychiatric Press; 1990.

[45] Ewing JA. Detecting alcoholism: the CAGE questionnaire. JAMA 1984;252:1905–7.

[46] Bohn MJ, Babor TF, Kranzler HR. The Alcohol Use Disorders Identification Test (AUDIT): validation of a screening instrument for use in medical settings. J Stud Alcohol 1995;56:423–31.

[47] D'Onofrio G. Web-based learning module for emergency physicians to assist with screening and intervention for alcohol problems in the ED. Available at: http://www.acep.org. Accessed August 14, 2006.

[48] D'Onofrio G, Bernstein E, Rollnick S. Motivating patients for change: a brief strategy for negotiation. In: Bernstein E, Bernstein J, editors. Case studies in emergency medicine and the health of the public. Boston: Jones and Bartlett; 1996. p. 295–303.

[49] Bernstein E, Bernstein J, Levenson S. Project ASSERT: an ED-based intervention to increase access to primary care, preventive services, and the substance abuse treatment system. Ann Emerg Med 1996;30:181–9.

[50] Monti PM, Spirit A, Myers M, et al. Brief intervention for harm reduction with alcohol-positive older adolescents in a hospital emergency department. J Consult Clin Psychol 1999;67:989–94.

[51] Longabaugh RH, Woolard RF, Nirenberg TD, et al. Evaluating the effects of a brief motivational intervention for injured drinkers in the emergency department. J Stud Alcohol 2001;62:806–16.

[52] Fleming MF, Barry KL, Manwell LB, et al. Brief physician advice for problem alcohol drinkers: a randomized controlled trial in community-based primary care practices. JAMA 1997;277:1039–45.

[53] Gentilello LM, Rivara FP, Donovan DM, et al. Alcohol interventions in a trauma center as a means of reducing the risk of injury recurrence. Ann Surg 1999;230:473–84.

[54] D'Onofrio G, Thomas MA, Degutis L. Project ASSERT: a 5 year evaluation of an ED-based screening, brief intervention and referral to treatment program. Acad Emerg Med 2005;12(1):60 [abstract].

[55] Substance Abuse and Mental Health Services Administration. The NSDUH Report: Driving Under the Influence (DUI) Among Young Persons. 2004. Available at: http://oas.samhsa.gov/2k4/youthDUI/youthDUI.htm. Accessed July 28, 2006.

[56] Marquet P, Delpla PA, Kerguelen S, et al. Prevalence of drugs of abuse in urine of drivers involved in road accidents in France: a collaborative study. J Forensic Sci 1998;43:806–11.

[57] Woolard R, Nirenberg T, Becker B, et al. Marijuana and prior injury among injured problem drinkers. Acad Emerg Med 2003;10:43–51.

[58] Woolard R, Nirenberg T, Becker B, et al. Marijuana and injury in the emergency department. Rhode Island Medicine and Health 2002;85:306–7.

[59] National Institute on Alcohol Abuse and Alcoholism. Reducing injury, ETOH & THC use among ED patients. National Institutes of Health.

[60] Nurco D, Hanlon TE, Kinlock MA. Recent research on the relationship between illicit drug use and crime. Behav Sci Law 1991;9:221–42.

[61] Arnsten JH, Demas PA, Grant RW, et al. Impact of active drug use on antiretroviral therapy adherence and viral suppression in HIV-infected drug users. J Gen Intern Med 2002;17:377–81.

[62] Stein MD, O'Sullivan PS, Ellis P, et al. Utilization of medical services by drug abusers in detoxification. J Subst Abuse 1993;5:187–93.

[63] Elsen M, Pallitto C, Bradner C, et al. Teen risk-taking: promising prevention programs and approaches. Washington: Urban Institute; 2000.

[64] Centers for Disease Control and Prevention. Youth Risk Behavior Surveillance System—United States, 2003. MMWR Surveill Summ 2004;53:1–29.

[65] Mott FL, Haurin RJ. Linkages between sexual activity and alcohol and drug use among American adolescents. Fam Plann Perspect 1988;20:128–36.

[66] Analysis of the Center on Disease Control and Prevention's 1997 YRBS dataDangerous liaisons: substance abuse and sex. New York: The Nation Center on Addiction and Substance Abuse at Columbia University (CASA); 1999.

[67] Santelli JS, Robin L, Brener N, et al. Timing of alcohol and other drug use and sexual risk behaviors among unmarried adolescents and young adults. Fam Plann Perspect 2001;33:200–5.

[68] National Household Survey on Drug Abuse. Academic performance and youth substance use. Available at: http://www.oas.samhsa.gov/2k2/academics/academics.htm. Accessed 28 July 2006.

[69] Mac Donald Z. The employment prospects of Scottish and English drug abusers. Department of Economics, Universigy of Leichester. Available at: http://www.le.ac.uk/economics/research/RePEc/lec/leecon/econ02-2.pdf. Accessed July 28, 2006.

[70] Prichard R. Expert commentary, substance abuse, October 2000. Available at: www.irmi. com/irmicom/expert/articles/2000/prichard10.aspx. Accessed August 14, 2006.

[71] The Drug and Alcohol Services Information System (DASIS) Report: trends in cocaine treatment admissions by state: 1992–2002. 2005. Available at: http://oas.samhsa.gov/ 2k5/CocaineTX/CocaineTX.htm. Accessed August 14, 2006.

[72] Bernstein J, Bernstein E, Tassiopoulos K, et al. Brief motivational intervention at a clinic visit reduces cocaine and heroin use. Drug Alcohol Depend 2005;77:49–59.

[73] Hughes PH, Storr CL, Brandenburg NA, et al. Physician substance use by medical specialty. J Addict Dis 1999;18:23–37.

[74] National Institute on Drug Abuse (NIDA) InfoFacts. Hospital visits. Available at: www.drugabuse.gov/Infofax/hospital.html. Accessed August 14, 2006.

[75] Office of Applied Studies. Mortality data from the Drug Abuse Warning Network (DAWN), 2002 Available at: http://dawninfo.samhsa.gov/. Accessed August 14, 2006.

[76] National Institute on Drug Abuse (NIDA) InfoFacts. Marijuana. Available at: http:// www.nida.nih.gov/Infofax/marijuana.html. Accessed August 14, 2006.

[77] Whalen LG, Grunbaum JA, Kinchen S, McManus T, Shanklin S, Kann L. Middle School Youth Risk Behavior Survey 2003, Centers for Disease Control and Prevention, 2005; 1–293. Available at: http://www.cdc.gov/HealthyYouth/YRBS/middleschool2003/pdf/ fullreport.pdf. Accessed July 28, 2006.

[78] National Institute on Drug Abuse (NIDA) InfoFacts. High school and youth trends. Available at: www.nida.nih.gov/InfoFax/HSYouthtrends.html. Accessed August 14, 2006.

[79] Substance Abuse and Mental Health Services Administration. The NSDUH report: nonmedical oxycodone users: a comparison with heroin users. 2005. Available at: www.oas. samhsa.gov/2k4/oxycodoneH/oxycodoneH.htm. Accessed August 14, 2006.

[80] Substance Abuse and Mental Health Services Administration. The DASIS report: characteristics of primary heroin injection and inhalation admissions: 2002. Available at: www.oas.samhsa.gov/2k4/heroin/heroin.cfm. Accessed August 14, 2006.

[81] Drug Abuse Warning Network. The Dawn report. Narcotic analgesics, 2002 update, September 2004. Available at: http://oas.samhsa.gov/2k4analgesics.pdf. Accessed July 28, 2006.

[82] Volkow ND. Confronting the rise in abuse of prescription drugs. NIDA notes 2005;19(5).

[83] Lee R, Bania T. ED management of current drugs of abuse. 2000. Available at: http://www.emedhome.com/. Accessed August 14, 2006.

[84] Gahlinger P. Club drugs: MDMA, gamma-hydorxybutyrate (GHB), rohypnol, and ketamine. Am Fam Physician 2004;69:2619–26.

[85] Drug Abuse Warning Network. Club drugs. Rockville (MD): Office of Applied Studies, Substance Abuse and Mental Health Services Administration. 2002. Available at: http://oas.samhsa.gov/2k4/clubDrugs/clubDrugs.pdf. Accessed August 14, 2006.

[86] SAMHSA. The National Survey on Drug Use and Health (NSDUH) Report. Stimulant use, 2003. Available at: www.oas.samhsa.gov/2k5/stimulants/stimulants.htm. Accessed August 14, 2006.

[87] Substance Abuse and Mental Health Services Administration (SAMHSA). The DASIS report. Heroin—changes in how it is used, 1992 2002. Available at: http://oas.samhsa. gov/2k4/heroinTrends/HeroinTrends.cfm. Accessed August 14, 2006.

[88] National Institute on Drug Abuse (NIDA) CEWG Meeting Report. Epidemiologic trends in drug abuse. Vol. 1 Proceedings of the Community Epidemiology Work Group Highlights and Executive Summary. US Department of Health and Human Services. Available at: http://www.drugabuse.gov/PDFCEWG/Vol11_1203.pdf. Accessed July 28, 2006.

[89] Gunnell D, Ho D, Murray V. Medical management of deliberate drug overdose: a neglected area for suicide prevention? Emerg Med J 2004;21:35–8.

[90] Gahlinger P. Club drugs: MDMA, gamma-hydroxybutyrate (GHB), rohypnol, and ketamine. Am Fam Physician 2004;69:2619–26.

[91] Schwartz R, Norman M. MDMA and the rave: a review. Pediatrics 1997;100:705–8.
[92] Milroy CM. Ten years of 'ecstasy'. J R Soc Med 1999;92:68–72.
[93] National Institute on Drug Abuse (NIDA) InfoFacts. MDMA (Ecstasy). Available at: http://www.nida.nih.gov/Infofax/ecstasy.html. Accessed August 14, 2006.
[94] Weber T. Raving in Toronto: peace, love, unity and respect in transition. J Youth Stud 1999;2:317–36.
[95] Green AR, Cross AJ, Goodwin GM. Review of the pharmacology and clinical pharmacology of 3, 4 methylenedioxymethamphetamine (MDMA or Ecstasy). Psychopharmacology (Berl) 1995;119:247–60.
[96] Weir E. Raves: a review of the culture, the drugs and the prevention of harm. CMAJ-JAMC 2000;162:13.
[97] Ropero-Miller JD, Goldberger BA. Recreational drugs current trends in the 90's. Clin Lab Med 1998;18:727–46.
[98] Chin RL, Sporer KA. Clinical course of g-hydroxybutyrate overdose. Ann Emerg Med 1998;31:716–22.
[99] Lee R, Bania T. ED management of current drugs of abuse. 2000. Available at: www.emedhome.com. Accessed August 14, 2006.
[100] Price G. IN-patient detoxification after GHB-dependence. Br J Psychiatry 2000;177:181.
[101] Addolorato G, Caputo F, Capristo E, et al. A case of gammahydroxybutyric acid withdrawal syndrome during alcohol addiction treatment: utility of diazepam administration. Clin Neuropharmacol 1999;22:60–2.
[102] Bowles TM, Sommi RW, Amiri M. Successful management of prolonged gammahydroxybutyrate and alcohol withdrawal. Pharmacotherapy 2001;21:254–7.
[103] Weiner AL, Vieira L. Ketamine abusers presenting to the emergency department: a case series. J Emerg Med 2002;18:447–51.
[104] Kohrs R, Durieux M. Ketamine: teaching an old drug new tricks. Anesth Analg 1998;87:1186–93.
[105] Pena BM, Krauss B. Adverse events of procedural sedation and analgesia in a pediatric emergency department. Ann Emerg Med 1999;34(4 pt 1):483–91.
[106] National Institute on Drug Abuse (NIDA) InfoFacts. Inhalants. Available at: www.nida.nih.gov/Infofax/inhalants.html. Accessed August 14, 2006.
[107] National Institute on Drug Abuse (NIDA) InfoFacts. LSD. Available at: www.nida.nih.gov/Infofax/lsd.html. Accessed August 14, 2006.
[108] Substance Abuse and Mental Health Services Administration. 2004. The NSDUH report: youth substance use and family income. Available at: http://oas.samhsa.gov/2k4/youthIncome/youthIncome.htm. Accessed August 14, 2006.
[109] Erikson TB, Aks SE, Koenigsberg M, et al. Drug use patterns at major rock concert events. Ann Emerg Med 1996;28:22–6.
[110] National Institute on Drug Abuse (NIDA). NIDA News Scan June 24, 2002. Journal of General Internal Medicine produces special issue on substance abuse. Available at: www.drugabuse.gov/Newsroom/02/NS-06.html. Accessed August 14, 2006.
[111] Pollack HA, Khoshnood K, Blankenship KM, et al. The Impact of needle exchange-based health services on emergency department use. J Gen Intern Med 2002;17:341–8.
[112] Substance Abuse and Mental Health Services Administration. 2003. Results from the 2002 National Survey on Drug Use and Health: national findings. Office of Applied Studies, NHSDA Series H-22, DHHS Publication No. SMA 03–3836. Rockville (MD); 2003. United States Department of Health and Human Services.
[113] Substance Abuse Treatment Episode Data Set (TEDS) Highlights 2002. Highlights 2002 National Admissions to Substance Abuse Treatment Services, SASIS Series: S-22, DHHS Publication No. (SMA) 04–3946. Rockville (MD); 2004. Available at: www.dasis.samhsa.gov/teds02/index.htm. Accessed February 14, 2005.
[114] National Institute on Drug Abuse (NIDA) InfoFacts. Heroin. Available at: www.nida.nih.gov/Infofax/heroin.html. Accessed August 14, 2006.

[115] National Institute on Drug Abuse (NIDA) InfoFacts. Drug addiction treatment methods. Available at: www.drugabuse.gov/infofax/treatmeth.html. Accessed August 14, 2006.

[116] National Institute on Drug Abuse (NIDA) InfoFacts. Crack and cocaine. Available at: www.nida.nih.gov/Infofax/cocaine.html. Accessed August 14, 2006.

[117] Stephens RS, Roffman RA, Curtin L. Comparison of extended versus brief treatments for marijuana use. J Consult Clin Psychol 2000;68:898–908.

[118] French MD, Roebuck MC, McGerary KA, et al. Using the drug abuse screening test (DAST-10) to analyze health services utilization cost for substance users in a community-based setting. Subst Use Misuse 2001;36:927–46.

[119] Skinner HA. The drug abuse screening test. Addict Behav 1982;7:363–71.

[120] Skinner HA, Blaine JD, Bryant K, et al. Future directions of research: next five years. In: Blaine JD, Horton AM, Towle L, editors. Diagnosis and severity of drug dependence and abuse. National Institute on Drug Abuse Technical Report, (NI 95–3884). Rockville (MD): 1995.

[121] Saunders B, Wilkinson C, Phillips M. The impact of a brief motivational intervention with opiate users attending a methadone program. Addiction 1995;90:415–24.

[122] Stotts AM, Schmitz JM, Rhoades HM, et al. Motivational interviewing with cocaine-dependent patients: a pilot study. J Consult Clin Psychol 2001;69:858–62.

[123] Donovan DM, Rosengren DB, Downey L, et al. Attrition prevention with individuals awaiting publicly funded drug treatment. Addiction 2001;96:1149–60.

[124] Booth RE, Kwiatkowski C, Iguchi MY, et al. Facilitating treatment entry among out-of-treatment injection drug users. Public Health Rep 1998;113(Suppl 1):116–28.

[125] Miller WR, Yahne CE, Tonigan JS. Motivational interviewing in drug abuse services: a randomized trial. J Consult Clin Psychol 2003;71:754–63.

[126] Dunn CW, Ries R. Linking substance abuse services with general medical care: integrated, brief interventions with hospitalized patients. Am J Drug Alcohol Abuse 1997;23:1–13.

[127] Dunn C, Deroo L, Rivara FP. The use of brief interventions adapted from motivational interviewing across behavioral domains: a systematic review. Addiction 2001;96:1725–42.

[128] Samet J, Larson H, Mary JO, et al. Linking alcohol- and drug-dependent adults to primary medical care: a randomized controlled trial of a multi-disciplinary health intervention in a detoxification unit. Addiction 2002;98:509–16.

[129] Treating tobacco use and dependence: a systems approach. A guide for health care administrators, insurers, managed care organizations, and purchasers, November 2000. US Public Health Service. Available at: http://www.surgeongeneral.gov/tobacco/systems.htm. Accessed August 14, 2006.

[130] New Public Health Service guideline calls on health professionals to make treating tobacco dependence a top priority. Press Release, June 27, 2000. Department of Health and Human Services. Available at: http://www.hhs.gov/news/press/. Accessed August 14, 2006.

[131] Centers for Disease Control and Prevention. State-specific prevalence of current cigarette and cigar smoking among adults—United States, 1998. MMWR Surveill Summ 1999;48:1034–9.

[132] Bernstein S. The impact of smoking-related illness in the ED: an attributable risk model. Am J Emerg Med 2000;20:161–4.

[133] Boudreaux E, Kim S, Hohrmann J, et al. Interest in smoking cessation among emergency department patients: a prospective multicenter study. Acad Emerg Med 2003;10:568–9.

[134] Lowenstein S, Tomlinson D, Koziol-McLain J, et al. Smoking habits of emergency department patients: an opportunity for disease prevention. Ann Emerg Med 1995;2:165–71.

[134a] Prochazka A, Koziol-McLain J, Tomlinson D, Lowenstein SR. Smoking Cessation counseling by emergency physicians: opinions, knowledge, and training needs. Acad Emerg Med 1995;2:211–6.

[135] Becker B, Bock B, Monteiro R, et al. Emergency department patients with acute respiratory illness: motivation to quit, risk perception, and physician intervention. Ann Emerg Med 2000;7:489.

[135a] Frank E, Winkleby MA, Altman DG, Rockhill B, Fortmann SP. Predictors of physicians smoking cessation advice. JAMA 1991;266:538–44.

[136] Treating tobacco use and dependence. Fact Sheet, June 2000. US Public Health Service. Available at: http://surgeongeneral.gov/tobacco/smokfact.htm. Accessed August 14, 2006.

[137] Abrams DB, Niaura RS. Planning evidence based treatment for tobacco dependence. In: Abrams DB, Niaura RS, Brown RA, et al, editors. The tobacco dependence treatment handbook. New York: The Guilford Press; 2003.

[138] Fiore MC, Novotny TE, Pierce JP, et al. Methods used to quit smoking in the United States: do cessation programs help? JAMA 1990;263:2760–5.

[139] Hughes JR. Pharmacotherapy for smoking cessation: unvalidated assumptions, anomalies, and suggestions for future research. J Consult Clin Psychol 1993;61:751–60.

[140] Cinciripini PM, et al. Tobacco addiction: implications for treatment and cancer prevention. J Natl Cancer Inst 1997;89:1852–67.

[141] Lichtenstein E, Glasgow RE. Smoking cessation: what have we learned over the past decade? J Consult Clin Psychol 1992;60:518–27.

[142] McBride CM, Emmons KM, Lipkus IM. Understanding the potential of teachable moments: the case of smoking cessation. Health Educ Res 2003;18:156–70.

[143] Jelley M, Prochazka AV. A smoking cessation intervention in family planning clinics. J Womens Health 1995;4:555–67.

[144] Demers RY, Neale AV, Adams R, et al. The impact of physician's brief smoking cessation counseling. J Fam Pract 1990;31:625–9.

[145] Kottke TE, Battista RN, DeFriese GH, et al. Attributes of successful smoking interventions in medical practice: a meta-analysis of 39 controlled trials. JAMA 1988;259:2883–9.

[146] Ockene JK, Kristeller J, Pbert L, et al. The physician-delivered smoking intervention projects: can short-term interventions produce long-term effects for a general outpatient population? Health Psychol 1994;13:278–81.

[147] USPHS. A clinical practice guideline for treating tobacco use and dependence: a US Public Health Service report. The Tobacco Use and Dependence Clinical Practice Guideline Panel, Staff, and Consortium Representatives. JAMA 2000;283:3244–54.

[148] Slama K, Karsenty S, Hirsch A. Effectiveness of minimal intervention by general practitioners with their smoking patients: a randomised controlled trial in France. Tob Control 1995;4:162–9.

[149] Wilson DH, Wakefield MA, Steven ID, et al. Sick of smoking: evaluation of a targeted minimal smoking cessation intervention in general practice. Med J Aust 1990;152:518–21.

[150] Severson HH, Andrews JA, Lichtensetin E, et al. Reducing maternal smoking and relapse: long term evaluation of a pediatric intervention. Prev Med 1997;26:120–30.

[151] Hebert JR, Kristeller J, Ockene J, et al. Patient characteristics and the effect of three physician-delivered smoking interventions. Prev Med 1992;21:557–73.

[152] Ockene JK. Physician-delivered interventions for smoking cessation: strategies for increasing effectiveness. Prev Med 1987;16:723–37.

[153] Cummings SR, Coates TJ, Richard RJ, et al. Training physicians in counseling about smoking cessation: a randomized trial of the Quit for Life program. Ann Intern Med 1989;110:640–7.

[154] Debusk RF, Houston-Miller N, Superko R, et al. A case-management system for coronary risk factor modification after acute myocardial infarction. Ann Intern Med 1994;120:721–9.

[155] Glasgow RE, Stevens VJ, Vogt TM, et al. Changes in smoking associated with hospitalization: quit rates, predictive variables, and intervention implications. Am J Health Promot 1991;6:24–9.

[156] Perkins KA. Maintaining smoking abstinence after myocardial infarction. J Subst Abuse 1988;1:91–107.

[157] Rigotti NA, McKool KM, Shiffman S. Predictors of smoking cessation after coronary artery bypass graft surgery. Ann Intern Med 1994;120:287–93.

[158] Richman PB, Dinowitz S, Nashed AH, et al. The emergency department as a potential site for smoking cessation intervention: a randomized, controlled trial. Acad Emerg Med 2000;7:348–53.

[159] Tatum JL, Jesse RL, Kontos MC, et al. Comprehensive strategy for the evaluation of triage of the chest pain patient. Ann Emerg Med 1997;29:116–25.

[160] Zalenski RJ, Rydman RJ, McCarren M, et al. Feasibility of a rapid diagnostic protocol for an emergency department chest pain unit. Ann Emerg Med 1997;29:99–108.

[161] Grijseels EW, Deckers JW, Hoes AW, et al. Optimal use of coronary care units: a review. Prog Cardiovasc Dis 1995;37:415–21.

[162] Graff L, Joseph T, Andelman R, et al. American College of Emergency Physicians information paper: chest pain units in emergency departments. A report from the Short-Term Observation Services Section. Am J Cardiol 1995;76:1036–9.

[163] Herlitz J, Bengtson A, Hjalmarson A, et al. Smoking habits in consecutive patients with acute myocardial infarction: prognosis in relation to other risk indicators and to whether or not they quit smoking. Cardiology 1995;86:496–502.

[164] Tosteson AN, Goldman L, Udvarhclyi IS, et al. Cost-effectiveness of a coronary care unit versus an intermediate care unit for emergency department patients with chest pain. Circulation 1996;94:143–50.

[165] Abrams DB, Biener L. Motivational characteristics of smokers at the worksite: a public health challenge. Int J Prev Med 1992;21:679–87.

[166] Marcus BH, Lewis BA, King TK, et al. Rationale, design, and baseline data for Commit to Quit II: An evaluation of the efficacy of moderate-intensity physical activity as an aid to smoking cessation in women. Prev Med 2003;36:479–92.

[167] Smith PM, Reilly KR, Miller NH, et al. Application of a nurse-managed inpatient smoking cessation program. Nicotine Tob Res 2002;4:211–22.

[168] Hughes JR, Brandon TH. A softer view of hardening. Nicotine Tob Res 2003;5:961–2.

[169] McCaig LF, Burt CW. National Hospital Ambulatory Medical Care Survey: 2002 Emergency Department Summary. Advance Data for Vital Health Statistics; number 340. Hyatsville (MD): National Center for Health Statistics; 2004. Available at: http://www.cdc.gov/nchs/data/ad/ad340.pdf. Accessed August 14, 2006.

[170] Centers for Disease Control. Cigarette smoking among adults—United States, 2000. MMWR Morb Mortal Wkly Rep 2002;51:642–5.

[171] D'Onofrio G, Pantalon MV, Degutis LC, et al. Development and implementation of an emergency practitioner-performed brief intervention for hazardous and harmful drinkers in the emergency department. Acad Emerg Med 2005;12:249–56.

[172] Longabaugh R, Minugh PA, Nirenberg TD, et al. Injury as a motivator to reduce drinking. Acad Emerg Med 1995;2:817–25.

[173] Rollnick S, Mason P, Butler C. Health behavior change: a guide for practitioners. Edinburgh: Churchill Livingstone; 1999.

[174] Miller WR, Rollnick S. Motivational interviewing: preparing people to change addictive behavior. 2nd edition. New York: Guilford Press; 2002.

[175] Graham DM, Maio RF, Blow FC, et al. Emergency physician attitudes concerning intervention for alcohol abuse/dependence delivered in the emergency department: a brief report. J Addict Dis 2000;19:45–53.

[176] Grol R. Improving the quality of medial care: building bridges among professional pride, payer profit and patient satisfaction. JAMA 2001;28:2578–86.

[177] D'Onofrio G, Nadel ES, Deguis LC, et al. Improving emergency medicine residents' approach to patients with alcohol problems: a controlled educational trial. Ann Emerg Med 2002;40:50–62.

[178] Connecticut General Statutes. P.A. 98–201. An ACT concerning substace abuse emergency rom screening and training for health care professionals. 1998.

[179] Rhodes KV, Lauderdale DS, Stocking CB, et al. Better health while you wait: a controlled trial of a computer-based intervention for screening and health promotion in the emergency department. Ann Emerg Med 2001;37:284–91.
[180] Gregor MA, Shope J, Blow F, et al. Feasibility of using an interactive laptop program in the emergency department to prevent alcohol misuse among adolescents. Ann Emerg Med 2003;42:276–84.
[181] Maio RF, Shope JT, Blow FC, et al. A randomized controlled trial of an emergency department-based interactive computer program to prevent alcohol misuse among injured adolescents. Ann Emerg Med 2005;45:430–2.
[182] D'Onofrio G, Mascia RL, Razzak J, et al. Utilizing health promotion advocates for selected health risk screening and intervention in the ED. Acad Emerg Med 2001;8:543 [abstract].

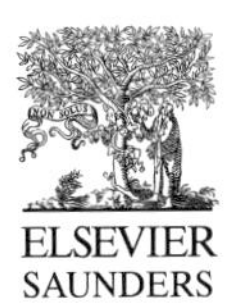

ELSEVIER
SAUNDERS

Emerg Med Clin N Am
24 (2006) 969–987

EMERGENCY
MEDICINE
CLINICS OF
NORTH AMERICA

Death, Dying, and Last Wishes

Catherine A. Marco, MD, FACEP[a],*,
Raquel M. Schears, MD, MPH, FACEP[b]

[a]Department of Emergency Medicine, Acute Care Services, St Vincent Mercy Medical Center,
2213 Cherry Street, Toledo, OH 43608-2691, USA
[b]Department of Emergency Medicine, Mayo Clinic/St Mary's Hospital, 200 First Street,
SW, G410, Rochester, MN 55905, USA

Numerous issues confront emergency physicians regarding end-of-life care in the emergency department (ED). Principles of bioethics can be helpful in developing a framework for the analysis and conclusions of ethical dilemmas. Some of the important issues and dilemmas frequently encountered in emergency medicine include issues surrounding resuscitation and resuscitation attempts, palliative care, symptom resolution, honoring advance directives and patient preferences, religious preferences, and spiritual beliefs. Effective communication and support techniques, including establishing the patient's wishes, goals, and values of medical treatment can be beneficial in carrying out those wishes. In many cases, definitive curative care is not possible or is not desired, and the goals of medical care at the end of life shift away from technologic care to measures that provide comfort and support to the patient and family.

Fundamental principles of medical ethics

The term "ethics" has been defined as the way of *understanding and examining the moral life* [1], and as *a theory or a system of moral values* [2]. The basic principles of medical ethics can be valuable in developing a framework for understanding ethical dilemmas. Codes of medical ethics have been established by many organizations and individuals as standards of moral and ethical medical care. The Hippocratic Oath is believed to be one of the oldest codes of medical ethics and its principles are still revered by

---

* Corresponding author. Department of Emergency Medicine, Acute Care Services, St Vincent Mercy Medical Center, 2213 Cherry Street, Toledo, OH 43608-2691.
E-mail address: cmarco2@aol.com (C.A. Marco).

0733-8627/06/$ - see front matter © 2006 Elsevier Inc. All rights reserved.
doi:10.1016/j.emc.2006.06.007 *emed.theclinics.com*

many. In recent years, more modern codes have been developed to provide guidelines for physicians in the application of ethical principles to clinical practice, including the American Medical Association (AMA) Code of Ethics (earliest version from 1847), The American College of Emergency Physicians (ACEP) Code of Ethics (1997), and The Society for Academic Emergency Medicine Code of Conduct (1999) [3–5]. Many ethical codes address common elements of ethical practice, such as beneficence (doing good), nonmaleficence (doing no harm), respect for patient autonomy, confidentiality, honesty, distributive justice, and respect for the law. Ethical dilemmas frequently arise in clinical practice when two ethical principles or values conflict. Ethical dilemmas may be resolved by using strategies such as physician judgment; the gathering of additional information; meetings with health care professionals, patients, and families; and the use of consultants, such as ethics, risk management, or social work advisors. Although the involvement of the institutional ethics committee or the judicial system may be helpful in some clinical settings, decisions in the emergency department frequently do not allow the time necessary for such consultations.

"Last wishes" as expressed by advance directives

The term *advance directive* refers to any document stating the patient's wishes regarding medical care, should he or she be unable to state his or her own wishes in the future. The *living will* is a document used by some terminally ill individuals, in which the treating physician accepts the provisions of the living will in advance. Many living wills state that no life-sustaining treatment be used in cases where meaningful recovery is unlikely. Living wills are often problematic, owing to uncertainty regarding definitions and timing. The *durable power of attorney* document designates a surrogate decision maker in the event the patient is no longer able to make medical decisions. Most states (at least 42) now have state-approved advance directives, often with specific documents to be completed by patients and physicians [6]. In 1991, the Federal Patient Self-Determination Act mandated that all patients who are admitted to hospitals have the opportunity to complete an advance directive.

Advance directives have many positive effects, the most important of which is facilitating the implementation of the specific wishes of the individual patient, even when the patient is unable to communicate those wishes. Without advance directives, physicians and surrogate decision makers often make incorrect assumptions regarding the preferences of patients [7–10]. Although some health care providers may be reluctant to discuss issues such as end-of-life care and advance directives, it has been demonstrated that many patients welcome the opportunity to discuss their wishes [11]. Most patients have definite opinions regarding resuscitation preferences, despite the lack of completion of legal advance directives [12].

Certain problems exist that prevent the universal application of advance directives. Even when advance directives are completed and available, there can be significant disagreement among physicians regarding which specific procedures are appropriate for individual patients [13]. Despite widespread advocacy and some legal mandates supporting the increased use of advance directives, only a minority of patients have completed these documents [14,15], and an even smaller minority present to the ED with documentation of the advance directive. Even in today's environment, where many recommend a change in policy away from standing orders for resuscitative efforts, many social and institutional policies still suggest resuscitation attempts for most patients. The development of national and state guidelines to address out-of-hospital care of patients with Do-Not-Attempt-Resuscitation (DNAR) orders is an important facet of the provision of appropriate medical care for these patients [16].

Studies conducted in other inpatient settings have demonstrated variable compliance with advance directives by medical personnel. In contrast, recent studies in the ED and prehospital environment have demonstrated that emergency medical personnel comply with advance directives more often than previously estimated. According to one recent survey, most emergency physicians (78%) withhold resuscitation attempts for patients who have a legal advance directive, indicating a willingness to honor patients' wishes regarding their own medical care [17]. Additionally, most prehospital providers (89%) state that they withhold resuscitation attempts for patients with legal advance directives [18]. These results suggest that advance directives may be especially helpful in prehospital and emergency department environments.

To resuscitate or not to resuscitate: that is the question!

In the United States, cardiopulmonary resuscitation is frequently attempted for patients in cardiac arrest. In many cases, this is appropriate and has some measurable likelihood of successful outcome. In many other cases, however, a successful outcome is extremely improbable and resuscitation attempts are unlikely to benefit the patient and may not be in accordance with the patient's wishes. Understanding the data regarding resuscitation, outcomes, factors predictive of outcomes, and alternatives are essential to appropriate medical decision making regarding resuscitation.

In the resuscitation arena, decisions must be made rapidly and decisions are based on information available to the emergency physician, which may be incomplete or erroneous. When making decisions regarding resuscitation, many factors must be considered, including the potential benefits of resuscitation (restoring life to the patient, providing a sense of closure and resolution of guilt for the survivors) and potential risks (resuscitation to a suboptimal quality of life and high resource use, and so forth).

It has been estimated that between 250,000 and 500,000 patients experience sudden cardiac death annually in the United States [19,20]. As a result, $58 million in Medicare expenditures are estimated to result from unsuccessful resuscitations annually in the United States [21]. Resuscitation attempts are by nature invasive, high-cost, labor-intensive, and carry a very low likelihood of successful outcome in most clinical settings. Traditionally, most emergency physicians attempt cardiopulmonary resuscitation for patients in cardiac arrest, unless a legal advance directive is available [17]. Since so few patients have completed legal advance directives, and only a fraction of those have the document available, the default option for many physicians is to attempt resuscitation.

Reported survival rates for patients with cardiac arrest vary in the literature and are dependent on many factors, including time elapsed since arrest (down time) [17,22,23], presenting electrical rhythm [24], early defibrillation [25,26], cardiac activity on bedside echocardiogram [27], underlying medical condition [28], response to prehospital advanced life support (ALS) protocols [29,30], age [31], and long-term care [32]. In summary, published reports have estimated survival for victims of cardiac arrest to hospital discharge between 0% and 16% [33–36]. Certain groups of patients have survival rates approaching 0%, for example, residents of long-term care facilities following unwitnessed arrests. Despite the relatively low success rate, current American Heart Association Guidelines and many hospital policies suggest or mandate resuscitation for all patients except those with prior DNAR orders, clear signs of death such as rigor mortis or dependent lividity, or if no physiological benefit can be expected after maximal therapy [37].

Some authors have recommended withholding of "futile" resuscitative efforts. The term "futility," although commonly used, has fallen out of favor among many ethicists. The term is fraught with difficulties in definition and inconsistencies in interpretation. Some authors have proposed a variety of different definitions and standards, for both the quantitative and qualitative aspects of futility. Proposed definitions include "quantitative futility" defined as the likelihood of benefit to the patient falling below a minimal threshold, and a "patient-centered" definition meaning failure to produce effects that the patient desires [38,39]. Health care professionals may have variable interpretations of the term "futile" as applied to medical interventions. For example, some may use the term "futile" to refer to interventions that carry an absolute impossibility of successful outcome, a low likelihood of success, a low likelihood of survival to discharge from the hospital, or a low likelihood of restoration of meaningful quality of life. Several reports have demonstrated that there is no consensus among physicians about the meaning of futility [40,41]. It may be preferable to avoid the term "futility" because of the continuing controversy over the meaning of the term. Instead, interventions should be referred to as medically "nonbeneficial," "ineffectual," or having a "low likelihood of success."

Solutions to dilemmas involving nonbeneficial interventions ("futility")

Dilemmas regarding nonbeneficial interventions often arise as a result of inadequate or ineffective communication between physician, patient, and family [42]. When a difference of opinion exists, initial efforts should be made to improve communication, education, and joint decision making. In many cases, this is sufficient to resolve conflicts.

Many authors, ethicists, and leaders agree that physicians are under no obligation to render treatments they believe will provide little or no benefit to the patient. There have been numerous ethical opinions supportive of the position of providing only those treatments judged to be of likely medical benefit. The AMA Council on Ethical and Judicial Affairs states that cardiopulmonary resuscitation (CPR) may be withheld, even if requested by the patient, "when efforts to resuscitate a patient are judged by the treating physician to be futile" [43]. Numerous other ethicists and authors support withholding interventions deemed unlikely to benefit patients [44,45].

Several national policies may be of guidance regarding nonbeneficial interventions. The ACEP adopted a policy statement that states that "physicians are under no ethical obligation to render treatments that they judge have no realistic likelihood of medical benefit to the patient." The policy also states that emergency physicians' judgments should be unbiased, based on scientific evidence and societal as well as professional standards, and that physicians should be sensitive to differences of opinion regarding the value of medical intervention in various situations [46].

The AMA Council on Ethical and Judicial Affairs recommends a process-based approach to addressing futility [47], to include such actions as the following:

1. Deliberation and resolution
2. Joint decision making with physician and patient or proxy
3. Assistance of a consultant or patient representative
4. Use of an institutional committee (ie, ethics committee)

Decisions regarding emergency interventions and treatments; the likelihood of benefit to the patient; and decisions to provide, limit, or withhold interventions should be made in the context of well-established data, patient and family wishes, and professional judgment [48,49]. Importantly, when certain interventions or therapies are withheld because they are judged to be unlikely to benefit the patient, it is crucial that the physician continue to care for the patient and maintain compassion, communication, delivery of information, counseling, and coordination of other services that may be helpful to the patient and family. Maintaining an active role in these aspects of care of the patient and loved ones may, in many cases, be of greater value than technologic interventions.

What do patients really want?

Numerous studies have demonstrated inaccurate beliefs among the general public regarding CPR and the expected outcome. Many laypersons erroneously believe that the success rate of CPR is between 40% and 60% [50–52]. Some authors believe that inaccurate knowledge is perpetuated by dramatically unrealistic portrayals of successful resuscitations in the media [53].

Physicians generally presume that most patients would desire resuscitative attempts, unless expressed otherwise. Physicians' decisions regarding resuscitation, however, are often influenced by such issues as perceived quality of life, age, down time, presenting rhythm, whether the arrest was witnessed, family preferences, fear of litigation, and other factors [54]. Such preferences regarding resuscitation attempts vary greatly and depend on numerous factors including age, state of health, and clinical setting [55,56]. Recent reports suggest that full resuscitative efforts are not necessarily desired by all patients and that trends toward societal consensus can be identified in a variety of hypothetical resuscitation scenarios [57,58].

Improving public education regarding resuscitation

Because of widespread inaccuracies among the general public's knowledge regarding resuscitation, public education to improve accurate knowledge to assist with medical decision making is an important step in bridging the gap between patient preferences and physician actions. It has been previously demonstrated that accurate knowledge regarding probability of survival influences patient preferences [59–61]. Additionally, a recent prospective interventional study demonstrated that education of the general public using an educational video can be effective in improving knowledge about resuscitation, and thus affecting personal preferences regarding resuscitation [62]. Additional community educational programs, in conjunction with improved accuracy in media portrayals, may be important steps in increasing public awareness of facts regarding resuscitation.

Training in CPR is another area of potential improvement in public education. Because bystander CPR is an important predictor of outcome, improved public training may be an important component of rapid institution of medical care and improved outcomes. Recent data demonstrate that certain populations are more likely to be trained in CPR [63], suggesting potential target populations for education in CPR.

The physician's role at the end of life

The role of the physician at the end of life is multifaceted and complex. Many presume that the primary goal of the physician is to preserve or restore life. Echoing this common belief, a noted author stated,

"There is a profound, unconscious, emotional rejection of death. Inasmuch as medicine is assumed to be curative, a patient's death brings to the physician a deep and unacceptable feeling of defeat." [64]

Physicians and other health care providers must work to overcome this traditional perspective of the physician's role. In many cases, curative therapies are not possible or desired and death is a natural step. Death may not be unwelcome to the patient and family. In such cases, the dying process should be accepted as such, by the patient, loved ones, and health care providers [65]. Aggressive medical interventions judged unlikely to benefit the patient need not be offered simply because the technologic capability exists. At the end of life, the role of the physician broadens as less tangible actions and interventions carry greater significance. The physician should address the numerous challenges that face patients and loved ones, which may include physical, emotional, social, cultural, and spiritual challenges [66]. Although some use phrases such as "withdrawal of care," *care* itself should never be withdrawn, even if technologic interventions or therapies are withdrawn or withheld. Comfort care should always be provided for patients near the end of life and may include pain management, management of other symptoms, such as shortness of breath, nausea, fatigue, and depression, as well as communication, empathy, reassurance, and solace to the patient and family [67].

Palliative care in emergency medicine

Symptom relief

When a friend or loved one experiences a terminal illness, the final stages can be very difficult [68]. Whereas some dying patients feel strongly about avoiding care that prolongs life without offering a cure, these patients still frequent the ED for many reasons. The desired goals, not the availability of any specific critical care technology, should be elicited from the patients and surrogates to help guide the plan of care [69]. Unfortunately, physician discomfort with death in the ED often propels burdensome interventions and intensive care admissions, which may overreach the goals of symptom relief in the dying process. Answering the question of "How do I help them as they are dying?" helps to acknowledge a process and develop an awareness of medical limitations.

Oddly enough, the need for medical "permission" to die and reassurance regarding terminal symptoms may motivate patients to seek ED care at the end of life, as opposed to an expectation for illness cure or symptom eradication. Improving the tolerability of the dying process, without rushing or prolonging death, is a practical challenge [70]. The most commonly reported symptoms include pain, anxiety, nausea, anorexia, weakness, fatigue, depression, delirium, and dyspnea [71–75].

Pain

Pain is a common disabling complaint at the end of life. It has been estimated that between 38% and 74% of cancer patients experience significant pain [76]. Unfortunately, approximately 50% of these patients receive inadequate analgesia [77]. Adequate pain relief for patients facing end-of-life illness must be addressed in a timely fashion without concern for addiction. Pain management guidelines, such as those recommended by the Agency for Health Care Policy and Research among others [78–80], are constructed to take the edge off pain without producing disabling side effects. There is a standard approach to pain management: round-the-clock dosing with an oral long-acting opioid; short-acting opioids to treat unexpected pain exacerbations; constipation prevention with routine laxatives; and anti-emetic therapy for the first week after beginning treatment with opioids. The best method of opioid delivery is individualized. For example, some patients prefer a long-acting patch because they don't like hourly reminders of their illness or don't want to wait for available caregivers to provide pain control. Narcotic administration can often be supplemented with the use of other anti-inflammatory agents if necessary.

Several barriers to appropriate analgesia may exist, including psychological and educational barriers [81]. Some physicians may be overly concerned about the potential for diminishing the patient's respiratory drive with narcotic administration. Most medicolegal commentaries accept as nonculpable, the potential circumstance in which the unintended, yet not wholly unexpected adverse effect occurs. For example, The AMA Council on Ethical and Judicial Affairs has written in policy, "Physicians have an obligation to relieve pain and suffering and to promote the dignity and autonomy of dying patients in their care. This includes providing effective palliative treatment even though it may foreseeably hasten death" [82].

Anxiety

Anxiety at the end of life is the partial product of the inescapability of death as the destiny for humankind and the shared refusal of physician and patient to being labeled as quitters. Fear of death and blame for it, uncertainty of its timing, the work involved in ordering one's affairs, survivor disquietude with dying, and physician concealment of prognosis [83] are also fodder for worry at life's end. The ED environment may contribute the context features of lack of privacy and absence of home-like surroundings, thus compounding misery and the feel of death, and leading to a view of disorderly conduct [67]. Others have argued a different ethic, which supports ED transport of even on-scene dead, with ongoing CPR, because of the concern for compassion, and acute bereavement care in survivors covictimized by their experience of home death [84].

Optimizing the environment may be one approach to anxiety control, whether prehospital or in the ED. Hospice programs and other alternatives to calling 911 for expected death and terminal symptom management are worthy, yet underused, strategies. The judicious use of medications such as anxiolytics (benzodiazepines) or sedatives (barbiturates) is often appropriate. In the ED, communication that facilitates the goals of symptom management and techniques that reassure patients and families involved in the dying experience should be emphasized [85].

Depression and delirium

Depression is a common symptom among patients near the end of life. It has been estimated to occur in 33% to 47% of dying patients [86,87]. Several scales exist to measure depression in terminally ill and frequently hospitalized patients [88,89]. Depression has been demonstrated to correlate with desire for early death among terminally ill patients [90]. While the sense of loss and sadness coexist for terminal patients, features of clinical depression (suicidal thoughts) can be palliated with antidepressants, anxiolytics, and psychiatric care.

Acute delirium must be separated from the process of normal detachment from life, common in dying patients. Delirium at the end of life has a variety of organic etiologies, but may be related to the effects of medications, hypoxia, and dehydration. Whereas reversible conditions should be treated, relative effects may require tolerance and surrogate reassurance. Delusional experiences and hallucinations in dying patients are also common. Discussing frightening content and affirming such experiences is part of preparing for death. If intolerable distress results from anxiety, depression, or delirium, pharmacologic management can be used with agents such as benzodiazepines or butyrophenones.

Weakness and fatigue

Weakness and fatigue are particularly common among oncology patients. Reversible conditions should be addressed, including anemia, medication side effects, insomnia, and malnutrition. Several agents are endorsed for management of fatigue, including corticosteroids, progestational agents, and psychostimulants [91]. Nonpharmacologic management would include endorsement of adequate rest, hydration, and nutrition; counseling; and psychosocial advocacy.

Nausea and anorexia

Nausea and anorexia are routinely present in dying patients. The etiology is multifactorial, with dehydration, malnutrition, narcotic administration, and drug interactions commonly implicated. Pharmacologic agents such prochlorperazine, promethazine, metoclopramide, and ondansetron, can be helpful in controlling nausea. Many antiemetics are available as suppositories, and smaller volume, high-nutrition meals may be more palatable to the nauseated patient. Anorexia is often more distressing to caregivers than to patients [92]. The understanding that dying rarely causes acute symptoms of hunger or thirst and reassurance that patients are still comfortable without food or fluid may be of value. The use of artificial hydration and nutrition are individual decisions and have no clear benefit, but also have not been demonstrated as prolonging the dying process in terminal patients.

Dyspnea

Shortness of breath is a commonly encountered complaint among patients with terminal conditions, and may occur in nearly three quarters of this population [93]. Traditional diagnostic measures such as oxygen saturation, respiratory rate, and arterial blood gas measurements do not correlate with symptomatology [94,95]. However, patient self-reports of functional impairment are more accurate in predicting worsening of the symptom. Appropriate management should be tailored to the etiology of dyspnea, correction of any reversible underlying cause, and symptomatic control in the event no reversible condition is identified. First-line pharmacologic therapy for dyspnea in these circumstances is opiates, followed by anxiolytic medications [96–98]. Oxygen and repositioning to improve respiratory mechanics, providing patients with education, and providing reassurance through close observation, have also demonstrated efficacy [93,99–101].

Restlessness and intractable distress

Restless behaviors and tangential thoughts are often noted in terminal patients. These signs and symptoms may benefit from alternative, complementary, and homeopathic medicine, including the use of chiropractors, acupuncture, or nutrition-based therapy. Spiritual healing, meditation, music/reading, and aromatherapy have not been studied extensively but are of interest to patients nearing death [102–105].

When traditional measures are unsuccessful at relieving symptoms, palliative sedation may be used as an effective means to provide patient comfort [106,107]. Palliative sedation, however, interferes with the patient's ability to communicate and interact. Therefore, decisions to provide palliative sedation although rare, should be made in accordance with patient's wishes, surrogate assent, and in conjunction with specialty consultation.

Rituals at the end of life

Throughout history, rituals have been an important aspect of spiritual and cultural life. In many cultures, rituals are performed at the time of important events signifying change, such as birth, puberty, marriage, and death. The significance of rituals to groups and individuals is vital, complex, and multifaceted. Rituals may use symbolism to help groups and individuals to interpret the meaning of daily life. Rituals may provide a sense of comfort and constancy amid change, an emotional guarantee of future well-being to the participants [108], and may also serve anxiolytic functions [109]. Particularly near the end of life, rituals (cultural, religious, or social) may serve important functions for the dying patient and the family and friends. End-of-life rituals can provide spiritual, religious, emotional, social, and physical well-being. Patients and families who wish to use rituals at the end of life should be encouraged to do so, provided that they are not disruptive or disrespectful of others.

The role of religion in end-of-life medical care

Interestingly, many profound advancements in technology have evolved during an era of increasing spiritual needs. It has been reported that increasing numbers of people report a belief in God or some similar spiritual force, and also report participation in prayer or other spiritual practices [110–112]. Thus, it may become a challenging but very important question to health care providers how to balance technology and religion in health care. The indiscriminate widespread use of technology, although done with good intentions, may result in the unintentional abandonment of other important needs, such as comfort, pain control, communication, spirituality, or other significant values [64]. In general, it is inappropriate for physicians to suggest specific religious persuasions to dying patients and their families. However, attention to religious issues that are important to each patient and family can be important in ensuring a meaningful end-of-life experience. Communication regarding religion, the patient's belief in God, desire to pray or participate in other religious observances, and desire to involve pastoral care services can be vital to meeting spiritual goals at the end of life.

Dignity at the end of life

References to human dignity began in the 1970s within discussions about foregoing life support as a mere means of prolonging the dying experience. Dignity was written into state statutes, federal mandates, and templates for advance directives. Dignity figured into the phraseology used in rights language (ie, "right to die with dignity"), in professional ethics codes (ACEP) for providing emergency care, and as justification for critical care access [5]. Dignity has more recently been touted as a "useless concept" as a result of failing to contribute more than what respect for autonomy achieves in medicolegal or ethical analysis [113]. However, one separate and further use of the term is instructive.

Lack of dignity is used to describe postmortem violation of the human body. Medical students and residents practicing procedures on the newly dead, without prior surrogate consent for these educational activities, opportune violation of the dignity of the dead person. However, obtaining surrogate permission is enough to render the same activity ethically acceptable. Thus, cadavers lose the legal protections of autonomy, in transit (from a person to an object), but not their ethical oneness with perceptible humanity. Likewise, it is postulated, the future of surrogate consent for organ donation from either anencephalics or the permanently vegetative may contend less with the legal definition of brain death than the real haunt of dignity (perceptible humanity).

Communication skills

Effective communication with patients and loved ones is an essential component of care at the end of life. Data from families of deceased patients confirm perceived lack of optimal physician communication [114]. An accurate understanding of the patient's goals and expectations of medical treatment can improve the physician's ability to provide the best care possible, in accordance with the patient's wishes. The delivery of accurate information, even if considered bleak, is useful to patients in developing realistic goals and expectations [115]. For example, while some patients wish to prolong life, others value dignity and pain relief, even at the price of a potentially shortened lifespan. Privacy, attentiveness, empathy, and spending adequate time together are essential to effective communication about life values and significant decisions. Other effective techniques include using nonverbal communication to demonstrate empathy, using eye contact, addressing patients by name, using understandable layperson language, and employing active listening techniques [116–121].

Procedures on recently deceased patients

The practice of learning from and performing procedures on recently deceased patients ("the newly dead") for educational purposes is controversial. In many areas, this was a longstanding tradition considered important to the hands-on education of students and residents. The most important argument supporting this practice is the recognized need for practice for students and housestaff, as well as experienced physicians [122]. The setting of the recently deceased patient provides the unique clinical setting in which there is literally *no* risk to the patient. In part as a result of this practice, trained physicians are able to competently perform these procedures on living patients, resulting in an overall benefit to society. However, informed consent had traditionally been rarely obtained in these settings [123].

Some consider performing procedures on deceased patients without informed consent to be disrespectful, deceptive, and unethical [124]. Recent literature suggests that most adults believe that consent from family members is appropriate before practicing procedures on the newly dead [125,126]. Several studies have demonstrated the feasibility of obtaining consent for certain postmortem procedures from family members [127,128]. However, other data have demonstrated that only a minority of families consented to a postmortem procedure [129,130]. The AMA recently instituted a policy regarding procedures on recently deceased patients, which states that consent should be obtained [131]. The Society for Academic Emergency Medicine recently published a position statement affirming that permission should be obtained from family before performing procedures on newly deceased patients [132].

Emergency physicians must operate within local and hospital policies, and make the choices they judge most appropriate in the specific clinical situations encountered. Factors to be considered when making such decisions include the teaching benefit to the student and his or her future patients, the overall benefit to society, disfigurement produced by the procedure(s), and the availability of the family and feasibility of informed consent.

Family presence during procedures and resuscitation

Traditionally, family members have not been permitted to witness resuscitation attempts. However, several recent reports have demonstrated positive results of allowing family members to witness procedures and resuscitation attempts [133,134]. Family presence during procedures may serve to allay the family's guilt or disappointment, and may be a helpful part of the grieving process. Many families simply wish to have the option of being present. Despite concerns that family members may be traumatized by witnessing procedures, or may interfere with medical care, data do not support such fears [135,136]. If family members are allowed to be present, a chaperone can be helpful to assist with communication and education about procedures and other medical issues.

Physician-assisted suicide and euthanasia

The difference between euthanasia and physician-assisted death (PAD) amounts to whether or not the physician actively administers an agent with the intent to end the life of the patient. If so, this defines euthanasia, which is illegal outside of The Netherlands. A famous US example of euthanasia, involved a retired pathologist, Dr Jack Kevorkian. He was indicted and acquitted numerous times for participating in patients' suicides by prescription, preceding his conviction for homicide. This latter act of euthanasia occurred when he delivered a lethal injection to a patient who had consented to the administration and subsequently died. In contrast, PAD depends on doctors to facilitate *indirectly* the competent wishes of patients to end their own lives [137]. Since 1994, PAD has been legal only in Oregon, under strict guidelines, which first require patients to receive expert palliative care, including psychosocial and spiritual counseling. Even then, the threshold permitting PAD is rarely crossed and only for symptoms of persistent "intolerable distress" [138,139].

Summary

There are numerous clinical and ethical issues related to care at the end of life. Basic principles of bioethics can be valuable in assessing ethical dilemmas. Recognition and effective management of symptoms can be of great comfort to the dying patient and family. Education of patients regarding end-of-life issues, such as resuscitation and advance directives, are crucial to improving the ability of health care providers to act in accordance with patients' wishes. Communication with patients and families is an essential skill that can improve experiences near the end of life for patients, families, and health care providers.

References

[1] Beauchamp TL, Childress TF. Principles of biomedical ethics. 4th edition. Oxford University Press, USA; 1994.

[2] The American Heritage dictionary of the English language. 4th edition. Boston, Massachusetts: Houghton Mifflin Company; 2000.

[3] AMA Code of Medical Ethics. Available at: http://www.ama-assn.org/ama/pub/category/2512.html. Accessed July 14, 2006.

[4] American College of Emergency Physicians. Code of ethics for emergency physicians. Dallas, TX: American College of Emergency Physicians; 1997.

[5] Larkin GL. A code of conduct for academic emergency medicine. Acad Emerg Med 1999; 6:45.

[6] Sabatino CP. Survey of state EMS-DNR laws and protocols. J Law Med Ethics 1999; 27:297–315, 294.

[7] Wenger NS, Phillips RS, Teno JM, et al. Physician understanding of patient resuscitation preferences: insights and clinical implications. J Am Geriatr Soc 2000;48:S44–51.

[8] Golin CE, Wenger NS, Liu H, et al. A prospective study of patient-physician communication about resuscitation. J Am Geriatr Soc 2000;48:S52–60.

[9] Ebell MH, Doukas DJ, Smith MA. The do-not-resuscitate order: a comparison of physician and patient preferences and decision-making. Am J Med 1991;91:255–60.

[10] Fischer GS, Tulsky JA, Rose MR, et al. Patient knowledge and physician predictions of treatment preferences after discussion of advance directives. J Gen Intern Med 1998;13: 447–54.

[11] Uhlmann RF, Pearlman RA. Perceived quality of life and preferences for life-sustaining treatment in older adults. Arch Intern Med 1991;151:495–7.

[12] Marco CA, Larkin GL. A time to die: patient-centered priorities in cardiac resuscitation. Acad Emerg Med 2001;8:475.

[13] Beach MC, Morrison RS. The effect of do-not-resuscitate orders on physician decision-making. J Am Geriatr Soc 2002;50:2057–61.

[14] Taylor DM, Ugoni AM, Cameron PA, et al. Advance directives and emergency department patients: owners rates and perceptions of use. Intern Med J 2003;33:586–92.

[15] The SUPPORT Principle Investigators. A controlled trial to improve care for seriously ill hospitalized patients. JAMA 1995;274:1591–8.

[16] Schears RM, Marco CA, Iserson KV. Do not attempt resuscitation (DNAR) in the out-of-hospital setting. Ann Emerg Med 2004;44:68–70.

[17] Marco CA, Bessman ES, Schoenfeld CN, et al. Ethical issues of cardiopulmonary resuscitation: current practice among emergency physicians. Acad Emerg Med 1997;4:898–904.

[18] Marco CA, Schears RM. Prehospital resuscitation practices: a survey of prehospital providers. J Emerg Med 2003;24:101–6.

[19] American Heart Association. 2002 heart and stroke statistical update. Dallas, TX: American Heart Association; 2002.

[20] Zheng ZJ, Croft JB, Giles WH, et al. Sudden cardiac death in the United States, 1989 to 1998. Circulation 2001;104:2158–63.

[21] Suchard JR, Fenton FR, Powers RD. Medicare expenditures on unsuccessful out-of-hospital resuscitations. J Emerg Med 1999;17:801–5.

[22] Vukmir RB. Witnessed arrest, but not delayed bystander cardiopulmonary resuscitation improves prehospital cardiac arrest survival. Emerg Med J 2004;21:370–3.

[23] Vukmir RB. Sodium bicarbonate study group: the influence of urban, suburban, or rural locale on survival from refractory prehospital cardiac arrest. Am J Emerg Med 2004;22:90–3.

[24] Aprahamian C, Thompson CM, Gruchow HW, et al. Decision making in prehospital sudden cardiac arrest. Ann Emerg Med 1986;15:445–9.

[25] The Public Access Defibrillation Trial Investigators. Public-access defibrillation and survival after out-of-hospital cardiac arrest. N Engl J Med 2004;351:637–46.

[26] Bunch TJ, White RD, Gersh BJ, et al. Long-term outcomes of out-of-hospital cardiac arrest after successful early defibrillation. N Engl J Med 2003;348:2626–33.

[27] Blaivas M, Fox JC. Outcome in cardiac arrest patients found to have cardiac standstill on the bedside emergency department echocardiogram. Acad Emerg Med 2001;8:616–21.

[28] Bedell SE, Delbanco TL, Cook EF, et al. Survival after cardiopulmonary resuscitation in the hospital. N Engl J Med 1983;309:569–76.

[29] Schoenenberger RA, von Planta M, von Planta I. Survival after failed out-of-hospital resuscitation: are further therapeutic efforts in the emergency department futile? Arch Intern Med 1994;154:2433–8.

[30] Bonnin MJ, Pepe PE, Kimball KT, et al. Distinct criteria for termination of resuscitation in the out-of-hospital setting. JAMA 1993;270:1457–62.

[31] Murphy DJ, Murray AM, Robinson BE, et al. Outcomes of cardiopulmonary resuscitation in the elderly. Ann Intern Med 1989;111:199–205.

[32] Awoke S, Mouton CP, Parrott M. Outcomes of skilled cardiopulmonary resuscitation in a long-term facility: futile therapy? J Am Geriatr Soc 1992;40:593–5.

[33] Engdahl J, Bang A, Lindqvist J, et al. Factors affecting short- and long-term prognosis among 1069 patients with out-of-hospital cardiac arrest and pulseless electrical activity. Resuscitation 2001;51:17–25.

[34] Callaham M, Madsen CD. Relationship of timeliness of paramedic advanced life support interventions to outcome in out-of-hospital cardiac arrest treated by first responders with defibrillator. Ann Emerg Med 1995;27:638–48.

[35] Stratton SJ, Niemann JT. Outcome from out-of-hospital cardiac arrest caused by nonventricular arrhythmias: contribution of successful resuscitation to overall survivorship supports the current practice of initiating out-of-hospital ACLS. Ann Emerg Med 1998;32:448–53.

[36] Varon J, Fromm RE. In-hospital resuscitation among the elderly: substantial survival to hospital discharge. Am J Emerg Med 1996;14:130–2.

[37] American Heart Association. Ethical aspects of CPR and ECC. Circulation 2000;102:1–12.

[38] Jecker NS, Schneiderman LJ. An ethical analysis of the use of 'futility' in the 1992 American Heart Association guidelines for cardiopulmonary resuscitation and emergency cardiac care. Arch Intern Med 1993;153:2195–8.

[39] Schneiderman LJ, Jecker NS, Jonsen AR. Medical futility: its meaning and ethical implications. Ann Intern Med 1990;112:949–54.

[40] Brody BA, Halevy A. Is futility a futile concept? J Med Philos 1995;20:123–44.

[41] Dull SM, Graves JR, Larsen MP, et al. Expected death and unwanted resuscitation in the prehospital setting. Ann Emerg Med 1994;23:997–1002.

[42] Goold SD, Williams B, Arnold RM. Conflicts regarding decisions to limit treatment: a differential diagnosis. JAMA 2000;283:909–14.

[43] AMA CEJA. Guidelines for the appropriate use of do-not-resuscitate orders. Council on Ethical and Judicial Affairs, American Medical Association. JAMA 1991;265:1868–71.

[44] Jecker NS, Schneiderman LJ. Futility and rationing. Am J Med 1992;92:189–96.

[45] Paris JJ, Reardon FE. Physician refusal of requests for futile or ineffective interventions. Camb Q Healthc Ethics 1992;2:127–34.

[46] Policy Statement ACEP. Nonbeneficial ("futile") emergency medical interventions. Dallas, TX: American College of Emergency Physicians; 1998.

[47] AMA. Council on Ethical and Judicial Affairs. Medical futility in end of life care. JAMA 1999;281:937–41.

[48] Marco CA, Larkin GL, Moskop JC, et al. The determination of "futility" in emergency medicine. Ann Emerg Med 2000;35:604–12.

[49] Marco CA, Larkin GL. Case studies in futility. Acad Emerg Med 2000;7:1147–51.

[50] Roberts D, Hirschman D, Scheltema K. Adult and pediatric CPR: attitudes and expectations of health professionals and laypersons. Am J Emerg Med 2000;18:465–8.

[51] Marco CA, Larkin GL. To be or not to be: factors predictive of resuscitation preferences. Acad Emerg Med 2001;8:420.

[52] Jones GK, Brewer KL, Garrison HG. Public expectations of survival following cardiopulmonary resuscitation. Acad Emerg Med 2000;7:48–53.

[53] Diem SJ, Lantos JD, Tulsky JA. Cardiopulmonary resuscitation on television: miracles and misinformation. N Engl J Med 1996;334:1578–82.

[54] Lockey AS, Hardern RD. Decision making by emergency physicians when assessing cardiac arrest patients on arrival at hospital. Resuscitation 2001;50:51–6.

[55] Rosenfeld KE, Wenger NS, Phillips RS, et al. Factors associated with change in resuscitation preference of seriously ill patients. The SUPPORT Investigators. Study to understand prognoses and preferences for outcomes and risks of treatments. Arch Intern Med 1996; 156:1558–64.

[56] Miller DL, Jahnigen DW, Gorbien MJ, et al. Cardiopulmonary resuscitation: how useful? Attitudes and knowledge of an elderly population. Arch Intern Med 1992;152:578–82.

[57] Hamel MB, Lynn J, Teno JM, et al. Age-related differences in care preferences, treatment decisions, and clinical outcomes of seriously ill hospitalized adults: lessons from SUPPORT. J Am Geriatr Soc 2000;48:S176–82.

[58] Marco CA, Schears RM. Societal preferences regarding cardiopulmonary resuscitation. Am J Emerg Med 2002;20:207–11.

[59] Murphy DJ, Burrows D, Santilli S, et al. The influence of the probability of survival on patients' preferences regarding cardiopulmonary resuscitation. N Engl J Med 1994;330: 545–9.

[60] Yamada R, Galecki AT, Goold SD, et al. A multimedia intervention on cardiopulmonary resuscitation and advance directives. J Gen Intern Med 1999;14:559–63.

[61] de Vos R, Koster RW, de Haan RJ. Impact of survival probability, life expectancy, quality of life and patient preferences on do-not-attempt resuscitation orders in a hospital. Resuscitation 1998;39:15–21.

[62] Marco CA, Larkin GL. Public education regarding resuscitation: effects of a multimedia intervention. Ann Emerg Med 2003;42:256–60.

[63] Larkin GL, Marco CA. Who knows CPR? A national survey (abstract). Presented at the Annual Meeting of the Society for Academic Emergency Medicine, Atlanta, Georgia, May 6–9, 2001.

[64] Urzua J. Modern medicine and the rejection of death. Anaesth Intens Care 1991;19:400–20.

[65] McCue JD. The naturalness of dying. JAMA 1995;273:1039–43.

[66] Rhymes JA. Barriers to effective palliative care of terminal patients. Clin Geriatr Med 1996; 12:407–16.

[67] Schears RM. Emergency physicians' role in end of life care. Emerg Med Clin North America 1999;17:539–59.

[68] DeSpelder LA, Strickland AL. The last dance: encountering death and dying. New York: McGraw-Hill; 2002.

[69] Pisetsky DS. Doing everything. Ann Intern Med 1998;128(10):869–70.

[70] Brody H, Campbell ML, Faber-Langendoen K, et al. Withdrawing intensive life-sustaining treatment–recommendations for compassionate clinical management. N Engl J Med 1997; 336(9):652–7.

[71] Potter J, Hami F, Bryan T, et al. Symptoms in 400 patients referred to palliative care services: prevalence and patterns. Palliat Med 2003;17:310–4.

[72] Reynolds K, Henderson M, Schulman A, et al. Needs of the dying in nursing homes. J Palliat Med 2002;5:895–901.

[73] Sutton LM, Demark-Wahnefried W, Clipp ED. Management of terminal cancer in elderly patients. Lancet Oncol 2003;4:149–57.

[74] Pantilat SZ. End of life care for the hospitalized patient. Med Clin North Am 2002;86: 749–70.

[75] Hall P, Schroder C, Weaver L. The last 48 hours of life in long-term care: a focused chart audit. J Am Geriatr Soc 2002;50:501–6.

[76] Cowan JD. The dying patient. Curr Oncol Rep 2000;2:331–7.

[77] Ripamonti C, Zecca E, Brunelli C, et al. Pain experienced by patients hospitalized at the National Cancer Institute of Milan: research project "towards a pain-free hospital." Tumori 2000;86:412–8.

[78] Agency for Health Care Policy and Research: Management of cancer pain: adults. Clin Pract Guide 1 Quick Ref Guide Clin 1994;(9):1–29.

[79] Kumar KS, Rajagopal MR, Naseema AM. Intravenous morphine for emergency treatment of cancer pain. Palliat Med 2000;14:183–8.

[80] Hagen NA, Elwood T, Ernst S. Cancer pain emergencies: a protocol for management. J Pain Symptom Manage 1997;14:45–50.

[81] Ducharme J. Acute pain and pain control: state of the art. Ann Emerg Med 2000;35: 592–603.

[82] American Medical Association Council on Ethical and Judicial Affairs. Code of Medical Ethics: current opinions with annotations. Chicago, Illinois: American Medical Association; 2002. p. 28.

[83] Annas GJ. Informed consent, cancer, and truth in prognosis. N Engl J Med 1994;330(3): 223–5.

[84] Bishai D, Siegel A. Moral obligations to families when there is a sudden death. J Clin Ethics 2001;12(4):382–7.

[85] Bedell SE, Cadenhead K, Graboys TB. The doctor's letter of condolence. N Engl J Med 2001;344(15):1161–2.

[86] Breibart W, Bruera E, Chochinov H, et al. Neuropsychiatric syndromes and psychological symptoms in patients with advanced cancer. J Pain Symptom Manage 1995;10:131–41.

[87] Stromgren AS, Goldschmidt D, Grownvold M, et al. Self-assessment in cancer patients referred to palliative care: a study of feasibility and symptom epidemiology. Cancer 2002;94:512–20.

[88] Lloyd-Williams M, Spiller J, Ward J. Which depression screening tools should be used in palliative care? Palliat Med 2003;17:40–3.

[89] Lloyd-Williams M, Friedman T, Rudd N. An analysis of the validity of the Hospital Anxiety and Depression scale as a screening tool in patients with advanced metastatic cancer. J Pain Symptom Manage 2001;22:990–6.

[90] Tiernan E, Casey P, O'Boyle C, et al. Relations between desire for early death, depressive symptoms and antidepressant prescribing in terminally ill patients with cancer. J R Soc Med 2002;95:386–90.

[91] Barnes EA, Bruera E. Fatigue in patients with advanced cancer: a review. Int J Gynecol Cancer 2002;12:424–8.

[92] Poole K, Froggatt K. Loss of weight and loss of appetite in advanced cancer: a problem for the patient, the carer, or the health professional? Palliat Med 2002;16:499–506.

[93] Hately J, Laurence V, Scott A, et al. Breathlessness clinics within specialist palliative settings can improve the quality of life and functional capacity of patients with lung cancer. Palliat Med 2003;17:410–7.

[94] Thomas JR, Von Gunten CF. Treatment of dyspnea in cancer patients. Oncology 2002;16: 745–50.

[95] Thomas JR, Con Gunten CF. Clinical management of dyspnoea. Lancet Oncol 2002;3: 223–8.

[96] LeGrand SB, Khawam EA, Walsh D, et al. Opioids, respiratory function, and dyspnea. Am J Hosp Palliat Care 2003;20:57–61.

[97] Johnson MJ, McDonagh TA, Harkness A, et al. Morphine for the relief of breathlessness in patients with chronic heart failure: a pilot study. Eur J Heart Fail 2002;4:753–6.

[98] Jennings AL, Davies AN, Higgins JP, et al. A systematic review of the use of opioids in the management of dyspnoea. Thorax 2002;57:939–44.

[99] Tarzian AJ. Caring for dying patients who have air hunger. J Nurs Scholarsh 2000;32: 137–43.

[100] Syrett E, Taylor J. Non-pharmacological management of breathlessness: a collaborative nurse-physiotherapist approach. Int J Palliat Nurs 2003;9:150–6.

[101] Luce JM, Luce JA. Perspectives on care at the close of life. Management of dyspnea in patients with far-advanced lung disease: "once I lose it, it's kind of hard to catch." JAMA 2001;285:1331–7.

[102] Halstead MT, Roscoe ST. Restoring the spirit at the end of life: music as an intervention for oncology nurses. Clin J Oncol Nurs 2002;6:332–6.

[103] Hadfield N. The role of aromatherapy massage in reducing anxiety in patients with malignant brain tumours. Int J Palliat Nurs 2001;7:279–85.

[104] Thompson EA, Reilly D. The homeopathic approach to symptom control in the cancer patient: a prospective observational study. Palliat Med 2002;16:227–33.

[105] Ernst E. A primer of complementary and alternative medicine commonly used by cancer patients. Med J Aust 2001;174:88–92.

[106] Cowan JD, Palmer TW. Practical guide to palliative sedation. Curr Oncol Rep 2002;4: 242–9.

[107] Morita T, Tsunoda J, Inoue S, et al. Terminal sedation for existential distress. Am J Hosp Palliat Care 2000;17:189–95.

[108] Fenn RK. The end of time: religion, ritual, and the forging of the soul. Cleveland, OH: The Pilgrim Press; 1997.

[109] Goldbloom RB. Prisoners of ritual. JAMC 1999;161:528–9.

[110] Lukoff D, Lu FG, Turner R. Cultural considerations in the assessment and treatment of religious and spiritual problems. Psychiatr Clin N America 1995;18:467–85.

[111] Waldfogel S, Wolpe PR. Using awareness of religious factors to enhance interventions in consultation-liaison psychiatry. Hosp Community Psychiatry 1993;44:473–7.

[112] Lukoff D, Lu F, Turner R. Towards a more culturally sensitive DSM-IV: psychoreligious and psychospiritual problems. J Nerv Ment Dis 1992;180:673–82.

[113] Macklin R. Dignity is a useless concept. BMJ 2003;327:1419–20.

[114] Marco CA, Buderer N, Thum D. End of life care: perspectives of families of deceased patients. Am J Hospice Pall Care 2005;22:26–31.

[115] Fallowfield LF, Jenkins VA, Beveridge HA. Truth may hurt but deceit hurts more: communication in palliative care. Palliat Med 2002;16:297–303.

[116] Olsen JC, Buenese ML, Falso W. Death in the emergency department. Ann Emerg Med 1998;31:758–65.

[117] Delbanco T. Enriching the doctor-patient relationship by inviting the patient's perspective. Ann Intern Med 1992;116:414–8.

[118] Quill T. Recognizing and adjusting to barriers in doctor-patient communication. Ann Intern Med 1989;111:51.

[119] Ong LM, de Haes JC, Hoos AM, et al. Doctor-patient communication: a review of the literature. Soc Sci Med 1995;40:903–18.

[120] Lipkin M Jr. Patient education and counseling in the context of modern patient-physician-family communication. Patient Educ Couns 1996;27:5–11.

[121] O'Mara K. Communication and conflict resolution in emergency medicine. Emerg Med Clin N Am 1999;17:451–9.

[122] Iserson KV. Law versus life: the ethical imperative to practice and teach using the newly dead emergency department patient. Ann Emerg Med 1995;25:91–4.

[123] Fourre MW. The performance of procedures on the recently deceased. Acad Emerg Med 2002;9:595–8.

[124] Goldblatt AD. Don't ask, don't tell: practicing minimally invasive resuscitative techniques on the newly dead. Ann Emerg Med 1995;25:86–90.

[125] Moore GP. Ethics seminars: the practice of medical procedures on newly dead patients. Is consent warranted? Acad Emerg Med 2001;8:389–92.

[126] Berger JT, Rosner F, Cassell EJ. Ethics of practicing medical procedures on newly dead and nearly dead patients. J Gen Intern Med 2002;17:774–8.

[127] McNamara RM, Monti S, Kelly JJ. Requesting consent for an invasive procedure in newly deceased adults. JAMA 1995;273:310–2.

[128] Brown MA, Fontane EL, Reeder TJ. Performing procedures on the newly deceased: survey of a rural community. Acad Emerg Med 2004;11:598–9.

[129] Olsen J, Spilger S, Windisch T. Feasibility of obtaining family consent for teaching cricothyrotomy on the newly dead in the emergency department. Ann Emerg Med 1995; 25:660–5.

[130] Manifold CA, Storrow A, Rodgers K. Patient and family attitudes regarding the practice of procedures on the newly deceased. Acad Emerg Med 1999;6:110–5.

[131] Performing procedures on the newly deceased for training purposes. Available at: http://www.ama-assn.org/apps/pf_online/pf_online?f_n=browse&doc=policyfiles/CEJA/E-8.181.HTM&&s_t=&st_p=&nth=1&prev_pol=policyfiles/CEJA/E-7.05.HTM&nxt_pol=policyfiles/CEJA/E-8.01.HTM&. Accessed December 14, 2006.

[132] The Society for Academic Emergency Medicine. Position on procedures on the newly dead. Acad Emerg Med 2004;11:962–7.

[133] Boyd R. Witnessed resuscitation by relatives. Resuscitation 2000;43:171–6.

[134] Eichhorn DJ, Meyers TA, Mitchell TG, et al. Opening the doors: family presence during resuscitation. J Cardiovascular Nurs 1996;10:59–70.

[135] Sachetti AD, Paston C, Carraccio C. Do family members disrupt care when present during invasive procedures in children? Acad Emerg Med 2004;11:594–5.

[136] Robinson SM, Mackenzie-Ross S, Campbell Hewson GL, et al. Psychological effect of witnessed resuscitation on bereaved relatives. Lancet 1998;352:614–7.

[137] Foley K, Hendin H. The case against assisted suicide: for the right to end of life care. Baltimore, MD: Johns Hopkins University Press; 2002.

[138] Cooke M, Gourlay L, Collette L. Informal caregivers and the intention to hasten AIDS-related death. Arch Intern Med 1998;158:69–75.

[139] Pierce SF. Allowing and assisting patients to die: the perspectives of oncology practitioners. J Adv Nurs 1999;30(3):616–22.

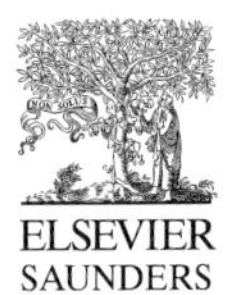

ELSEVIER
SAUNDERS

Emerg Med Clin N Am
24 (2006) 989–1017

EMERGENCY
MEDICINE
CLINICS OF
NORTH AMERICA

Communicable Respiratory Threats in the ED: Tuberculosis, Influenza, SARS, and Other Aerosolized Infections

Richard E. Rothman, MD, PhD*,
Yu-Hsiang Hsieh, PhD,
Samuel Yang, MD

*Department of Emergency Medicine, The Johns Hopkins University School of Medicine,
1830 East Monument Street, Suite 6-100, Baltimore, MD 21205, USA*

Communicable diseases are infections that are caused by microorganisms that can be transmitted from one infected person to another [1]. In spite of improvements in methods to prevent, detect, and decrease transmission of these infections, communicable diseases still represent a significant public health threat. The relative burden of communicable diseases varies globally, accounting for 10% of the overall global disease burden, but nearly 50% of deaths in developing countries [2]. The recent occurrence of emerging and biological threats has heightened awareness of the potential devastation associated with an unexpected infectious disease outbreak [3].

Respiratory infections are the most common communicable infectious diseases [2]. Transmission can occur by a number of routes including contact transmission (direct or indirect exposure to infected patients), droplet transmission (contact with contagious large respiratory droplets that do not stay suspended in the air), and airborne transmission (contact with small, less than 5 micromolar particles that can remain suspended in the air for extended periods of time and be disseminated and inhaled by susceptible hosts) [4]. Airborne transmissible respiratory infections represent the most significant public health risk, as the route of transmission puts large numbers of persons at risk and introduces the greatest potential for hospital outbreaks and epidemics. The most common of these include influenza, tuberculosis, and measles, which together account for approximately 25% of infectious causes of death worldwide [2]. Also included in this discussion are emerging and biothreat agents, which follow the same route of

* Corresponding author.
E-mail address: rrothman@jhmi.edu (R.E. Rothman).

transmission. Most prominent examples include severe acute respiratory syndrome (SARS) and pneumonic plague (smallpox is discussed in the chapter by Saks and Karras elsewhere in this issue).

Emergency departments (EDs) serve as the frontline for patients with communicable respiratory diseases because of the acute nature of these illnesses and because the ED serves as the principal site of health care for many of those at highest risk for these diseases (see Fig. 1). A discussion of each of these contagious respiratory agents follows with attention to epidemiology, pathogenesis, diagnosis, and treatment. Emphasis will be given to the pivotal role of the ED as a public health prevention arena for communicable aerosolized respiratory infectious diseases, with attention to the three critical arms of prevention: primary (education and disease prevention), secondary (early identification of disease in patients at risk), and tertiary (reduction of illnesses in patients with diseases) [5].

Five communicable respiratory threats

Tuberculosis

Epidemiology and pathophysiology

Tuberculosis (TB) is caused by *Mycobacterium tuberculosis,* which is a slow-growing, acid-fast bacillus. It is the second most common cause of infectious disease–related deaths worldwide, after HIV/AIDS [6], with 8.8 million incident cases per year and 1.7 million deaths per year [7]. In the United States, the disease burden is lower but still significant, with approximately 15 million people infected overall [8]. Although public health preventive measures over the past decade have resulted in a favorable trend in the incidence of TB in the United States (with a peak of 10.5 cases per 100,000 in 1992, to 5.1 cases per 100,000 in 2003), rates of decline have recently slowed [8]. This slowing in the rate of decline, along with the recent emergence of multidrug-resistant tuberculosis (MDRTB) [9], makes this disease one of the leading public health threats to our nation.

TB is spread by tiny 1- to 5-μm airborne droplet nuclei, which can remain airborne for hours after expectoration caused by coughing, sneezing, or talking. The infectious nuclei are inhaled and lodge in the distal alveoli where host defenses are activated. A variety of potential subsequent events follow, based on pathogen load and host responsiveness. In most cases, cell-mediated immunity results in immediate destruction of the organism. In some cases, however, initial infection is established when the organism is transported to regional lymph nodes. Here, further cell-mediated immune response results in containment of infection, or in those with less-effective immune systems, development of immediate disease (ie, primary active TB). For the majority of infected individuals who successfully contain the infection, bacteria remain contained in granulomas or tubercles where replication of the organism is limited. This latent infectious state generally lasts

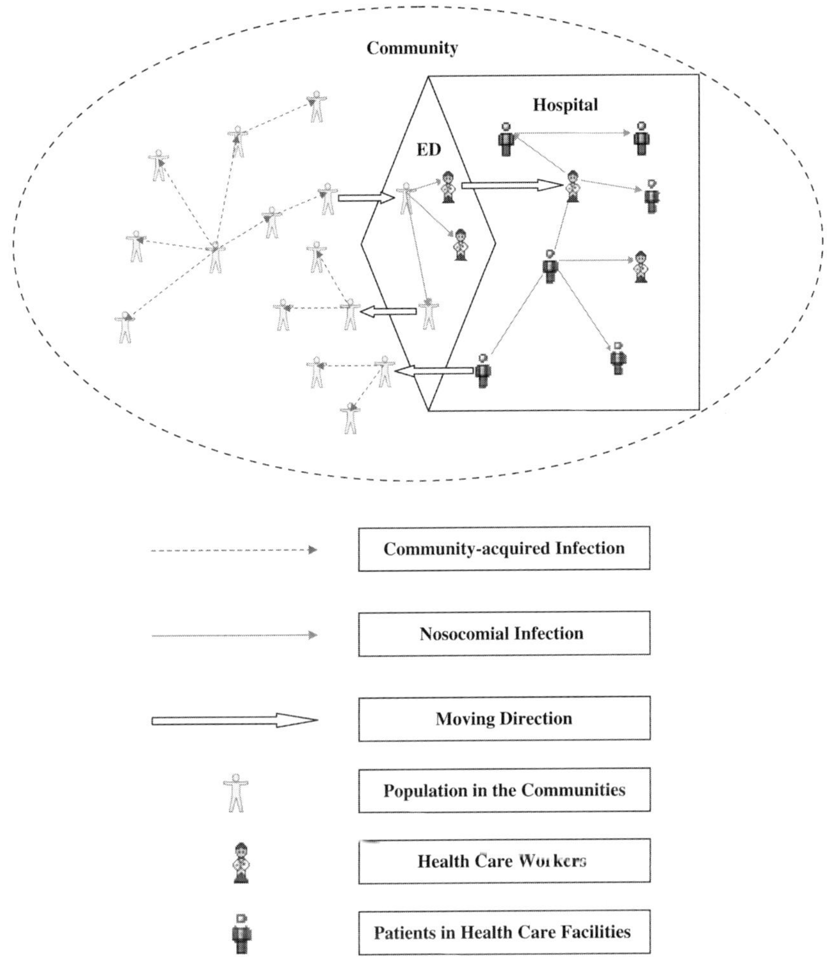

Fig. 1. Emergency department (ED) as potential bridge between community and nosocomial aerosolized respiratory infections.

for the life of the infected patient. In others, reactivation of infection occurs when the host's immune response is no longer capable of containment. Those at highest risk for reactivation include the very young, the elderly, and patients with chronic immunocompromising diseases, particularly HIV [10]. For immunocompetent individuals, the overall lifetime risk of reactivation of TB is 10%; for those with HIV the risk of reactivation is significantly higher, estimated to be about 7% per year.

Clinical presentation, diagnosis, and treatment

ED diagnosis and public health control measures are challenging because clinical presentation of TB can be highly variable and culturing the organism takes days to weeks. Primary TB is most frequently asymptomatic and identifiable only by a positive skin test (PPD, purified protein derivative). In rare cases, active disease may develop, which is clinically similar to reactivation TB. Signs and symptoms of reactivation TB can be either pulmonary only (80% of cases) or systemic.

Early recognition of TB in the clinical area requires maintaining a high level of clinical vigilance. Populations recognized to be at increased risk of infection include foreign-born persons from areas where TB is common (eg, Asia, Africa, Latin America, and countries that were part of the former Soviet Union), medically underserved patients, low-income populations, racial and ethnic minority groups (eg, African Americans, Hispanics, Asians and Pacific Islanders, and Native Americans), the residents of long-term care facilities (eg, correctional facilities and nursing homes), injection drug users (IDUs), migrant farm workers, homeless persons, and persons who may have had a personal or occupational exposure to TB [11].

The most common symptoms of TB are fever, productive cough, and dyspnea. Other symptoms include night sweats, malaise, fatigue and weight loss, hemopytysis, and pleuritic chest pain. In one ED-based study of a series of patients who later were identified as having contagious TB, cough was present in only 64% of cases and was the chief complaint in less than 20% of cases. Furthermore, only 36% of patients reported any pulmonary complaints at triage [12]. TB can involve nearly every organ system but the most common extrapulmonary sites infected are the lymph nodes, central nervous system (CNS), bones, and joints. CNS presentations are usually subacute with findings including indolent headache, fever, and occasionally altered mental status. Although TB can affect nearly every joint, the spine is the most commonly affected site (Pott's disease). Disseminated TB can involve multiple organ systems, including the lungs. Diagnosis should be suspected in those with a miliary pattern on chest radiographs.

Patients with suspected TB should be isolated in negative pressure isolation rooms as early as possible until TB has been ruled out with certainty. Definitive diagnosis is not possible in the ED, since culture is the gold standard and requires several weeks for growth. A presumptive diagnosis of TB can be made by Ziehl-Neelson staining, which identifies acid-fast bacilli; sensitivity of this method is only 50% to 80%, however, and requires obtaining multiple positive sputum samples for confirmation. New laboratory-based molecular diagnostics such as polymerase chain reaction hold promise for rapid definitive diagnosis, but are not yet accepted as routine for clinical decision making [13]. Chest radiographs should be obtained on patients with suspected TB. Classic radiographic findings are upper-lobe infiltrates, cavitary infiltrates, and hilar or paratracheal adenopathy. It is critical to keep in mind, however, that radiographic findings with TB are highly variable, with atypical findings more common in those with immunosuppressive states, such as advanced HIV [14].

Disposition and treatment decisions for ED patients with suspected or confirmed TB should be made in consultation with infectious disease specialists. Hospital epidemiologist and public health services should be notified for all new cases (suspected or confirmed) and respiratory isolation patients should be maintained. Outpatient treatment is considered acceptable in those instances in which compliance and home isolation can be assured. Admission with inpatient respiratory isolation should be arranged for any patient with uncertain diagnosis, question regarding outpatient medication compliance, concern for MDRTB, or other obvious clinical parameters requiring hospitalization (ie, hypoxemia). Beginning treatment (which is beyond the scope of this review) consists of three- or four-drug therapy until drug susceptibility can be confirmed.

Disease burden in the ED

Emergency departments are particularly vulnerable to the threat of TB, and represent high-risk sites for potential propagation of disease. Contributing factors include characteristics of the patient populations served, ED infrastructure, and the inherent nonspecific clinical features and highly contagious nature of the disease [15–17]. As described above, those groups at highest risk for TB (eg, the homeless, the uninsured, immigrants, IDUs, and HIV/AIDS patients) often use the ED as their principal or sole site of care [18–20]. Busy inner-city waiting rooms and overcrowded conditions with long wait times and lack of adequate isolation rooms and personal protective equipment further contribute to the potential spread of TB [21]. One recent retrospective study from an urban teaching hospital found that 44 active TB patients made 66 contagious ED visits over a 30-month period that went unrecognized before diagnosis [12]; a similar retrospective study found that nearly 50% of newly diagnosed TB cases had an antecedent visit within 6 months of diagnosis [22]. Several studies from high-risk urban EDs have demonstrated delayed disease recognition with reports of lengthy ED stays (median 13 hours) [23], and significant delays in time to isolation (median time of 8 hours from triage to isolation) [24].

Increased risk of TB infection among health care workers (HCWs) versus the general population is evident. The results are principally derived from the evaluation of PPD conversion studies, with one recent review reporting an overall incidence of PPD positivity 100 times higher in HCWs versus that found in the general population [25]. Risk of TB infection significantly increases when clinical procedures that produce large amounts of aerosol are performed, such as induced sputum or intubation [26]. ED staff reportedly have PPD conversion rates up to six times higher than other hospital workers, with rates of conversion ranging from 1% to 12% [27]. Principal explanations for the high rates of ED HCW PPD conversion include the high frequency of atypical presentations for patients with TB at initial presentation, the lack of consistent implementation of triage screening for TB, and the lack of availability of adequate infection control facilities in EDs [21].

Public health interventions

Interventional approaches to TB control can be primary, secondary, or tertiary. Consistent application of simple public health measures can convert the ED from a site that represents a high-risk venue for further disease transmission, to one that can improve disease prevention, recognition, and control. The principles of TB control described in the 1994 Centers for Disease Control and Prevention (CDC) guidelines for hospitals and other health care facilities encompass three areas of intervention: administrative, engineering, and use of personal protective equipment (PPE) [28]. Although there are no specific guidelines for TB control provided by the American College of Emergency Physicians (ACEP), most texts use the CDC guidelines as a standard [28].

Administrative interventions include development of methods to ensure early isolation of persons with suspected disease, development of hospital-wide TB control plans, and maintenance of an active PPD skin-testing program among HCWs. Engineering controls focus on handing of air: negative-pressure respiratory isolation rooms, UV light fixtures, and HEPA (high-efficiency particulate air) filters [29]. PPE involves routine use of the N-95 particulate respirator for HCWs who are in close contact with suspected cases. Several studies conducted since 1994 have demonstrated that adherence to these guidelines significantly increases identification of cases and reduces disease transmission in HCWs [16,23]. For example, the introduction of TB control measures including engineering upgrades and improved access to PPE in one inner-city ED resulted in a nearly sixfold diminution in PPD conversion among HCWs [16]. Similar administrative and facilities improvement in another high-risk ED resulted in decreased wait times and increased rates of appropriate isolation for ED patients with suspected TB [23].

Development of methods for rapid identification of cases of TB at ED triage has met with mixed results. One study that evaluated the use of a simple triage guideline found that the sensitivity and specificity of their screening tool was only 63% and 78%, respectively [30]. Explanations for the relatively low sensitivity of the tool included lack of consistent compliance with guideline implementation and failure of a subset of patients to report key risk factors and symptoms at ED triage (which were elicited later during the ED evaluation). An alternate TB screening tool that was retrospectively derived from a population of culture-positive cases had a much higher sensitivity (96%) [31]. The final decision instrument involved assigning a 1-point score to each of several variables (abnormal chest x-ray, temperature greater than 101°F, homeless/shelter dwelling, and TB history), with a positive screen assigned to any patient with more than 2 points. The principal limitation of this method, which restricts applicability for triage decision making, is the need for chest radiographic findings to assign a score. However, the tool may be appropriate for determining need for isolation.

A tertiary public health intervention for TB control involves routine PPD testing in ED patients. The one study conducted to date to evaluate the feasibility of this approach reports promising findings. Sixty percent of eligible patients consented to testing, and more than half returned for follow-up, which is comparable to that seen in other public health venues [32]. Optimal strategies for targeted screening found that it is possible to identify a "high-risk" group, which would identify nearly 90% of cases while testing only about 50% of the ED population. Although promising, further research is required to evaluate the cost-effectiveness of this strategy.

General principles for management of patients with suspected TB for emergency physicians include maintaining a high index of suspicion and immediately providing a mask (to decrease rates of transmission) to any patients with TB risk factors or suspected symptoms. Early chest radiography should then be performed and implementation of full airborne precautions should be established for any patients with suggestive findings on radiographs or high clinical suspicion of disease. High-risk clinical procedures that will aerosolize *M tuberculosis* should be minimized as much as possible in the ED unless isolation facilities with proper ventilation are available [33].

Influenza

Epidemiology and pathophysiology

Influenza is a seasonal disease that occurs in the winter months, with the vast majority of cases reported from November through March. Annual outbreaks and sporadic pandemics result in significant morbidity and mortality. Globally, epidemics of influenza result in 3 to 5 million cases of severe illness and approximately 250,000 to 500,000 deaths each year. In the United States, influenza accounts for more than 100,000 hospitalizations and nearly 40,000 deaths each year, the majority occurring in susceptible populations, the elderly, or the very young [34].

During the past century, three pandemics (global epidemics) of influenza have occurred. The "Spanish flu" in 1918 to 1919 was responsible for 40 million deaths worldwide, and 650,000 in the United States. More recent pandemics, which have had less impact in the United States, include the "Asian flu" 1957 to 1958 (34,000 deaths in the United States), and the "Hong Kong flu" 1968 to 1969 (70,000 US deaths) [35]. In contrast to the annual epidemics of influenza, deaths during influenza pandemics frequently occur in young, otherwise healthy, individuals [36].

Influenza is a single-stranded RNA virus, which belongs to the family Orthomyxoviridae. There are three major types of influenza viruses (A, B, and C), which are structurally similar but vary antigenically. Only Types A and B cause infections in humans. Influenza A is more common and virulent than B and is divided into subtypes based on viral surface antigens hemagglutinin and neuraminidase. "Antigenic drift" is produced by point mutations in the viral antigen that occur during viral replication and result in slightly different, new strains of influenza for which there is diminished immunologic recognition. "Antigenic shift" is a sudden major change in the surface peptides that occurs when two different strains of influenza infect the same individual simultaneously. This results in mixing of the surface antigens and a new subtype of influenza for which humans have little or no protective immunity. All of the recent influenza pandemics were caused by antigenic shift [37].

In 1997, the avian strain A (H5N1), the first avian virus known to have been transmitted directly from birds to humans [38], began to appear in several Asian nations [39,40]. This strain has proven to be highly virulent with nearly 200 deaths reported to date worldwide. Although several family clusters of avian influenza suggest that human-to-human transmission may have occurred, there is no evidence that efficient transmission can occur via this route [41–43]. Significant public health concern exists regarding reassortment of avian influenza with the human virus, which could then produce a strain of flu that would be both extremely virulent and contagious, potentially triggering the next pandemic [44].

Influenza A and B can be transmitted from person to person via a number of routes including (1) direct or indirect contact with contaminated articles; (2) droplet (>10 μm) transmission produced by release of contagious droplets produced by coughing or sneezing by an infected host, resulting in contact with the nasal mucosa, conjunctiva, or mouth of another person; or (3) airborne transmission leading to inhalation of small (<5 μm) nuclei that remain suspended in the air and can be disseminated by air currents [4]. Evidence exists that transmission may begin 1 to 6 days before the onset of symptoms, and that viral shedding and human infectivity may persist for several weeks, particularly among those who are immunocompromised.

Clinical presentation, diagnosis, and treatment

In adults the classic presentation of influenza is abrupt onset of high fever, myalgia, headache, and malaise, with accompanying respiratory symptoms (cough, sore throat, and rhinitis). In children, otitis media, nausea, and vomiting are also common [45]. Unfortunately, these signs and symptoms are highly nonspecific, making ED diagnosis challenging. One recent systematic review reported that no individual or combination of clinical signs and symptoms can reliably confirm or exclude the diagnosis of influenza [46]. Data from a recent ED-based study supporting this conclusion noted that more than 50% of laboratory-confirmed cases of influenza had atypical or nonclassic symptoms on presentation (particularly among those with comorbid conditions) [47]. Therefore, it is recommended that physicians be aware of both local and national epidemiologic data to determine if influenza is in a particular community, and then have a low index of suspicion for consideration of this disease [46]. With increasing concern about other acute communicable respiratory illnesses, emergency physicians should also be aware of new and evolving algorithms that may help clinicians differentiate common influenza from avian influenza, SARS, anthrax, or other emergent biothreats [48].

Suspected cases of influenza can either be managed empirically or have rapid testing performed to assist with treatment decision making. The value of diagnostic testing has been well described and includes limiting use of unnecessary antibiotics, more specific use of antivirals, identification of atypical cases of disease, decreased length of ED stay, and improved surveillance by local and state health departments regarding presence, subtype, and strain of influenza [47,49]. Clinical data supporting routine testing is more compelling in children than adults [50,51], although testing is advised by the CDC during suspected influenza outbreaks as part of the broader surveillance and public health strategy aimed at controlling the spread of disease in a health care facility. Laboratory tests currently available include rapid antigen testing, polymerase chain reaction (PCR), immunofluorescence, serology, and viral culture from various types of respiratory specimens (nasopharyngeal swab, throat swab, nasal wash, nasal aspirate, sputum, and bronchial wash) or serum. Commercially available rapid tests can provide results in the ED within 30 minutes. Performance characteristics of the tests are variable, but generally sensitivity is greater than 70% and specificity is greater than 90%. The CDC recognizes the limited sensitivity of the rapid test and recommends that samples should always be sent for viral culture, which is considered gold standard confirmation with viral culture [45].

Definitive laboratory diagnosis of influenza is not absolutely required for management [46], and many ED texts recommended using laboratory testing only in those instances where testing would influence treatment decisions [52]. Thus, in the midst of a known influenza outbreak, a patient with typical signs and symptoms who can be managed with empiric therapy need not be subjected to testing. Instances in which laboratory testing may be indicated include cases in which the diagnosis is in doubt (because of early or late seasonal presentation or atypical clinical presentation) or in those cases where treatment decisions may be aided by a definitive test (eg, those patients in whom complications of untreated influenza are more likely) [53]. The most common complications associated with influenza are primary influenza viral pneumonia and secondary bacterial pneumonia. Other less frequent complications include encephalopathy, transverse myelitis, Reye's syndrome, myositis, myocarditis, and pericarditis.

General guidelines regarding treatment issued by the CDC in 2004 to 2005 are as follows: CDC encourages the use oseltamivir or zanamivir for treatment as supplies allow, in part to minimize the development of adamantane resistance (used for prophylaxis) among circulating influenza viruses. Treatment with antiviral medication is advised for (1) any person experiencing a potentially life-threatening influenza-related illness, and (2) any person at high risk for serious complications of influenza and who is within the first 2 days of illness. Prompt diagnosis and treatment also has the beneficial effect of reducing the duration of host infectivity. (Pregnant women should consult with their primary providers regarding use of influenza antiviral medications. Further details and the most up-to-date treatment and prophylaxis recommendations can be found on the CDC Web site).

Disease burden in the ED

During flu season, influenza is one of the leading causes of ED visits, especially among children and among adults aged 65 and older [54]. Several US- and Canadian-based studies that evaluated emergency medical system (EMS) diversion as a proxy for ED overcrowding have reported high correlations between influenza season and EMS diversion [55,56]. Another study, conducted in Europe during peak flu season, found that approximately one third of all ED visits for children younger than 1 year of age were attributable to influenza [57]. Although several nosocomial outbreaks of influenza in health care workers have been documented, there has been relatively little research describing transmission in the ED. One study conducted in an acute-care hospital during the 1986 to 1987 flu season found that one third of Influenza A cases identified could be traced to the ED, and that the estimated nosocomial influenza attack rate was 0.3 per 100 hospital admissions [58]. The ED thus represents a high-risk location for nosocomial transmission.

Public health interventions

Several interventions help to decrease the likelihood of individuals contracting influenza and lessen the likelihood and burden of a public health crisis associated with an influenza outbreak. The principal known preventive measure is routine and widespread use of vaccination [59]. Current CDC recommendations for populations to vaccinate include adults aged 65 years and older; persons aged 2 to 64 years with underlying chronic medical conditions; all women who will be pregnant during the influenza season; residents of nursing homes and long-term care facilities; children aged 2 to 18 years on chronic aspirin therapy; health care workers involved in direct patient care; and out-of-home caregivers and household contacts of children aged younger than 6 months [60].

Several studies lend support for using the ED settings for routine influenza immunization [61]. Data demonstrate high rates of ED visits for unimmunized individuals who are at high risk for influenza (eg, nursing home patients and the elderly) as well as moderate to high rates of physician and patient acceptability for ED-based immunization [62–66]. One recent randomized clinical trial comparing on-site ED-based vaccination to education and referral demonstrated that ED-based vaccination was significantly more efficacious both for pediatric patients as well as their accompanying family members [67]. Other potential vaccination strategies that remain relatively unexplored include use of EMS [68] either as a routine preventive measure or in the event of an epidemic outbreak. In the wake of the flu vaccine shortage, and in preparation for future inevitable influenza outbreaks, the ACEP issued a policy statement in 2004 highlighting ED priorities during suspected or known influenza outbreaks (Box 1) [69].

Severe Acute Respiratory Syndrome (SARS)

Epidemiology and pathophysiology

The first documented cases of SARS occurred in November of 2002, in the Guangdong Province of China, initially presenting as an atypical pneumonia [70,71]. Over the next several months, a surge in cases of pneumonia were reported in the surrounding regions, with a disproportionate number of hospital workers affected and several unexpected deaths [72]. Months

---

Box 1. Use of the emergency department during outbreaks of influenza (approved by the ACEP board of directors November 2004)

1. Ensure that emergency care and critical providers, including emergency medical services (EMS) personnel, nurses, and ancillary staff involved in direct patient care, are immunized against influenza.
2. Implement rapid screening, identification, and appropriate respiratory infection control interventions for all individuals arriving in the ED.
3. End the practice of boarding admitted patients in the ED when no inpatient beds are available. Hospitals operating at full capacity may be required to distribute boarded patients to inpatient hallways, solariums, admission units, and other spaces outside the ED, but this practice is preferable to packing seriously ill influenza patients together in the hallways of an ED.
4. Implement regional protocols to monitor hospital inpatient and ED capacity, as well as ambulance diversion status.
5. Adopt regional protocols to govern when, how, why, and for how long crowded hospital Eds can divert inbound ambulances.
6. Require hospitals and communities that are severely affected by influenza to postpone elective admissions until the crisis abates.
7. Provide federal and state emergency funding to compensate hospitals and EDs for the unreimbursed costs of meeting this grave public health challenge.

From American College of Emergency Physicians. Emergency Department Utilization During Outbreaks of Influenza. Policy #400558, approved November 2004; with permission.

after the initial case of this atypical pneumonia, a physician from Guangdong traveled to Hong Kong, infecting up to 16 others during a brief hotel stay. This triggered a global pandemic with outbreaks in Hong Kong, Singapore, Vietnam, and Canada [73,74]. In spite of early evidence that these illnesses represented an emerging infectious disease (based on number of cases, lack of responsiveness to standard therapy, and high transmissibility), hospitals were generally slow to implement respiratory isolation procedures. It was not until several hundred more cases were reported that the World Health Organization (WHO) issued a global health alert, resulting in establishment of an international laboratory reporting network and standardized protocols for infection containment [75]. These measures contributed to the definitive identification of SARS (a novel previously uncharacterized Coronavirus) as the causative pathogen [73,76].

The peak period of the SARS pandemic occurred in late 2002 and early 2003, during which time cases were reported in more than 25 countries spanning five continents. Although the exact number of cases is unknown, it is estimated that there have been more than 8000 probable cases, and 774 deaths as of July 2003, at which time human-to-human transmission was essentially contained [77,78]. The largest number of SARS cases have occurred in mainland China, Hong Kong, Taiwan, and Canada (where a significant outbreak occurred in the city of Toronto). In the United States, there have been 29 cases of probable SARS, all of which have been linked with preceding international travel to an endemic area [79,80]. There have been no US SARS-attributable deaths to date. Sporadic cases of SARS continue to be reported. Four cases were reported in Guangdong in late 2003; three separate laboratory-related incidents were reported in Singapore, Taiwan, and China, one of which resulted in a small contained community outbreak [81].

Clinical presentation, diagnosis, and treatment

Clinical symptoms associated with SARS typically emerge 2 to 10 days after an exposure, with a mean incubation period of 5 days in most infected individuals. Initial clinical presentation and the clinical course of patients with SARS is variable and generally nonspecific, making diagnosis challenging [82]. Since definitive diagnosis relies on advanced laboratory testing, ED consideration of SARS must rely on having a high clinical suspicion, which should be guided by history (focusing on potential exposure), characteristic clinical features, and laboratory and radiographic findings as described in the following paragraphs.

During the first stage of infection, patients infected with SARS typically present with flu-like symptoms. The most common finding on initial presentation is fever (greater than 38°C), although exceptions occur in the elderly and in those with chronic underlying illness. Other clinical features occurring in more than 50% of cases include chills, rigors, cough, and myalgias. Less frequent but also commonly appearing are rhinorrhea, dyspnea, watery nonbloody diarrhea, and headache [74,83–85].

Common laboratory findings associated with SARS including lymphopenia, thrombocytopenia, derangements in clotting profiles, and various electrolyte abnormalities. The majority of patients with SARS have abnormal radiographs. The most common chest x-ray finding in a patient with SARS is a unilateral infiltrate early on, followed by bilateral interstitial or confluent infiltrates. These findings are usually indistinguishable from viral or atypical pneumonias. One study suggests that the presence of an air-space opacity on chest radiographs may be a helpful early diagnostic clue to SARS [86].

For public health surveillance purposes, WHO defines a clinical case of SARS as an individual with (1) a history of fever, or documented fever ≥38°C (100.4°F); (2) one or more symptoms of lower respiratory tract illness (cough, difficulty breathing, shortness of breath); (3) radiographic evidence of lung infiltrates consistent with pneumonia or acute respiratory distress syndrome (ARDS), or autopsy findings consistent with the pathology of pneumonia or ARDS without an identifiable cause; and (4) no alternative diagnosis that can fully explain the illness [87].

Laboratory testing for SARS should include both respiratory and blood samples. Laboratory diagnosis can be made by any one of three assays according to WHO standards: (1) any of one nucleic acid test for the SARS-CoV in two specimens or two nucleic acid tests in one specimen; (2) seroconversion by ELISA or IFA (immunofluoresence assay); or (3) isolation of the SARS-CoV using validated testing methods and appropriate quality assurance mechanisms [87].

Approximate 20% to 30% of SARS cases require treatment in the intensive care unit. The case fatality rate of SARS is estimated at approximately 10% to 15% globally, with increased rates seen in older patients with comorbid disease [83] The clinical course of disease can be mild to fulminant. Respiratory decompensation typically occurs in a week to 10 days, although some patients may have a more rapid progression requiring intubation at the time of initial presentation. In one of the largest SARS cohorts from Hong Kong, a triphasic progression of disease was described: phase 1 is a brief period of malaise, fever, and flu-like symptoms, which resolves with antibiotics; phase 2 occurs several days later and is characterized by recurrent fevers, diarrhea, oxygen desaturation, and progression of x-ray findings; only a small subset of patients (approximately 20%) progress to phase 3, which is marked by severe sepsis and multiorgan system failure, most notably ARDS [85].

Disease burden in the ED

Transmission of SARS from infected patients to health care workers, visitors, and other patients was well documented during the SARS pandemic [88]. Early on it was recognized that overcrowded, understaffed emergency departments with limited resources represent extremely high-risk sites for disease transmission [89–94]. One study that tracked 322 SARS patients in Beijing, China, found that of all heath care workers, ED staff had the highest attack rate (11.9%) [95]. Another detailed epidemiologic investigation from Toronto found that transmission of SARS to ED staff who had contact with SARS patients ranged from 0% to 22%, with a calculated attack rate of 13.6 per 1000 nursing hours, exceeding that found in the ICU [94]. Factors believed to contribute to the high rates of contagion in the ED included difficulty with early identification and isolation of patients (particularly those with atypical symptoms), use of aerosol treatments for patients with respiratory symptoms in the ED, and poor compliance with basic (ie, hand washing) and other recognized public health control measures for reducing transmission of respiratory infections [96]. Implementation and adherence with systematic preventive measures resulted in significant reduction of disease transmission throughout the world, and are discussed further below [92,97].

Public health interventions

The 2003 SARS pandemic forced a widespread shift in thinking regarding the role of the ED, from that of emergent treatment and stabilization of patients with acute illnesses, to central coordination of a public health response plan in the face of an emerging pandemic [92,98]. Recognition that EDs serve as the primary portal of entry for patients with a highly contagious and potentially lethal disease was paramount to the development of rationale and well-organized infection control programs [99].

One recent comprehensive literature review describes the cumulative experiences of hospitals and health care organizations [100]. SARS was found to be spread principally by the respiratory droplet route, making PPE use the mainstay of infection control. While use of N95 masks offers theoretical advantages over surgical masks, no studies have documented significant additional benefits in patient care settings. Importantly, consistent compliance with PPE has been proven to decrease risk of disease transmission. Indirect evidence from "super-spreading" events in hospitals has suggested that SARS may be aerosolized [101,102]. Infectious disease experts advise that special care should be taken to decrease aerosol-generating procedures as much as possible and to observe additional precautions when these procedures are necessary. Recommended environmental interventions include placing surgical masks on patients with suspected SARS at triage and during transport, limiting the movement of patients with suspected SARS, and making use of physical isolation measures, including warding and use of negative-pressure isolation rooms when available [103]. Successful policies for containment of SARS in EDs demand strict attention and enforcement of ED operational protocols (including procedures for recycling of supplies and equipment, and guidelines for optimization of patient and staff traffic) [97]. The SARS outbreak exemplified the need for modified ED staffing owing to the increased demands of patient care that occurred during the period of the greatest disease threat and burden [98].

Secondary prevention measures for SARS have involved methods for early disease detection. Early detection requires a reliable definition of cases. The WHO definition of SARS cases, although useful for epidemiologic purposes, was found to be insufficiently sensitive for assessing patients in ED triage areas. Consequently, physicians had to develop clinical prediction rules that could more accurately identify patients with SARS during an acute outbreak [104–107]. One group from Taiwan derived a simple SARS decision rule that relied on combinations of symptoms and laboratory findings. The scores were reported to have greater than 90% sensitivity and were found to be highly reliable when validated in a separate cohort [105,107]. A more recent study from Hong Kong, which included nearly one third of the SARS cases from 2003, reported similar results with key variables including exposure history, symptoms, and laboratory values [104]. Although determination of which prediction rule will be most effective is not known, these studies provide compelling support for integration of ED-based decision guidelines in future respiratory outbreaks. Potential gains include early identification and isolation of high-risk patients, reduction of disease transmission in the ED, and optimization of use of limited resources. Principal limitations of these decision tools include lack of proven reliability in nonendemic areas and the need for validation with each new outbreak, based on potential strain and geographic variation that may alter clinical presentation.

Future challenges

Dr Anthony Fauci, director of the National Institutes of Allergy and Infectious Diseases, suggests that SARS teaches a valuable lesson: it demonstrates the ever-present threat of emerging and reemerging infectious diseases [108]. Dr Fauci and Dr Julie Gerberding, director of the CDC, emphasize the importance of a strong public health preparedness and response system, which in addition to use of personal and environmental infection control parameters includes a system capable of early detection [109].

As the frontline of the health care system, the nation's EDs are receiving renewed recognition as pivotal sites for early detection surveillance systems. A number of national surveillance systems were put in place largely in response to the 2003 SARS outbreak. Effective disease control will require a reliable national surveillance program, as well as consistency in local hospital-based education, and practice of proven risk-reduction measures.

Biothreat (BT) agents

General principles

A civilian target in a bioterrorism act has the potential to create a large number of casualties, civil panic, and disruption. Early detection and preattack preparedness is central to any response. Timely, coordinated intervention triggered by early recognition will result in improved patient outcome, disease containment, preservation of the medical infrastructure, and effective law enforcement responses. This is evidenced by the lowest fatality rate ever recorded for inhalational anthrax following the 2001 bioterrorist attacks in the United States.

Serving in the frontline, emergency physicians play a critical role in responding to such an attack. Early recognition requires prior knowledge of typical clinical syndromes of the various bioterrorism agents. However, diagnosis of index cases may be difficult as clinical presentations of the BT agents are generally nonspecific, and laboratory confirmations are often delayed for these otherwise rare disease entities. ED-based syndromic surveillance systems with autonomous sensing and reporting capabilities can provide early warning and earlier recognition of suspicious patterns. Epidemiologic patterns peculiar to a biological attack, which can help differentiate it from a natural outbreak of disease, include (1) an extraordinary number of patients arriving from a similar geographical area with similar symptoms and acuity; (2) rapid rise and fall of epidemic curves over a short period of time (hours to days); (3) steady rise in cases instead of peaks and troughs seen in natural outbreaks; (4) rapidly fatal cases; (5) a lower attack rate in people who were indoors than in those who were outdoors; and (6) increased infected and dying animals [110].

Once a bioterrorist attack is suspected, the first order of business is to initiate early protective infection control measures (eg, contact, droplet, or airborne precautions) and identify the causal agent. Local- and state-level health care authorities should be notified immediately. As soon as the attack has been confirmed, prompt therapy, postexposure prophylaxis, and vaccination should be initiated. Advance preparation for EDs will be essential in mitigating the effects of a bioterrorist attack. Key components of a bioterrorism response plan should include (1) specific guidelines for plan activation and notification of proper authorities; (2) facility protection from contamination and secondary transmission; (3) methods of decontamination; (4) expansion of service capacity; (5) ensuring an adequate cache of medical supplies; (6) staff education and training; (7) incident command system for controlled management; and (8) coordination and communication with the surrounding community [111].

The CDC has divided biological agents that are critical biothreat agents into categories based on their risks for causing mass casualties [112]. Category A agents, the highest priority, represent organisms that pose a risk to national security because they can be easily disseminated or transmitted person-to-person, have a high risk of mortality, and have the potential to cause public panic and social disruption. These agents include *Bacillus anthracis* (anthrax), *Variola major* (smallpox), *Yersinia pestis* (plague), *Francisella tularensis* (tularemia), viral hemorrhagic agents, and *Clostridium botulinum* toxin. Other potential agents of concern but posing a less imminent threat were assigned to categories B or C. A comprehensive review of the individual BT is beyond the scope of this discussion.

The principal route of delivery of most BT agents is by the inhalation of aerosols, which in some cases may result in pulmonary manifestations, such as cough and sputum production, and can be easily mistaken for common respiratory illnesses. The spectrum of potential pulmonary consequences that result from these biothreat agents is broad and reflects the variety of agents that could be involved. Category A agents, which can be easily aerosolized for weaponization, include inhalational anthrax, pneumonic plague, inhalational tularemia, and viral hemorrhagic fever. Only a subset of these agents, specifically *Y pestis* and the viral hemorrhagic fever viruses, have the potential for secondary human-to-human spread through respiratory droplets or airborne transmission. Of note, despite its general lack of prominent respiratory symptoms, smallpox can also be highly contagious via droplet or airborne transmission of the virus. Other significant aerosolizable category B agents with pulmonary manifestations include *Coxiella burnetti* (Q fever), *Brucella* species (brucellosis), and *Burkholderia mallei* (glanders); however, only *B mallei* has the potential for human-to-human transmission. From the ED perspective, it is critical that patients who are suspected to be infected with such communicable agents be cared for in respiratory isolation for disease containment. Need for isolation should be determined by suspicion before definitive diagnosis. With these exigencies in mind, we will focus our discussion on pneumonic plague as an example of a communicable respiratory biothreat agent.

Yersinia pestis (plague)

Epidemiology and pathogenesis

Plague is a zoonosis with a rodent host and a flea vector, which is caused by the gram-negative bacillus, *Yersinia pestis*. Transmission to humans is from the bite of an infected rodent flea. The bacilli multiply intracellularly resulting in painful swollen regional lymph nodes called buboes. Septicemic plague and pneumonic plague can occur secondarily as a complication of hematogenous dissemination of bubonic plague. The vector is not essential for infection; however, inhalation of aerosolized bacillus from cough or deliberate dissemination can result in primary pneumonic plague.

Historically, plague was responsible for three pandemics, killing millions of people throughout the centuries. The most recent pandemic originated in China and spread worldwide at the turn of the twentieth century [113]. From 1987 to 2001, 36,876 plague cases were reported in 24 countries [114]. In the Western Hemisphere, the incidence of plague is highest in the Andes and the southwestern United States [115]. From 1916 to 1947, 390 cases of plague were reported in the United States, 84% of which were bubonic, 13% septicemic, and 2% pneumonic. Concomitant case fatality rates were 14%, 22%, 57%, respectively. Although pneumonic plague has rarely been the dominant manifestation of the disease, large outbreaks of pneumonic plague have occurred [116].

Advances in living conditions, public health, and antibiotic therapy make future pandemics improbable. However, outbreaks following use of plague as a biological weapon represent plausible threats. In World War II, plague-infected fleas bred by the billions were released over Chinese cities and resulted in multiple epidemics [117]. Of greater concern is that the biological weapons program by the former Soviet Union has reportedly developed techniques to aerosolize plague directly, eliminating the dependence on fleas as vectors [118]. In 1997, the WHO reported that in the worse case scenario, if 50 kg of *Y pestis* were released as an aerosol over a city of 5 million people, 150,000 cases of pneumonic plague would result, with 36,000 expected deaths [119].

Clinical presentation, diagnosis, and treatment

Inhalation of aerosolized *Y pestis* following a biothreat attack would result in primary pneumonic plague, which can be distinguished from secondary pneumonic plague by the absence of buboes. Infected patients may experience chest pain, progressive tachypnea and dyspnea, productive cough (sputum may be watery, frothy, blood-tinged, hemorrhagic, or purulent), and hypoxia. Prominent gastrointestinal symptoms, such as nausea, vomiting, and diarrhea, may be present. Pneumonic plague is a fulminant process with rapid progression to exudative pulmonary consolidation and respiratory failure [120]. Many patients with pneumonia develop profound septic shock with multiorgan system failure. Inhalation of infectious aerosol may also produce plague pharyngitis, with focal suppuration and prominent cervical buboes. Plague pneumonia is almost always fatal if treatment is not initiated within 24 hours of the onset of symptoms.

Early diagnosis of individual cases requires a high index of suspicion, especially in areas without endemic, zoonotic plague. Clinical suspicion of pneumonic plague in the context of a bioterrorist attack may be based on presentation of many patients with rapidly progressive pneumonia with hemoptysis. There are no pathognomonic radiographic characteristics of primary pneumonic plague. In primary infections radiographic signs usually begin as localized unilateral alveolar infiltrates that quickly advance to patchy, diffuse, and bilateral pneumonitis; in secondary pneumonic cases infiltrates are mostly bilateral, involving lower lung fields [121]. Early presumptive diagnosis can be made by Gram, Wright-Giemsa, or direct fluorescent antibody (DFA) staining of peripheral blood, sputum, or lymph node aspirates that will reveal a bipolar "safety pin" morphology that distinguishes plague bacilli from other gram-negative organisms. The first clinical or laboratory suspicion of plague should lead to immediate notification of the hospital epidemiologist or infection control specialist, hospital and reference laboratories, local and state health departments, and the CDC. Confirmation of *Y pestis* is made by culture, serology, or PCR.

Parenteral aminoglycosides (eg, streptomycin or gentamicin) are considered first-line plague therapy [120]. Doxycycline or ciprofloxacin are recommended for postexposure prophylaxis or in mass casualty settings. All persons developing a fever (>38.5°C) or new cough should be promptly treated with parenteral antibiotics. Close contacts with untreated pneumonic plague should receive postexposure antibiotics for 7 days. A vaccine is available, but it is not protective against pneumonic plague [122].

Public health interventions

The available evidence indicates that person-to-person transmission of pneumonic plague is through respiratory droplet, not droplet nuclei. Accordingly, routine protection from respiratory droplets, including mask, eye protection, gowns, and gloves should be used by medical personnel attending infected patients who have not been on antibiotics for at least 48 hours. Exposed persons who refuse to take antibiotic prophylaxis but who are not symptomatic do not require isolation but need to be watched and treated when the first sign of cough or fever occurs. Microbiology laboratory personnel should practice biosafety level 3 precautions when handling potentially infectious samples during high-risk laboratory procedures.

Measles

Despite recent attention toward emerging and biothreat pathogens, viruses that have coexisted with the human population for hundreds of years continue to have a profound, worldwide impact. Measles virus is one such virus. It is highly contagious via the respiratory route. Although effective vaccines have been available for more than 40 years, measles remains one of the most frequent causes of vaccine-preventable childhood death, with the greatest mortality seen in poor regions of the world where adequate vaccine coverage has not been achieved [123]. Even in developed nations, endemic outbreaks of measles can be reestablished following an importation from foreign countries if high immunization coverage is not sustained. In addition to disease surveillance for outbreak control, emergency physicians can play a pivotal role in outbreak prevention by identifying underimmunized individuals who often use the ED as their principal source of primary care.

Epidemiology and pathophysiology

In 2001, the WHO estimated a global incidence of 39.9 million measles cases, 777,000 deaths, and 28 million disability-adjusted life years [124]. About half of these deaths occurred in Africa, in which fewer than 50% of children aged 1 year have received at least one dose of measles vaccine. Factors that contribute to the high case-fatality rates in developing countries include crowding, poor nutritional state, occurrence of infection at young age, underlying immune deficiency disorders, and limited access to health care. In 2001, the WHO and United Nations Children's Fund (UNICEF) established the goal of reducing measles deaths by 50% by 2005 (compared with 1999 estimates) through mass vaccination campaigns worldwide [124]. As a result, global measles mortality decreased by 39% between 1999 and 2003, with the largest gains (46%) occurring in the African regions [125]. In the United States, routine measles vaccination has been part of a childhood immunization program since 1963, resulting in a downward trend in the incidence of disease. However, resurgence occurred between 1989 and 1991 because of low vaccination coverage. Since 1997, the incidence of measles in the United States has been sustained at record low levels of approximately 100 cases per year [126]. Unfortunately, efforts toward measles eradication in the US have been challenged by the continued high prevalence of measles outside our borders, as evidenced by identification of imported viral genotypes among the majority of incident US cases [127]. Efforts to ensure high immunization rates among people in both developed and developing countries must be sustained to control measles worldwide.

Clinical presentation, diagnosis, and treatment

Infection is acquired via the respiratory tract. Primary viremia occurs 2 to 3 days after exposure. Subsequent infection of the reticuloendothelial system results in secondary viremia with skin and respiratory tract manifestations after an incubation period of 10 to 12 days. The clinical prodrome is characterized by fever and is followed by the onset of cough, coryza, and conjunctivitis. Koplik's spots, lesions on the buccal mucosa, occur 1 to 2 days before the onset of rash. The measles rash occurs 2 to 4 days after the prodrome, and is usually first noted on the face and neck, before gradually spreading downward and outward to the trunk and extremities. Maculopapular lesions are generally discrete, but may become confluent. Fine desquamation may occur, and the rash fades in the same order that it appears, from head to extremities.

The diagnosis of measles can usually be made on clinical grounds. Isolation of the measles virus is not recommended as a routine. However, as with influenza, virus isolates are important for molecular epidemiologic surveillance to help determine the geographic origin of the virus. A serologic test, most commonly by enzyme-linked immunoassay, can be used to establish the diagnosis. A fourfold rise in titer of IgG antibody to measles virus, or a positive result of serological testing for measles IgM antibody is considered diagnostic.

Complications from measles can involve every organ system, and the rates of complication vary by age and underlying conditions. Complications are more common among children under age 5 and adults over 20 years of age. Pneumonia is the most common fatal complication associated with measles, occurring in 56% to 86% of measles-related deaths [128]. Pneumonia may be caused by the measles virus alone or secondary viral or bacterial infection [129]. The prevalence of measles virus pneumonia is higher in pregnant women and patients who are immunocompromised as a result of hematologic malignancy, AIDS, or immunosuppressive therapy [130]. Chest radiographic findings may include infiltrates, consolidations, hilar lymph node enlargement, and pleural effusions.

Treatment of the primary disease is mainly supportive. Bacterial superinfection should be promptly treated with appropriate antimicrobials, but prophylactic antibiotics to prevent superinfection are of no known value and are therefore not recommended. Vitamin A administration has been shown to reduce mortality, severity, and duration of complications in children with measles [131]. Immunocompromised children and infants younger than 1 year of age who are susceptible and have been exposed to measles may be given passive immunization within 6 days of exposure.

Public health interventions

Transmission of measles is primarily person-to-person via large respiratory droplets; however, airborne transmission via aerosolized droplet nuclei has been documented. Maximum communicability occurs from onset of prodrome through the initial 3 to 4 days of rash [132]. Although suspected patients should be placed in respiratory isolation to preclude airborne transmission, isolation and quarantine procedures may be of limited value given that exposure usually occurs before diagnosis is made, and the availability of passive immunization or vaccination of susceptible contacts has obviated quarantine.

The measles virus is an RNA virus belonging to the genus *Morbillivirus* in the family Paramyxoviridae. It has only one serotype and can, therefore, be prevented with a single monovalent vaccine. Measles vaccine is one of the safest and most effective of all vaccines [133]. It is a live attenuated vaccine, which is frequently given in a combined product with rubella vaccine (as MR vaccine) or with rubella and mumps vaccine (as MMR vaccine). Immunization produces a nontransmissible, asymptomatic infection. Approximately 5% of children who receive only one dose of MMR vaccine will remain susceptible owing to primary vaccine failure, but after a second immunization, more than 99% of vaccinees develop serologic evidence of measles immunity, which can be lifelong [134]. Recent experience has demonstrated that prevention of endemic outbreaks with single-dose vaccination is not possible even with high vaccination coverage, a two-dose vaccine schedule is thus recommended [135]. The first dose of MMR should be given on or after a child's first birthday, and the second dose may be given as soon as 1 month after the first, but should routinely be given at age 4 to 6 years. Postexposure prophylaxis with vaccination within 72 hours or passive immunization within 6 days of exposure should be given to susceptible contacts (ie, persons exposed and not fully vaccinated). All health care workers are at high risk for exposure and should be adequately vaccinated.

Prevention and control of vaccine-preventable disease outbreaks require that disease transmission be interrupted by sustained high levels of immunization (greater than 95% for measles). As part of the effort to ensure high immunization rates, EDs may be well suited to capture nonimmunized children because they are often the primary sources of medical care for many of the urban poor who are considered the highest risk for underimmunization. Several studies have evaluated EDs as potential sites for routine vaccination and for accelerated vaccine delivery during outbreaks, with limited success [136,137]. Major barriers with measles vaccination have included high costs, lack of continuity, and difficulty in determining the true immunization status of patients [138,139]. Until these barriers are effectively addressed, ED providers can contribute to measles control by screening and referring underimmunized children to private or public health clinics in the community for vaccination. As with all emerging or reemerging infectious diseases, ED-based surveillance (which relies on early recognition and reporting of suspected cases) plays a key role in outbreak control.

Evolving approaches to prevention in the ED

Primary and secondary prevention are recognized as the most effective measures for containing infectious disease outbreaks. The role of EDs in instituting these preventive measures is rapidly evolving in response to increasing awareness of the critical role EDs serve as the initial encounter site for most patients with acute communicable infectious illnesses. Evidence and support for ED-based primary prevention strategies such as influenza vaccination or prophylaxis exists [67], although practical challenges regarding such issues as education, counseling, and sustainable funding present ongoing challenges. Secondary preventive measures using clinical decision rules to rapidly identify and sequester patients with diseases have also been demonstrated to be effective in ED settings [31,104], but are by no means failsafe; recognized limitations of decision guidelines include difficulties with ensuring routine and consistent application, and need to establish generalizability.

Disease surveillance is another method of secondary prevention that is recognized as a critical tool in prevention and control of communicable disease outbreaks (both natural and bioterrorist) [140]. The methodology involves continuous systematic collection, analysis, and interpretation of health-related data for timely dissemination to essential parties, who can then use this information for evaluating, planning, and implementing the most effective public health preventive measures [141]. Syndromic surveillance has been recognized to be especially applicable to airborne respiratory infections that can be insidious and highly contagious.

The ED serves as a rich, yet relatively untapped surveillance site that could contribute to control of respiratory infectious disease outbreaks. There are a large number of ED variables to track and evaluate, including ED ambulance diversion rates, numbers of ED patient visits by chief complaint, and ED discharge diagnosis and hospital/ICU admission rates [56,142]. The best-known ED-based surveillance network for infectious diseases, *EMERGEncy ID Net*, was established in the mid-1990s as a cooperative research and operational program involving the CDC, the National Center for Infectious Diseases, and about 12 university-based EDs throughout the United States [143]. The surveillance network monitoring activities are varied, but have shown the capacity to effectively monitor various infectious disease outbreaks, including methicillin-resistant skin infections and respiratory *M tuberculosis*. Public health surveillance based on ED data is further discussed in the chapter by Varney and Hirshon elsewhere in this issue.

Development and testing of novel molecular techniques for rapid real-time detection of infectious diseases is another evolving public heath approach for ED evaluation of aerosolized infectious diseases [144]. Rapid laboratory-based disease surveillance systems have the potential to detect infected individuals even before the onset of symptoms. This could represent one step ahead of traditional clinical syndromic surveillance. Although promising, further technical advancement in automation, optimization of detection, sensitivity and specificity is required before their true impact can be determined.

References

[1] Nelson K. Epidemiology of infectious disease: general principles. In: Nelson K, Williams C, Graham N, editors. Infectious disease epidemiology: theory and practice. Gaithersburg, MD: Aspen Publishers; 2000. p. 17–49.

[2] World Health Organization. World Health Organization: report on infectious diseases—removing obstacles to healthy development. Geneva, Switzerland: World Health Organization; 1999.

[3] Noah D, Fidas G. The global infectious disease threat and its implications for the United States. Washington, DC: US Central Intelligence Agency; 2000.

[4] Bridges C, Kuehnert M, Hall C. Transmission of influenza: implications for control in health care settings. Clin Infect Dis 2003;37(8):1094–101.

[5] Mausner J, Bahn A. Epidemiology: an introductory text. Philadelphia, PA: Saunders; 1974.

[6] Frieden T, Sterling T, Munsiff S, Watt C, Dye C. Tuberculosis. Lancet 2003;362(9387): 887–99.

[7] WHO. Global tuberculosis control—surveillance, planning, financing. WHO report 2005. Geneva, Switzerland: World Health Organization; 2005. WHO/HTM/TB/2005.349.

[8] CDC. Trends in tuberculosis—United States, 2004. MMWR Morb Mortal Wkly Rep 2005; 54(10):245–9.

[9] Blower S, Gerberding J. Understanding, predicting and controlling the emergence of drug-resistant tuberculosis: a theoretical framework. J Mol Med 1998;76(9):624–36.

[10] De Cock K, Chaisson R. Will DOTS do it? A reappraisal of tuberculosis control in countries with high rates of HIV infection. Int J Tuberc Lung Dis 1999;3(6):457–65.

[11] Coberly J, Chaisson R. Tuberculosis. In: Nelson K, Williams C, Graham N, editors. Infectious disease epidemiology: theory and practice. Gaithersburg, MD: Aspen Publishers; 2000. p. 411–37.

[12] Sokolove P, Rossman L, Cohen S. The emergency department presentation of patients with active pulmonary tuberculosis. Acad Emerg Med 2000;7(9):1056–60.

[13] Schluger N. The diagnosis of tuberculosis: what's old, what's new. Semin Respir Infect 2003;18(4):241–8.

[14] Sepkowtiz K. Tuberculosis control in the 21st century. Emerg Infect Dis 2001;7(2):259–62.

[15] Sepkowitz K. Occupationally acquired infections in health care workers. Part I. Ann Intern Med 1996;125(10):826–34.

[16] Behrman A, Shofer F. Tuberculosis exposure and control in an urban emergency department. Ann Emerg Med 1998;31(3):370–5.

[17] Dorevitch S, Forst L. The occupational hazards of emergency physicians. Am J Emerg Med 2000;18(3):300–11.

[18] Baker D, Stevens C, Brook R. Regular source of ambulatory care and medical care utilization by patients presenting to a public hospital emergency department. JAMA 1994; 271(24):1909–12.

[19] Baker D, Stevens C, Brook R. Determinants of emergency department use: are race and ethnicity important? Ann Emerg Med 1996;28(6):677–82.

[20] D'Amore J, Hung O, Chiang W, et al. The epidemiology of the homeless population and its impact on an urban emergency department. Acad Emerg Med 2001;8(11):1051–5.

[21] Moran G, Fuchs M, Jarvis W, et al. Tuberculosis infection—control practices in United States emergency departments. Ann Emerg Med 1995;26(3):283–9.

[22] Long R, Zielinski M, Kunimoto D, et al. The emergency department is a determinant point of contact of tuberculosis patients prior to diagnosis. Int J Tuberc Lung Dis 2002;6(4): 332–9.

[23] Stricof R, DiFerdinando GJ, Osten W, et al. Tuberculosis control in New York City hospitals. Am J Infect Control 1998;26(3):270–6.

[24] Moran G, McCabe F, Morgan M, et al. Delayed recognition and infection control for tuberculosis patients in the emergency department. Ann Emerg Med 1995;26(3):290–5.

[25] Menzies D, Fanning A, Yuan L, et al. Tuberculosis among health care workers. N Engl J Med 1995;332(2):92–8.

[26] Beggs C, Noakes C, Sleigh P, et al. The transmission of tuberculosis in confined spaces: an analytical review of alternative epidemiological models. Int J Tuberc Lung Dis 2003;7(11): 1015–26.

[27] Liss G, Khan R, Koven E, et al. Tuberculosis infection among staff at a Canadian community hospital. Infect Control Hosp Epidemiol 1996;17(1):29–35.

[28] CDC. Guidelines for preventing the transmission of Mycobacterium tuberculosis in health-care facilities, 1994. MMWR Recomm Rep 1994;43(RR-13):1–132.

[29] Sehulster L, Chinn R, HICPAC. Guidelines for environmental infection control in health-care facilities. Recommendations of CDC and the Healthcare Infection Control Practices Advisory Committee (HICPAC). MMWR Recomm Rep 2003;52(RR-10):1–42.

[30] Sokolove P, Lee B, Krawczyk J, et al. Implementation of an emergency department triage procedure for the detection and isolation of patients with active pulmonary tuberculosis. Ann Emerg Med 2002;35(4):327–36.

[31] Redd J, Susser E. Controlling tuberculosis in an urban emergency department: a rapid decision instrument for patient isolation. Am J Public Health 1997;87(9):1543–7.

[32] Kirsch T, Chanmugam A, Keyl P, et al. Feasibility of an emergency department-based tuberculosis counseling and screening program. Acad Emerg Med 1999;6(3):224–31.

[33] Talan D. Infectious disease issues in the emergency department. Clin Infect Dis 1996;23(1): 1–12.

[34] World Health Organization. Influenza. March 2003. Available at: http://www.who.int/ mediacentre/factsheets/2003/fs211/en/. Accessed July 1, 2005.

[35] Cox N, Subbarao K. Global epidemiology of influenza: past and present. Annu Rev Med 2000;51:407–21.

[36] CDC. Respiratory hygiene/cough etiquette in healthcare settings. December 17, 2003. Available at: http://www.cdc.gov/flu/professionals/infectioncontrol/resphygiene.htm. Accessed July 1, 2005.

[37] Scholtissek C. Source for influenza pandemics. Eur J Epidemiol 1994;10(4):455–8.

[38] CDC. Isolation of avian influenza A (H5N1) viruses from humans—Hong Kong, May– December 1997. MMWR Morb Mortal Wkly Rep 1997;46(50):1204–7.

[39] Monto A. The threat of an avian influenza pandemic. N Engl J Med 2005;352(4):323–5.

[40] Stohr K. Avian influenza and pandemics–research needs and opportunities. N Engl J Med 2005;352(4):405–7.

[41] Buxton Bridges C, Katz J, Seto W, et al. Risk of influenza A (H5N1) infection among health care workers exposed to patients with influenza A (H5N1), Hong Kong. J Infect Dis 2000; 181(1):344–8.

[42] Katz J, Lim W, Bridges C, et al. Antibody response in individuals infected with avian influenza A (H5N1) viruses and detection of anti-H5 antibody among household and social contacts. J Infect Dis 1999;180(6):1763–70.

[43] Ungchusak K, Auewarakul P, Dowell S, et al. Probable person-to-person transmission of avian influenza A (H5N1). N Engl J Med 2005;352(4):333–40.

[44] Kaye D, Pringle C. Avian influenza viruses and their implication for human health. Clin Infect Dis 2005;40(1):108–12.

[45] Harper S, Fukuda K, Uyeki T, et al. Prevention and control of influenza—recommendations of the Advisory Committee on Immunization Practices (ACIP). MMWR Recomm Rep 2004;53(RR-6):1–40.

[46] Call S, Vollenweider M, Hornung C, et al. Does this patient have influenza? JAMA 2005; 293(8):987–97.

[47] Monmany J, Rabella N, Margall N, et al. Unmasking influenza virus infection in patients attended to in the emergency department. Infection 2004;32(2):89–97.

[48] Cinti S, Saravolatz L, Nafziger D, et al. Differentiating inhalational anthrax from other influenza-like illnesses in the setting of a national or regional anthrax outbreak. Arch Intern Med 2004;164(6):674–6.

[49] Bonner A, Monroe K, Talley L, et al. Impact of the rapid diagnosis of influenza on physician decision-making and patient management in the pediatric emergency department: results of a randomized, prospective, controlled trial. Pediatrics 2003;112(2):363–7.

[50] Benich HW Jr. A cost-benefit analysis of testing for influenza A in high-risk adults. Ann Fam Med 2004;2(1):33–40.

[51] Rothberg M, He S, Rose D. Management of influenza symptoms in healthy adults. J Gen Intern Med 2004;18(10):808–15.

[52] Polis M, Haile-Mariam T. Viruses. In: Marx J, Hockberger R, Walls R, editors. Rosen's emergency medicine: concepts and clinical practice. 5th edition. St Louis: Mosby; 2002. p. 1812 33.

[53] Sharma V, Dowd M, Slaughter A, et al. Effect of rapid diagnosis of influenza virus type a on the emergency department management of febrile infants and toddlers. Arch Pediatr Adolesc Med 2002;156(1):41–3.

[54] Menec V, Black C, MacWilliam L, et al. The impact of influenza-associated respiratory illnesses on hospitalizations, physician visits, emergency room visits, and mortality. Can J Public Health 2003;94(1):59–63.

[55] Glaser C, Gilliam S, Thompson W, et al. Medical care capacity for influenza outbreaks, Los Angeles. Emerg Infect Dis 2002;8(6):569–74.

[56] Schull M, Mamdani M, Fang J. Community influenza outbreaks and emergency department ambulance diversion. Ann Emerg Med 2004;44(1):61–7.

[57] Ploin D, Liberas S, Thouvenot D, et al. Influenza burden in children newborn to eleven months of age in a pediatric emergency department during the peak of an influenza epidemic. Pediatr Infect Dis J 2003;22(10 Suppl):S218–22.

[58] Weingarten S, Friedlander M, Rascon D, et al. Influenza surveillance in an acute-care hospital. Arch Intern Med 1988;148(1):113–6.

[59] Nicholson K, Wood J, Zambon M. Influenza. Lancet 2003;362(9397):1733–45.

[60] CDC. Updated interim influenza vaccination recommendations—2004–05 influenza season. MMWR Morb Mortal Wkly Rep 2004;53(50):1183–4.

[61] Polis M, Smith J, Sainer D, et al. Prospects for an emergency department-based adult immunization program. Arch Intern Med 1987;147(11):1999–2001.

[62] Polis M, Davey V, Collins E, et al. The emergency department as part of a successful strategy for increasing adult immunization. Ann Emerg Med 1988;17(10):1016–8.

[63] Rodriguez R, Baraff L. Emergency department immunization of the elderly with pneumococcal and influenza vaccines. Ann Emerg Med 1993;22(11):1729–32.

[64] Wrenn K, Zeldin M, Miller O. Influenza and pneumococcal vaccination in the emergency department: is it feasible? J Gen Intern Med 1994;9(8):425–9.

[65] Kapur A, Tenenbein M. Vaccination of emergency department patients at high risk for influenza. Acad Emerg Med 2000;7(4):354–8.

[66] Slobodkin D, Zielske P, Kitlas J, et al. Demonstration of the feasibility of emergency department immunization against influenza and pneumococcus. Ann Emerg Med 1998;32(5):537–43.

[67] Pappano D, Humiston S, Goepp J. Efficacy of a pediatric emergency department-based influenza vaccination program. Arch Pediatr Adolesc Med 2004;158(11):1077–83.

[68] Mosesso VJ, Packer C, McMahon J, et al. Influenza immunizations provided by EMS agencies: the MEDICVAX Project. Prehosp Emerg Care 2003;7(1):74–8.

[69] The American College of Emergency Physicians (ACEP). Emergency department utilization during outbreaks of influenza. Available at: http://www.acep.org/webportal/PracticeResources/PolicyStatementsByCategory/PublicHealth/EmergencyDepartmentUtilizationOutbreaksInfluenza.htm. Accessed July 1, 2005.

[70] Xu R, He J, Evans M, et al. Epidemiologic clues to SARS origin in China. Emerg Infect Dis 2004;10(6):1030–7.

[71] Rosling L, Rosling M. Pneumonia causes panic in Guangdong province. BMJ 2003;326(7386):416.

[72] Zhong N, Zheng B, Li Y, et al. Epidemiology and cause of severe acute respiratory syndrome (SARS) in Guangdong, People's Republic of China, in February, 2003. Lancet 2003;362(9393):1353–8.

[73] Ksiazek T, Erdman D, Goldsmith C, et al. A novel coronavirus associated with severe acute respiratory syndrome. N Engl J Med 2003;348(20):1953–66.

[74] Poon L, Guan Y, Nicholls J, et al. The aetiology, origins, and diagnosis of severe acute respiratory syndrome. Lancet Infect Dis 2004;4(11):663–71.

[75] Stöhr K. A multicentre collaboration to investigate the cause of severe acute respiratory syndrome. Lancet 2003;361(9370):1730–3.

[76] Kuiken T, Fouchier R, Schutten M, et al. Newly discovered coronavirus as the primary cause of severe acute respiratory syndrome. Lancet 2003;362(9380):263–70.

[77] WHO. Summary of probable SARS cases with onset of illness from 1 November 2002 to 31 July 2003. 26 September 2003. Available at: http://www.who.int/csr/sars/country/2003_08_15/en/. Accessed March 15, 2005.

[78] Peiris J, Guan Y, Yuen K. Severe acute respiratory syndrome. Nat Med 2004;10(12 Suppl):S88–97.

[79] Peck A, Newbern E, Feikin D, et al. Lack of SARS transmission and US SARS case-patient. Emerg Infect Dis 2004;10(2):217–24.

[80] Isakbaeva E, Khetsuriani N, Beard R, et al. SARS-associated coronavirus transmission, United States. Emerg Infect Dis 2004;10(2):225–31.

[81] Fleck F. SARS outbreak over, but concerns for lab safety remain. Bull World Health Organ 2004;82(6):470.

[82] Jernigan J, Helfand R, Parashar U. Accurate clinical prediction of severe acute respiratory syndrome: are we there yet? Ann Intern Med 2004;141(5):396–8.

[83] Peiris J, Yuen K, Osterhaus A, et al. The severe acute respiratory syndrome. N Engl J Med 2003;349(25):2431–41.

[84] Christian M, Poutanen S, Loutfy M, et al. Severe acute respiratory syndrome. Clin Infect Dis 2004;38(10):1420–7.

[85] Hoffmann C, Kamps B. SARS reference: clinical presentation and diagnosis. October 17, 2003. Available at: http://www.sarsreference.com/sarsref/diag.htm. Accessed Jun 24, 2005.

[86] Wong K, Antonio G, Hui D, et al. Severe acute respiratory syndrome: radiographic appearances and pattern of progression in 138 patients. Radiology 2003;228(2):401–6.

[87] WHO. WHO guidelines for the global surveillance of severe acute respiratory syndrome (SARS). Updated recommendations, October 2004. Geneva, Switzerland: Department of Communicable Disease Surveillance and Response, WHO; 2004. WHO/CDS/CSR/ARO/2004.1.

[88] Chan-Yeung M, Seto W, Sung J. Severe acute respiratory syndrome: patients were epidemiologically linked. BMJ 2003;326(7403):1393.

[89] Chen Y, Huang L, Chan C, et al. SARS in hospital emergency room. Emerg Infect Dis 2004;10(5):782–8.

[90] Chang W, Kao C, Chung M, et al. SARS exposure and emergency department workers. Emerg Infect Dis 2004;10(6):1117–9.

[91] Ooi S, Tambyah P. Transmission of severe acute respiratory syndrome in an emergency department. Am J Med 2004;116(7):486–9.

[92] Tham K. An emergency department response to severe acute respiratory syndrome: a prototype response to bioterrorism. Ann Emerg Med 2004;43(1):6–14.

[93] Man C, Yeung R, Chung J, et al. Impact of SARS on an emergency department in Hong Kong. Emerg Med (Fremantle) 2004;15(5–6):418–22.

[94] Varia M, Wilson S, Sarwal S, et al. Investigation of a nosocomial outbreak of severe acute respiratory syndrome (SARS) in Toronto, Canada. CMAJ 2003;169(4):285–92.

[95] Li L, Cheng S, Gu J. SARS infection among health care workers in Beijing, China. JAMA 2003;290(20):2662–3.

[96] Borgundvaag B, Ovens H, Goldman B, et al. SARS outbreak in the Greater Toronto Area: the emergency department experience. CMAJ 2004;171(11):1342–4.

[97] Farquharson C, Baguley K. Responding to the severe acute respiratory syndrome (SARS) outbreak: lessons learned in a Toronto emergency department. J Emerg Nurs 2003;29(3):222–8.

[98] Lateef F. SARS changes the ED paradigm. Am J Emerg Med 2004;22(6):483–7.

[99] Marley C, Levsky M, Talbot T, et al. SARS and its impact on current and future emergency department operations. J Emerg Med 2004;26(4):415–20.

[100] Gamage B, Moore D, Copes R, et al. Protecting health care workers from SARS and other respiratory pathogens: a review of the infection control literature. Am J Infect Control 2005;33(2):114–21.

[101] Christian M, Loutfy M, McDonald L, et al. Possible SARS coronavirus transmission during cardiopulmonary resuscitation. Emerg Infect Dis 2004;10(2):287–93.

[102] Dwosh H, Hong H, Austgarden D, et al. Identification and containment of an outbreak of SARS in a community hospital. CMAJ 2003;168(11):1415–20.

[103] Ho A, Sung J, Chan-Yeung M. An outbreak of severe acute respiratory syndrome among hospital workers in a community hospital in Hong Kong. Ann Intern Med 2003;139(7):564–7.

[104] Leung G, Rainer T, Lau F, et al. A clinical prediction rule for diagnosing severe acute respiratory syndrome in the emergency department. Ann Intern Med 2004;141(5):333–42.

[105] Su C, Chiang W, Ma M, et al. Validation of a novel severe acute respiratory syndrome scoring system. Ann Emerg Med 2004;43(1):34–42.

[106] Wang T, Jang T, Huang C, et al. Establishing a clinical decision rule of severe acute respiratory syndrome at the emergency department. Ann Emerg Med 2004;43(1):17–22.

[107] Chen S, Su C, Ma M, et al. Predictive model of diagnosing probable cases of severe acute respiratory syndrome in febrile patients with exposure risk. Ann Emerg Med 2004;43(1):1–5.

[108] Fauci A, Touchette N, Folkers G. Emerging infectious diseases: a 10-year perspective from the National Institute of Allergy and Infectious Diseases. Emerg Infect Dis 2005;11(4):519–25.

[109] Gerberding J. Faster... but fast enough? Responding to the epidemic of severe acute respiratory syndrome. N Engl J Med 2003;348(20):2030–1.

[110] Karwa M, Currie B, Kvetan V. Bioterrorism: Preparing for the impossible or the improbable. Crit Care Med 2005;33(1 Suppl):S75–95.

[111] Schultz C, Mothershead J, Field M. Bioterrorism preparedness. I: The emergency department and hospital. Emerg Med Clin North Am 2002;20(2):437–55.

[112] Khan A, Levitt A, Sage M. Biological and chemical terrorism: strategic plan for preparedness and response: recommendations of the CDC Strategic Planning Workgroup. MMWR Recomm Rep 2000;49(RR04):1–14.

[113] McGovern T, Friedlander A. Plague. In: Sidell F, Takafuji E, Franz D, editors. Medical aspects of chemical and biological warfare. Washington DC: TMM Publications; 1989. p. 479–502.

[114] World Health Organization. Human plague in 2000 and 2001. Wkly Epidemiol Rec 2003; 78(16):130–5.

[115] Dennis D. Plague as an emerging disease. In: Scheld W, Craig W, Hughes J, editors. Emerging infections 2. Washington DC: ASM Press; 1998. p. 169–83.

[116] CDC. Fatal human plague—Arizona and Colorado, 1996. MMWR Morb Mortal Wkly Rep 1997;46(27):617–20.

[117] Williams P, Wallace D. Unit 731: Japan's secret biological warfare in World War II. New York: The Free Press; 1989.

[118] Alibek K. Biohazard. New York: Random House; 1999.

[119] World Health Organization. Public health response to biological and chemical weapons: WHO guidance (2004). Geneva, Switzerland: World Health Organization; 2004.

[120] Inglesby T, Dennis D, Henderson D, et al. Plague as a biological weapon: medical and public health management. Working Group on Civilian Biodefense. JAMA 2000;283(17): 2281–90.

[121] Alsofrom D, Mettler FJ, Mann J. Radiographic manifestations of plague in New Mexico, 1975–1980. A review of 42 proved cases. Radiology 1981;139(3):561–5.

[122] Olson J, Relman D. Bioterrorism preparedness: what practitioners need to know. Infect Med 2001;18:497–514.

[123] World Health Organization. Global measles mortality reduction and regional elimination, 2000–2001 – Part I. Wkly Epidemiol Rec 2002;77(7):50–5.

[124] World Health Organization. WHO-UNICEF joint statement on strategies to reduce measles mortality worldwide. Geneva, Switzerland: World Health Organization; 2001.

[125] CDC. Progress in reducing measles mortality—worldwide, 1999–2003. MMWR Morb Mortal Wkly Rep 2005;54(8):200–3.

[126] CDC. Measles—United States, 2000. MMWR Morb Mortal Wkly Rep 2002;51(6):120–3.

[127] Rota P, Liffick S, Rota J, et al. Molecular epidemiology of measles viruses in the United States, 1997–2001. Emerg Infect Dis 2002;8(9):902–8.

[128] Duke T, Michael A, Mgone J, et al. Etiology of child mortality in Goroka, Papua New Guinea: a prospective two-year study. Bull World Health Organ 2002;80(1):16–25.

[129] Hussey G, Clements C. Clinical problems in measles case management. Ann Trop Paediatr 1996;16(4):307–17.

[130] Kim E, Lee K, Primack S, et al. Viral pneumonias in adults: radiologic and pathologic findings. Radiographics 2002;22:S137–49.

[131] Hussey G, Klein M. A randomized, controlled trial of vitamin A in children with severe measles. N Engl J Med 1990;323(3):160–4.

[132] Simpson R. Infectiousness of communicable diseases in the household (measles, chickenpox, and mumps). Lancet 1952;2(12):549–54.

[133] Duclos P, Ward B. Measles vaccines: a review of adverse events. Drug Saf 1998;19(6): 435–54.

[134] Watson J, Hadler S, Dykewicz C, et al. Measles, mumps, and rubella—vaccine use and strategies for elimination of measles, rubella, and congenital rubella syndrome and control

of mumps: recommendations of the Advisory Committee on Immunization Practices (ACIP). MMWR Recomm Rep 1998;47(RR-8):1–57.

[135] Puvimanasinghe J, Arambepola C, Abeysinghe N, et al. Measles outbreak in Sri Lanka, 1999–2000. J Infect Dis 2003;187(Suppl 1):S241–5.

[136] Lindegren M, Atkinson W, Farizo K, et al. Measles vaccination in pediatric emergency departments during a measles outbreak. JAMA 1993;270(18):2185–9.

[137] Olson C. Vaccination in pediatric emergency departments. JAMA 1993;270(18):2222–3.

[138] Bell L. Providing primary care to children in the emergency department: a problem or a missed opportunity? Pediatr Emerg Care 1991;7(2):124.

[139] Robinson P, Gausche M, Gerardi M, et al. Immunization of the pediatric patient in the emergency department. Ann Emerg Med 1996;28(3):334–41.

[140] Foldy S, Biedrzycki P, Barthell E, et al. Syndromic surveillance using regional emergency medicine Internet. Ann Emerg Med 2004;44(3):242–6.

[141] Nelson K. Surveillance. In: Nelson K, Williams C, Graham N, editors. Infectious disease epidemiology: theory and practice. Gaithersburg, MD: Aspen Publishers; 2000. p. 97–117.

[142] Henning K. What is syndromic surveillance? MMWR Morb Mortal Wkly Rep 2004; 53(Suppl):5–11.

[143] Talan D, Moran G, Mower W, et al. EMERGEncy ID NET: an emergency department-based emerging infections sentinel network. Ann Emerg Med 1998;32(6):703–11.

[144] Yang S, Rothman R. PCR-based diagnostics for infectious diseases: uses, limitations, and future applications in acute-care settings. Lancet Infect Dis 2004;4(6):337–48.

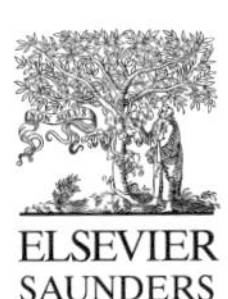

ELSEVIER
SAUNDERS

Emerg Med Clin N Am
24 (2006) 1019–1033

EMERGENCY
MEDICINE
CLINICS OF
NORTH AMERICA

Emergency Medicine and the Public's Health: Emerging Infectious Diseases

Mark A. Saks, MD, MPH[a],*,
David Karras, MD, FACEP, FAAEM[b]

[a]*Department of Emergency Medicine, Drexel University College of Medicine,
245 North 15th Street, Mail Stop 1011, Philadelphia, PA 19101, USA*
[b]*Department of Emergency Medicine, Temple University School of Medicine,
3401 North Broad Street, Philadelphia, PA 19140, USA*

Public health and medicine seem to have distinctly different roles regarding infectious diseases. Public health initiatives are typically aimed at the population or community-based level. They often focus their efforts on harm reduction and disease prevention. Medicine is focused on the diagnosis and treatment of individual patients with specific diseases. However, public health initiatives combined with medical advances have immeasurably improved the health of individuals and communities from the Middle Ages, when those with plague were quarantined, to the modern sciences of sanitation, water purification, and health education. It is clear that medicine and public health efforts must continue to be work in conjunction in the prevention, treatment, and cure of communicable disease.

The optimism of the "antibiotic era" in the mid-twentieth century has been diluted in recent years as forces have combined to create conditions facilitating the emergence and widespread distribution of previously unknown disease entities. In a 1992 report, the Institute of Medicine (IOM) cited increased globalization and global travel, climate change, destruction of natural habitat, rapid global food distribution, human population growth, and a change in the patterns and volume of human migration as factors favoring the emergence and spread of infectious diseases [1]. The emergency department (ED) is uniquely situated at the crossroads between medicine, public health, and the global forces responsible for the rapid spread of infectious diseases. As a 24-hour-a-day portal to the health care system, the ED serves a disproportionate number of poor, uninsured, and recent immigrants.

---

* Corresponding author.

E-mail address: msaks@drexelmed.edu (M.A. Saks).

doi:10.1016/j.emc.2006.06.005   *emed.theclinics.com*

While it has long been a safety net for those who fail outpatient therapy and for patients without primary care physicians, the ED is increasingly seen as a frontline center for disease surveillance and early identification of outbreaks. Additionally, given the close contact patients have with each other and with ED staff, concerns have been raised about the ED as a propagating source of infection.

We have chosen several representative emerging infections to discuss in more detail as they relate to the practice of emergency medicine. These are grouped into the following categories: those that were previously unknown; those spread to new areas by global forces; and those that we must reconsider as fears of bioterrorism increase. Respiratory infections represent a significant class of emerging disease and are discussed in detail in the chapter by Rothman, Hsieh, and Yang, elsewhere in this issue.

Previously unknown entities

Ebola hemorrhagic fever

The subject of numerous movies and books, Ebola virus is among the most feared infectious agents in the world. Far from the media's images of brave scientists in bright yellow containment suites, Ebola typically impacts rural African villagers and jungle wildlife with astounding mortality rates. The first known Ebola virus infection occurred in Sudan and the Democratic Republic of Congo (formerly Zaire) in 1976, causing near chaos [2]. By the time the outbreak was controlled, it had decimated hundreds of Africans with a high rate of transmission to health care workers and missionaries [3]. Although 20 years passed between the first and second Ebola outbreaks, epidemics have occurred almost yearly since the late 1990s.

Ebola virus belongs to the Filoviridae family, a group of single-stranded, enveloped RNA viruses. There are four known Ebola subtypes: Zaire, Sudan, Ivory Coast, and Reston. The first three are highly lethal in both humans and primates with mortality rates approaching 90%; the last causes disease in primates but is apparently nonpathogenic in humans [4]. Since 1976, there have been at least 20 documented Ebola virus outbreaks, including three US outbreaks of Ebola Reston among imported research monkeys [2,5]. A natural reservoir of Ebola in primates has long been suspected since human outbreaks are usually preceded by outbreaks in wild primates [6]. A recent study of wild chimpanzees found that 13% had Ebola antibodies indicating that Ebola virus is endemic in large areas and that nonlethal Ebola infection can occur in primates [7]. However, primates are not generally considered the primary reservoir because the disease is so lethal to them [6]. Serology studies of more than 30,000 animals, implicated bats as a possible reservoir since only they were able to support Ebola virus replication and circulation of high virus titers without causing disease [8]. Interestingly, hunters have higher Ebola antibody levels than farmers and presumably more contact with the virus by virtue of their time in the forest [9].

The most likely route of infection is via direct contact with mucous membranes through close personal contact or fomite ingestion, while respiratory and aerosol transmission may be secondary mechanisms of infection [3,10]. Often, dissemination occurs within medical facilities as a result of improper isolation or disposal of contaminated equipment [11]. In a recent outbreak, 30% of physicians who provided care contracted the disease [10]. Acutely ill patients have a very high viremia and the risk of transmission to caregivers increases as the patient's illness worsens [2]. Children may be relatively spared from Ebola infections because family members shield them from exposure to their sickest relatives [12].

Ebola virus–mediated hemorrhagic fever is an acute febrile illness that progresses rapidly. After an incubation period of 4 to 10 days, patients develop nonspecific symptoms such as malaise, myalgia, sore throat, headache, nausea, vomiting, and abdominal pain [2]. Initially, conjunctival injection may be the only clinical finding [3]. It is believed that Ebola infection triggers exaggerated cytokine release that combines with hepatic dysfunction and massive viremia to cause increased vascular permeability manifested by petechial hemorrhages, mild hypotension, and flushing [12]. Disseminated intravascular coagulopathy (DIC) then develops with prominent maculopapular rashes and generalized mucous membrane hemorrhage, primarily within the gastrointestinal tract [13]. The clinical picture resembles septic shock and death usually comes 5 to 14 days after the first symptoms appear [14,15].

Laboratory studies may show early leucopenia, as the severity of disease increases neutrophilia. Atypical lymphocytes, marked thrombocytopenia, and platelet dysfunction are also seen [16]. Patients can exhibit elevated liver transaminases with normal or slightly elevated alkaline phosphatase and bilirubin levels [2]. Coagulation profiles, fibrinogen degradation products, and D-dimer values become more abnormal as the disease progresses. The disease should be suspected in cases that meet the following criteria: a temperature over 101°F for less than 3 weeks, severe illness with no predisposing factors for hemorrhage, and at least two of the following: hemorrhagic rash, epistaxis, hematemesis, hemoptysis, or blood in the stools [17]. Care should be taken to rule out other pathogens that can cause similar disease syndromes such as malaria, meningococcal disease (Waterhouse-Friedrichsen's syndrome), leptospirosis, rickettsial disease, and fulminant viral hepatitis [18]. Ebola virus infection can be identified with reverse transcriptase polymerase chain reaction (RT-PCR) and antigen-capture ELISA in conjunction with the Centers for Disease Control and Prevention (CDC) [19].

The CDC has classified Ebola virus as an "agent of highest concern" for its potential use as a biological weapon and for the major health impact and social disruption that would result from a domestic outbreak [20]. There have been several cases of travelers who have inadvertently imported other hemorrhagic fevers into countries where it is not endemic [21]. Emergency physicians should consider Ebola hemorrhagic fever in travelers recently returned from Africa presenting with fever and signs of hemorrhage, especially if the traveler spent time in rural areas [22]. Once Ebola is suspected, high-level barrier nursing and respiratory isolation should be initiated immediately. Suspected cases must be reported immediately to infection control personnel and public health departments who can identify and monitor high-risk contacts.

Treatment of Ebola hemorrhagic fever is supportive. Because of DIC and resulting hemorrhagic complications, invasive procedures such as central lines should be avoided whenever possible. Red blood cells, platelets, and clotting factor transfusions may be necessary [14]. Fluids should be used judiciously because of a propensity to develop pulmonary edema. Passive transfer of antibodies (IgG) shows some efficacy in animal models, but has not been proven to be of benefit in humans [14]. Antiviral drugs and interferon have not been found to be effective in treating Ebola infection. Vaccine development appears to be promising, although no vaccine currently exists [12].

Hantavirus

In early spring 1993, public health officials in New Mexico were notified of the unusual case of a healthy 19-year-old man and a 21-year-old woman living in the same household who both died of adult respiratory distress syndrome. Over the next 2 weeks, state and Indian Health Service investigators identified 24 similar cases of a febrile prodrome followed by the rapid development of pulmonary edema, pleural effusions, lactic acidosis, and, in 12 fatal cases, severe cardiopulmonary shock and death [23]. All of the identified cases were people living in or near the "Four Corners" region, where New Mexico, Arizona, Utah, and Colorado converge in the southwest desert. Initial testing for known toxins and bacterial or viral pathogens was negative, but laboratory studies of serum and tissue samples quickly revealed an acute infection with a species of Hantavirus previously unrecognized in North America [24]. This virus was named Sin Nombre virus (SNV), or "virus without a name," and the resulting disease was termed Hantavirus pulmonary syndrome (HPS).

Hantaviruses, rodent-borne members of the Bunyaviridae family, were previously known to cause hemorrhagic fevers throughout Europe and Asia where their epidemiology is largely defined by the distribution of their rodent hosts [25]. In the Four Corners outbreak, the SNV virus was associated with the deer mouse *Peromyscus maniculatus* in which the virus establishes a chronic infection [26]. However, many other species of deer mouse found throughout the Americas have been shown to carry SNV or similar hantaviruses [25]. As a result of chronic viremia, the mouse continually sheds virus into the environment in the form of contaminated fomites such as urine, feces, fur, saliva, and other infectious particles. Humans acquire SNV most frequently by inhalation of infectious aerosols, but any contact with infected particles can lead to transmission [27].

Most Hantavirus exposures occur in and around the patients' homes, especially when the individuals are handling rodents, storing food in areas contaminated by mouse droppings, and cleaning buildings with large mouse populations [28,29]. The risk of human disease is proportional to the frequency with which people come into contact with infectious mice. Preventive efforts, therefore, focus on three areas: properly disposing of rodent excreta, avoiding rodents in outdoor settings, and controlling rodent populations [30]. Person-to-person transmission to health care workers and other close contacts of infected individuals has been documented. In many cases, however, the mechanism of transmission is not known [31]. In the 10 years since the Four Corners outbreak, 349 cases of Hantavirus have been confirmed in the United States [32]. The vast majority of domestic cases have occurred west of the Mississippi River, but SNV infection and Hantavirus have been described in the southeast and northeast United States [33–36].

The pathophysiology of HPS is not well defined. The virus is widely distributed in the endothelium of the lungs, kidneys, heart, pancreas, adrenal glands, and skeletal muscle [24]. Pulmonary injury, either from direct viral-mediated damage or secondary to inflammatory mediators results in pulmonary capillary leak and alveolar edema, impairing gas exchange and rapidly leading to respiratory failure [37]. After a short incubation period of 1 to 2 weeks, clinical presentation typically begins with nonspecific, flu-like symptoms. Fever and myalgia are universal complaints, often accompanied by headache, cough, nausea and vomiting, chills, malaise, and diarrhea [24]. Thrombocytopenia may be seen in this prodromal phase [38]. Within 2 to 8 days, patients typically develop a nonproductive cough and noncardiogenic pulmonary edema associated with tachypnea, tachycardia, tissue hypoperfusion, and hypotension indicative of shock. At this point, laboratory studies reveal thrombocytopenia, leukocytosis, hemoconcentration, the absence of granulations in neutrophils, and more than 10% of lymphocytes with immunoblastic morphology [32]. The presence of four out of five of these laboratory abnormalities has been reported by Koster and colleagues [39] to have a sensitivity of 96% and a specificity of 99% for HPS. Chest radiographs typically demonstrate bibasilar interstitial infiltrates that rapidly progress to diffuse alveolar edema. Dyspnea is not characteristic until just before respiratory failure [37]. Definitive diagnosis requires demonstration of Hantavirus-specific IgA, IgM, and IgG [40].

In HPS patients with shock, hemodynamic monitoring shows a characteristic pattern of low cardiac index (CI), a low stroke volume (SV), and a high systemic vascular resistance (SVR), which is useful in differentiating HPS from classic septic shock [32,37]. Patients require a high degree of pulmonary support, have severe hypoxemia with uniformly low lung compliance, and may develop persistently elevated blood lactate levels. The overall mortality rate of HPS is approximately 50% with early or rapidly deteriorating cardiopulmonary dysfunction signaling highest risk of mortality [37]. Specific indicators of poor outcome include shock, cardiac arrhythmias, serum lactate greater than 4.0 mmol/L, and a cardiac index less than 2.5 L/min/m^2. Survivors tend to require aggressive therapy for only a few days, then recover fully without residual deficits [41]. Experimental treatment with venoarterial extracorporeal membrane oxygenation (ECMO) was been used with good efficacy in patients previously believed to have a 100% mortality rate, especially when initiated early [41]. Ribavirin has shown some effectiveness in vitro, but clinical trials do not support its use [32]. There are no Food and Drug Administration (FDA)-approved antiviral drugs, vaccines, or immunotherapeutic agents available for the treatment of SNV.

Severe HPS may present like cardiogenic shock as a result of acute myocardial infarction, Acute Respiratory Distress Syndrome (ARDS), or bacterial pneumonia. HPS should be considered on the basis of an infectious history and fever (unlike cardiogenic shock), a lack of initial respiratory symptoms (unlike ARDS), and a lack of a lobar infiltrate with negative sputum Gram stain and cultures (unlike bacterial pneumonia) [41,42]. The presence of thrombocytopenia, leukocytosis, hemoconcentration, the absence of granulations in neutrophils, and more than 10% of lymphocytes with immunoblastic morphology should further raise suspicions of HPS [39]. Finally, one should consider Hantavirus when diagnosing an unexplained acute respiratory distress syndrome or bilateral interstitial pulmonary infiltrates [28]. Early patient isolation and notification of public health officials of suspected HPS cases in the ED is essential.

Fears of bioterrorism

Smallpox

Smallpox is an infection caused by variola virus, a member of the *Orthopoxvirus* genus. It is generally spread though direct respiratory transmission or, less commonly, though contact with infected bodily fluids or contaminated fomites. There is historical evidence of spontaneous smallpox outbreaks in ancient Egypt, Mesopotamia, India, and China. However, smallpox did not become a leading cause of morbidity and mortality until the seventeenth and eighteenth centuries when it accounted for approximately 400,000 European deaths per year [43]. In the late 1700s, control of smallpox became a priority of the medical community and novel approaches to its prevention were developed. In 1796, Dr Edward Jenner noted that farmers who had contracted cowpox did not contract smallpox, even after they were inoculated with infectious material. He developed a procedure, later known as vaccination, involving inoculation of material from cowpox pustules into local children. The children developed lasting smallpox immunity.

The current smallpox vaccine is a live-attenuated vaccine derived from vaccinia virus, another *Orthopoxvirus* that confers immunity to variola virus (Wyeth Laboratories, Marietta, PA). The vaccine is introduced into the basal cells of the epidermis through three jabs with a bifurcated needle in the mid to outer deltoid region of the arm. Immunity develops through a combined cellular and humoral response and is effective within 2 to 3 days of vaccination [44]. Because smallpox has no natural hosts and vaccine can be delivered quickly and cheaply by minimally trained workers, vaccination programs were extremely effective [45]. In the United States, vaccination was phased out beginning in 1972 and discontinued for health care workers in 1976 [46]. In 1980, the World Health Assembly declared that smallpox had been eradicated worldwide [47]. However, stocks of the virus continue to be preserved at two sites: the CDC in Atlanta and the Research Institute for Viral Preparations in Moscow.

In 2002, the United States reversed its vaccination policy and announced an ambitious "preevent" smallpox vaccination plan. The vaccine was to be given first to selected troops, government personnel, and health care teams and then expanded to other medical providers and first responders. In the plan's final phase, the vaccine would be offered to the general public [48,49]. Implementation of this plan was met with strong resistance from the medical community because of concerns about vaccine safety, the uncertain risk of smallpox exposure, and issues of compensation and liability [50].

The side-effect profile of the current smallpox vaccine reflects its live-attenuated nature and affects both vaccinated patients and their close contacts [51]. Among the half-million military personnel vaccinated after 2002, there were 30 suspected cases of contact transfer of vaccinia, known as heteroinoculation [52]. Adverse reactions have been well characterized. The most common responses after vaccination are pain, erythema, edema, and ultimately scarring at the site of vaccination, as well as regional lymphadenopathy. Systemic symptoms including fevers, malaise, and headache are common vaccine reactions, usually occurring 7 to 10 days after vaccination [53]. Less common findings include lymphangitis and the development of proximal or single distal satellite lesions as a result of the spread of vaccinia virus from the primary vaccination site to another site, known as autoinoculation. Bacterial superinfection of the vaccine site may present as an impetiginous lesion or a typical cellulitis, and responds to antibiotic therapy. Most cellulitis after vaccination, however, is viral in origin and does not require specific therapy. Generalized vaccinia, a mild systemic infection with development of numerous single blisters that rapidly resolve, is a benign complication that is seen in about 1% of vaccines [44]. Although these adverse events are not serious, they are the cause of substantial missed work and school days [53].

Of greater concern are postvaccination neurologic and cardiac complications, especially among "first time" vaccine recipients, including those not vaccinated before 1976. Encephalomyelitis is estimated to occur nine times and cause three fatalities per million vaccinations [54]. Myocarditis and pericarditis occur between 140 and 600 times per million vaccinees [55]. There are numerous case reports of angina, myocardial infarction, and other cardiac diseases presenting following vaccination [52]. While there are no screening criteria to reduce the risk of vaccine-related coronary events, the CDC has advised against vaccination of people with a history of angina, cardiac disease, or stroke [56,57].

Smallpox vaccination is potentially harmful for immunocompromised individuals. Patients with malignancies, chronic inflammatory diseases, or other forms of immunocompromise are at elevated risk of developing severe local and systemic vaccine reactions. Patients with eczema and atopic dermatitis are at risk of developing eczema vaccinatum, characterized by widespread eruption of vaccinia lesions [44]. Therefore, those with eczema or atopic dermatitis and their immediate family members should not be vaccinated unless smallpox is an immediate risk. Progressive vaccinia, also known as vaccinia necrosum or disseminated vaccinia, is the most severe complication of smallpox vaccination. In progressive vaccinia, the virus progresses rapidly from the site of inoculation and induces a severe viral cellulitis, often leading to limb amputation or death [44]. Pregnant woman have the risk of developing fetal vaccinia and pregnancy loss. The CDC therefore recommends urine pregnancy testing on the day of vaccination and avoiding immunization in household contacts of pregnant women. There are at least 103 pregnant women who received vaccination despite negative urine tests, although none developed fetal vaccinia [58].

In the event of widespread smallpox vaccination, ED physicians will need to become proficient in postvaccination care. Local, wound-related complaints can usually be managed with supportive care and analgesics. Normal local vaccine reactions should be differentiated from superimposed bacterial infection. Individuals who receive vaccines should routinely be instructed to use meticulous hygiene and to keep the vaccination site covered and dry until the scabbing has resolved. Postvaccinial myopericarditis should be considered by ED physicians in the differential diagnosis of patients with chest pain within 30 days of smallpox vaccination [55]. For cases of severe generalized or progressive vaccinia, vaccinia immune globulin is available from the CDC and may be effective. However, it has no role in the treatment of encephalitis, myocarditis, or pericarditis. The role of antiviral therapy has not been established.

Smallpox itself has not been seen in the United States since 1949, but its recognition is critical to mitigating a potentially devastating outbreak. Smallpox has an incubation period of 7 to 17 days after initial exposure, during which the patient is asymptomatic and not infectious. This is followed by a 2- to 4-day prodrome of malaise, myalgia, and fevers. Because the patient at this stage may shed virus but has not yet developed the characteristic skin lesions, health care workers, particularly those in the ED, may be unwittingly exposed to the disease [56]. Skin lesions typically develop after 4 days and arise synchronously. The lesions are firm, deep-seated vesicles or well-circumscribed pustules with umbilicated centers that erupt diffusely but are most prominent over the face and hands, including the palms and soles. The vesicles then begin to weep and eventually scab and fall off, leaving deep craters. A person remains contagious until all of the scabs have fallen off and healed completely. Images of smallpox lesions can be accessed on the CDC Web site (www.cdc.gov/smallpox) [59].

It is vital that emergency physicians be able to differentiate smallpox from other diseases presenting with vesicular eruptions, notably chickenpox and shingles. Unlike the lesions of chickenpox that appear and evolve in crops, smallpox lesions are all in the same stage of development. Individuals with smallpox appear acutely ill and toxic, while those with chickenpox and shingles are generally well-appearing except for mild systemic symptoms and pain or pruritis at the site of the lesions. Suspected smallpox cases can be confirmed with PCR identification of variola DNA. Any confirmed case of smallpox would be considered an outbreak and would be a public health emergency requiring immediate notification of public health authorities.

Patients with suspected disease should be immediately placed in contact and respiratory isolation, and their contacts should be vaccinated as per recommendations of the CDC and local health authorities. Postexposure vaccination is believed to be fully effective at preventing smallpox if administered within 2 to 3 days of exposure. Later administration within a week of exposure confers partial immunity and greatly reduces morbidity and mortality.

Disease spread by global forces

West Nile virus

In late summer 1999, two seemingly unique clusters of deaths were noted in the metropolitan New York City area. The first involved an unusually high number of deaths in wild crows and in various exotic birds housed at the Bronx Zoo. Autopsies revealed that they died of meningoencephalitis and myocarditis, however serology was negative for common avian and equine encephalitis viruses and tissue samples were sent to the CDC for further investigation. Concurrently, two patients in a Queens hospital were reported to the New York City Department of Health as having an unusual type of meningoencephalitis associated with muscle weakness. An ensuing investigation revealed eight patients in nearby hospitals with similar symptoms. Initial cerebrospinal fluid (CSF) testing implicated St Louis encephalitis virus and citywide telephone hotlines, surveillance, and mosquito-control programs were initiated [60]. During the first season a total of 59 cases were identified, 7 of these were fatal [61].

By early fall, PCR and DNA testing of the avian isolates and comparison to human tissue samples revealed a close similarity to West Nile virus

(WNV), a single-stranded RNA flavivirus that is a member of the Japanese encephalitis virus family [60]. West Nile virus was known to be endemic across the Middle East, Africa, and Europe, causing occasional outbreaks of mild disease, but had never been isolated from the Western Hemisphere [62]. Migration of infected birds is believed to be responsible for the introduction of the virus to the United States [63]. Detailed genetic analysis implicated the responsible serotype as closely isolated to one associated with an outbreak in migratory Israeli birds from 1997 to 2000 [64]. It is also possible that the virus arrived via a mosquito trapped in an airliner or in the blood of an international traveler [65].

During the next several summers, it became clear that the outbreak of 1999 was not an isolated incident. The number of states reporting cases has increased steadily each year with a changing distribution in the northeastern United States. In 2004, the geographic focus of the disease shifted dramatically westward with California, Arizona, and Colorado accounting for the vast majority of reported illnesses and deaths from West Nile disease. In that year, a total of 2470 human cases of West Nile disease were reported to the CDC, associated with 87 fatalities [66]. Only Washington, Alaska, and Hawaii have yet to report the presence of West Nile virus.

Most cases of West Nile are transmitted to humans though the bite of an infected mosquito. Therefore, people at highest risk of infection are those that spend much of their time outdoors, such as landscapers, farmers, and construction workers. Because mammals do not develop high levels of viremia, human-to-human transmission is believed to be rare [67]. However, West Nile transmission has been reported to occur through blood transfusion, organ transplantation, and via maternal-fetal transfer by crossing the placenta or during breastfeeding [68–70]. Two cases of occupational exposure in lab workers have also been reported [71].

Most human WNV infections are subclinical. Based on serology studies during the 1999 outbreak, it is estimated that only 20% of people infected with the virus developed symptoms and that only half of them sought medical attention [72]. Patients most frequently complain of sudden onset fevers with accompanying fatigue, malaise, myalgias, anorexia, headaches, nausea, and vomiting. Lymphadenopathy or an erythematous macular, papular, or morbilliform rash on the neck, trunk, or extremities may be noted in a minority of patients. Neurologic syndromes ranging from a mild headache to aseptic meningitis to encephalitis are common and usually indistinguishable from other viral syndromes [73]. Encephalitis is the most common neurologic diagnosis (seen in 63%), followed by meningitis alone (29%) and headache only (8%). Severe neurologic deficits develop in less than 1% of infected persons but can be life threatening, especially in those over the age of 50 years and those with diabetes mellitus or immunosuppression [61,74]. WNV-related meningoencephalitis carries a mortality of up to 15%. Patients may have severe muscle weakness that can be confused with Guillain-Barre syndrome [68].

Poor prognostic factors include profound weakness, coma, immunosuppression, advanced age, and the presence of comorbid conditions.

The complete blood count shows no significant abnormalities while cerebrospinal fluid analysis is typical of viral infection, with pleocytosis and an elevated protein concentration. Computed axial tomography (CAT) scans of the brain typically show no signs of acute disease [61]. Typical of encephalitis, magnetic resonance imaging (MRI) may be normal initially or show an enhancement of the leptomeninges and the periventricular area or a characteristic pattern of deep gray matter nuclei [61,75]. Laboratory criteria required for the definitive diagnosis of West Nile Disease (WND) include isolation of virus-specific IgM, a fourfold or greater change in virus-specific serum antibody, or the isolation of virus or viral antigen from tissue of body fluid [73]. The CDC defines a "probable" WND case as any patient with encephalitis or meningitis occurring during a period when transmission is likely with suggestive serology. A case is not confirmed until the above serologic criteria are met.

Treatment of WND is primarily supportive. There is no disease-specific treatment and trials of interferon alfa and ribavirin have failed to demonstrate in vivo effectiveness [76]. Prevention of transmission therefore remains of paramount importance. Prevention efforts focus on health education campaigns, decreasing the number of mosquito breeding grounds, and use of insect repellant sprays. Vaccines are not yet available.

Because there are no bedside diagnostic tests for WND or pathognomonic signs or symptoms, it is unlikely that the illness will be diagnosed while the patient is in the ED. In the majority of symptomatic patients with WND who have mild, flu-like symptoms, no further treatment or evaluation is required if the patient is otherwise healthy. However, among ill-appearing patients, efforts should be made to exclude other potential causes of febrile illness while a definitive diagnosis is made following admission. WND should be considered in any patient with apparent encephalopathy and muscle weakness [68]. Additionally, the diagnosis should be entertained in elderly, diabetic, and immunocompromised patients who present with neurologic and flu-like symptoms during the peak WNV transmission periods of the late summer and fall.

The lesson of WND is that the ED is on the front lines of disease surveillance and that emergency physicians must remain alert for unusual illness clusters. The prompt reporting of two cases of an atypical meningoencephalitis triggered an early response to the initial West Nile outbreak. Public health authorities were able to initiate surveillance programs that undoubtedly reduced the morbidity and mortality of that and subsequent outbreaks.

Summary

As global forces continue to shape the emergence and distribution of novel infectious diseases, we must apply the lessons learned from Ebola virus, West Nile virus, Hantavirus, and smallpox to these new entities. Because the ED serves a disproportionate number of poor, uninsured, and recently immigrated, it will continue to play a major role in the identification, isolation, and treatment of these diseases. We must remember that the ED is on the frontlines for disease surveillance and early outbreak identification. Emergency physicians and other ED personnel are at increased risk of contracting and propagating disease. ED practitioners must be familiar with the presentation, management, and public health impact of new diseases and be prepared to interact with local, state, and national public health authorities on a regular and continuing basis. Only by combining medical advances with public health awareness will ED physicians successfully rise to the challenge of protecting the public against emerging infectious disease.

References

[1] Institute of Medicine. Emerging infections: microbial threats to health in the United States. Washington, DC: National Academy Press; 1994.

[2] Colebunders R, Borchert M. Ebola haemorrhagic fever—a review. J Infect 2000;40:16–20.

[3] Lee LM, Henderson DK. Emerging viral infections. Curr Opin Infect Dis 2001;14(4):467–80.

[4] Rollin PE, Williams RJ, Bressler DS, et al. Ebola (subtype Reston) virus among quarantined nonhuman primates recently imported from the Philippines to the United States. J Infect Dis 1999;179:S108–14.

[5] Vogel J. Ebola outbreaks may have had independent sources. Science 2004;303:298–9.

[6] Thacker PD. An Ebola epidemic simmers in Africa: in remote region, outbreak shows staying power. JAMA 2003;290(3):317–9.

[7] Leroy EM, Telfer P, Kumulungui B, et al. A serological survey of Ebola virus infection in Central African nonhuman primates. J Infect Dis 2004;190:1895–9.

[8] Swanepoel R, Leman PA, Burt FJ. Experimental inoculation of plants and animals with Ebola virus. Emerg Infect Dis 1996;2:321–5.

[9] Busico KM, Marshall KL, Ksiazek TG, et al. Prevalence of IgG antibodies to Ebola virus in individuals during an Ebola outbreak, Democratic Republic of the Congo, 1995. J Infect Dis 1999;179:S98–101.

[10] Peters CJ, LeDuc JW. An introduction to Ebola: the virus and the disease. J Infect Dis 1999; 179:S9–16.

[11] Centers for Disease Control and Prevention. Outbreak of Ebola hemorrhagic fever—Uganda, August 2000–January 2001. MMWR 2001;50(5):73–7.

[12] Dowell SF. Ebola hemorrhagic fever: why were children spared? Pediatr Infect Dis J 1996; 15(3):189–91.

[13] Varkey P, Poland GA, Cockerill FR, et al. Confronting bioterrorism: physicians on the front line. Mayo Clin Proc 2002;77(7):661–72.

[14] Bray M, Mahanty S. Ebola hemorrhagic fever and septic shock. J Infect Dis 2003;118: 1613–7.

[15] Richards GA, Murphy S, Jobson R, et al. Unexpected Ebola virus in a tertiary setting: clinical and epidemiological aspects. Crit Care Med 2000;28(1):240–4.

[16] Sanchez A, Lukwiya M, Bausch D, et al. Analysis of human peripheral blood samples from fatal and nonfatal cases of Ebola (Sudan) hemorrhagic fever: cellular responses, virus load, and nitric oxide levels. J Virol 2004;78(19):10370–7.

[17] Borio L, Inglesby T, Peters CJ, et al. Hemorrhagic fever viruses as biological weapons: medical and public health management. JAMA 2002;287(18):2391–405.

[18] Drosten C, Kümmerer BM, Schmitz H, et al. Molecular diagnostics of viral hemorrhagic fevers. Antiviral 2003;57:61–87.

[19] Towner JS, Rollin PE, Bausch DG, et al. Rapid diagnosis of Ebola hemorrhagic fever by reverse transcription-PCR in an outbreak setting and assessment of patient viral load as a predictor of outcome. J Virol 2004;78(8):4330–41.

[20] Centers for Disease Control and Prevention. Recognition of illness associated with the intentional release of a biologic agent. MMWR 2001;50:893–7.

[21] Isaäcson M. Viral hemorrhagic fever hazards for travelers in Africa. CID 2001;33: 1707–12.

[22] Ryan ET, Wilson ME, Kain KC. Illness after international travel. N Engl J Med 2002;347(7): 505–16.

[23] Centers for Disease Control and Prevention. Outbreak of acute illness—Southwestern United States. MMWR 1993;42:421–4.

[24] Duchin JS, Koster FT, Peters CJ, et al. Hantavirus pulmonary syndrome: a clinical description of 17 patients with a newly recognized disease. N Engl J Med 1994;330(14):949–55.

[25] Mills JN, Yates TL, Ksiazek TG, et al. Long-term studies of Hantavirus reservoir populations in the Southwestern United States: rationale, potential, and methods. Emerg Infect Dis 1999;5(1).

[26] Childs JE, Ksiazek TG, Spiropoulou CF, et al. Serologic and genetic identification of *Peromyscus maniculatus* as the primary rodent reservoir for a new Hantavirus in the Southwestern United States. J Infect Dis 1994;169:1271–80.

[27] Tsai TF. Hemorrhagic fever with renal syndrome: mode of transmission to humans. Lab Anim Sci 1987;37:428–30.

[28] Centers for Disease Control and Prevention. Hantavirus pulmonary syndrome—Panama, 1999–2000. MMWR 2000;283(17):2232–3.

[29] Armstrong LR, Zaki SR, Goldoft MJ, et al. Hantavirus pulmonary syndrome associated with entering or cleaning rarely used, rodent-infested structures. J Infect Dis 1995;171(4): 864–70.

[30] Centers for Disease Control and Prevention. Update: Hantavirus pulmonary syndrome—United States, 1999. MMWR 1999;48(24):521–5.

[31] Wells RM, Estani SS, Yadon ZE, et al. An unusual Hantavirus outbreak in southern Argentina: person-to-person transmission? Emerg Infect Dis 1997;3(2):171–4.

[32] Ferres M, Vial P. Hantavirus infection in children. Curr Opin Pediatr 2004;16(1):70–5.

[33] Doyle TJ, Bryan RT, Peters CJ. Viral hemorrhagic fevers and Hantavirus infections in the Americas. Infect Dis Clin North Am 1998;12(1):95–110.

[34] Centers for Disease Control and Prevention. Hantavirus pulmonary syndrome—Vermont 2000. MMWR 2001;50:603–5.

[35] White DJ, Means RG, Birkhead GS, et al. Human and rodent Hantavirus infection in New York State: public health significance of an emerging infectious disease. Arch Intern Med 1996;156(7):722–6.

[36] Wasser WG, Rossi CA, Glass GE. Hantavirus antibodies in New York. Ann Intern Med 1997;127(2):166–7.

[37] Hallin GW, Simpson SQ, Crowell RE, et al. Cardiopulmonary manifestations of Hantavirus pulmonary syndrome. Crit Care Med 1996;24(2):251–8.

[38] Mertz G, Hjelle B, Bryan R. Hantavirus infection. Adv Intern Med 1997;42:369–421.

[39] Koster F, Foucar K, Hjelle B, et al. Rapid presumptive diagnosis of Hantavirus cardiopulmonary syndrome by peripheral blood smear review. Am J Clin Pathol 2001;116:665–72.

[40] Bostik P, Winter J, Ksiazek TG, et al. Sin Nombre Virus (SNV) Ig isotype antibody response during acute and convalescent phases of Hantavirus pulmonary syndrome. Emerg Infect Dis 2000;6(2).

[41] Crowley MR, Katz RW, Kessler R, et al. Successful treatment of adults with severe Hantavirus pulmonary syndrome with extracorporeal membrane oxygenation. Crit Care Med 1998;26(2):409–14.

[42] Peters CJ, Ali S, Sherif R. Hantaviruses in the United States. Arch Intern Med 1996;156(7): 705–7.

[43] Eyler JM. Smallpox in history: the birth, death, and impact of a dread disease. J Lab Clin Med 2003;142(4):216–20.

[44] Wollenberg A, Engler R. Smallpox, vaccination and adverse reactions to smallpox vaccine. Curr Opin Allergy Clin Immunol 2004;4(4):271–5.

[45] Johnson RT. Smallpox: the threat of bioterrorism and the risk of the vaccine. Neurology 2003;60(8):1228–9.

[46] Centers for Disease Control and Prevention. Recommendations of the Public Health Service Advisory Committee on Immunization Practices: smallpox vaccination of hospital and health personnel. MMWR 1976;25:8–9.

[47] Fenner F, Henderson DA, Arita I, et al. Smallpox and its eradication. Geneva: World Health Organization; 1998. p. 122–67. Available at: http://www.who.int/emc/diseases/smallpox/ Smallpoxeradication.html. Accessed February 14, 2006.

[48] Centers for Disease Control and Prevention. Vaccinia (smallpox) vaccine: recommendations of the Advisory Committee on Immunization Practices (ACIP), 2001. MMWR 2001; 50(R10):1–25.

[49] Institute of Medicine. Review of the Centers for Disease Control and Prevention's smallpox vaccination program implementation—Letter Report #1. Washington, DC: National Academy of Sciences; 2003.

[50] Benin AL, Dembry L, Shapiro ED, et al. Reasons physicians accepted or declined smallpox vaccine February through April, 2003. J Gen Intern Med 2004;19:85–9.

[51] Jefferson T. Editorial: bioterrorism and compulsory vaccination. BMJ 2004;329:524–5.

[52] Centers for Disease Control and Prevention. Secondary and tertiary transfer of Vaccinia virus among US military personnel—United States and worldwide, 2002–2004. MMWR 2004; 53(05):103–5.

[53] Thorne CD, Hirshon JM, Himes CD, et al. Emergency medicine tools to manage smallpox (vaccinia) vaccination complications: clinical practice guideline and policies and procedures. Ann Emerg Med 2003;42(5):665–81.

[54] Aragón TJ, Ulrich S, Fernyak SE, et al. Risks of serious complications and death from smallpox vaccination: a systematic review of the United States experience, 1963–1968. BMC Public Health; 2003. Available at: http://biomedcentral.com/1471-2458/3/26. Accessed February 14, 2006.

[55] Arness MK, Eckart RE, Love SS, et al. Myopericarditis following smallpox vaccination. Am J Epid 2004;160(7):642–51.

[56] Aragón TJ, Fernyak SE. The risks and benefits of pre-event smallpox vaccination: where you stand depends on where you sit. Ann Emerg Med 2003;42(5):681–4.

[57] Centers for Disease Control and Prevention. Cardiac adverse events following smallpox vaccination—United States, 2003. MMWR 2003;52(12):248–50.

[58] Centers for Disease Control and Prevention. Women with smallpox vaccine exposure during pregnancy reported to the National Smallpox Vaccine in Pregnancy Registry—United States, 2003. MMWR 2003;52(17):386–8.

[59] Centers for Disease Control and Prevention. Smallpox: Images. Available at: http:// www.bt.cdc.gov/agent/smallpox/smallpox-images/. Accessed February 14, 2005.

[60] Centers for Disease Control and Prevention. Outbreak of West Nile-like virus—New York, 1999. MMWR Morb Mortal Wkly Rep 1999;48:845–9.

[61] Nash D, Mostashari F, Fine A, et al. The outbreak of West Nile virus infection in the New York City area in 1999. N Engl J Med 2001;344:1807–14.

[62] Hubalek Z, Halouzka J. West Nile Fever—a reemerging mosquito borne viral disease in Europe. Emerg Infect Dis 1999;5:643–50.

[63] Rappole JH, Derickson SR, Hubalek Z. Migratory birds and spread of West Nile virus in the Western Hemisphere. Emerg Infect Dis 2000;6:319–28.

[64] Lanciotti RS, Roehrig JT, Deubel V, et al. Origin of the West Nile virus responsible for an outbreak of encephalitis in the Northeastern United States. Science 1999;286:2333–7.
[65] Tyler KL. Editorial: West Nile Virus encephalitis in America. N Engl J Med 2001;344(24): 1858–9.
[66] Centers for Disease Control and Prevention. West Nile Virus-Statistics, Surveillance, and Control. http://www.cdc.gov/ncidod/dvbid/westnile/surv&control04Maps.htm. Accessed March 10, 2005.
[67] Goetz AM, Goldrick B. West Nile virus: a primer for infection control professionals. Am J Infect Control 2004;32(2):101–5.
[68] Petersen L, Marfin AA. West Nile virus: a primer for the clinician. Ann Intern Med 2002; 137(3):173–9.
[69] Iwamoto M, Jernigan DB, Guasch A, et al. Transmission of West Nile virus from an organ donor to four transplant recipients. N Engl J Med 2003;348:2196–203.
[70] Centers for Disease Control and Prevention. Possible West Nile virus transmission to an infant through breast-feeding—Michigan, 2002. MMWR 2002;51:877–8.
[71] Sampathkumar P. West Nile virus: epidemiology, clinical presentation, diagnosis, and prevention. Mayo Clin Proc 2003;78(9):1137–44.
[72] Mostashari F, Bunning ML, Kitsutani PT, et al. Epidemic West Nile encephalitis, New York 1999: results of a household-based seroepidemiological survey. Lancet 2001;358:261–4.
[73] Centers for Disease Control and Prevention. West Nile Virus-Information and Guidance for Clinicians. http://www.cdc.gov/ncidod/dvbid/westnile/clinicians/pdf/wnv-clinicaldescription.pdf. Accessed February 14, 2005.
[74] Hammerschlag MR. West Nile virus: from epidemic to endemic. Infect Med 2003;20(8): 374–5.
[75] Gea-Banacloche J, Johnson RT, Bagic A, et al. West Nile virus: pathogenesis and therapeutic options. Ann Intern Med 2004;140(7):545–53.
[76] Solomon T, Ooi MH, Beasley DW, et al. West Nile encephalitis. BMJ 2003;326:865–9.

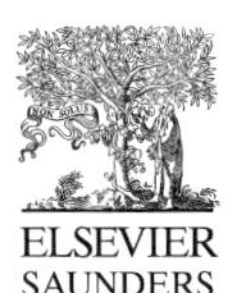

ELSEVIER
SAUNDERS

Emerg Med Clin N Am
24 (2006) 1035–1052

EMERGENCY
MEDICINE
CLINICS OF
NORTH AMERICA

Update on Public Health Surveillance in Emergency Departments

Shawn M. Varney, Lt Col, USAF, MC[a],*,
Jon Mark Hirshon, MD, MPH[b,c]

[a]59 MDW/MCED, 2200 Bergquist Drive, Suite 1, Lackland AFB,
TX 78236-5500, USA
[b]Division of Emergency Medicine, Department of Emergency Medicine
and Department of Epidemiology and Preventive Medicine,
University of Maryland School of Medicine, Baltimore, MD, USA
[c]The Charles McC. Mathias, Jr. National Study Center for Trauma and EMS,
University of Maryland School of Medicine, 701 West Pratt Street,
Fifth Floor, Baltimore, MD 21201, USA

The systematic collection and analysis of health data are important actions required to help understand the health needs of a population. When it is done to investigate a problem to contribute to generalizable knowledge, it is defined as research [1]. If these activities are done through the collection of health data in an ongoing manner to influence the health of the public, it can be considered public health surveillance. Considering that in 2003 there were an estimated 113.9 million emergency department (ED) visits nationwide [2], EDs are an ideal location to collect de-identified information on the acute health needs and patterns of the population of the United States. The systematic collection of data from multiple EDs can also serve as a barometer of the overall status of the US health system. While there are a number of logistical and infrastructural barriers that can impede the development of surveillance systems, the potential benefits from these systems are significant. The ability to analyze data; distribute results; and influence policy, funding, and patients' behavior are important outgrowths of public health surveillance in emergency departments.

* Corresponding author. Department of Emergency Medicine, 59 MDW/MCED, 2200 Bergquist Drive, Suite 1, Lackland AFB, TX 78236-5500.
E-mail address: shawn.varney@lackland.af.mil (S.M. Varney).

doi:10.1016/j.emc.2006.06.004   *emed.theclinics.com*

What is public health surveillance?

Definition of surveillance

The Centers for Disease Control and Prevention (CDC) has defined public health surveillance as "the ongoing systematic collection, analysis and interpretation of health data essential to the planning, implementation and evaluation of public health practices, closely integrated with the timely dissemination of these data to those who need to know. The final link in the surveillance chain is the application of these data to prevention and control" [3]. Surveillance systems are used to prepare, execute, and assess public health intervention programs and relay the acquired information to decision makers. In the present age of heightened security awareness and threats of bioterrorism, surveillance systems play an additional role in the early detection of health use anomalies. Through the rapid recognition of multiple patients with similar symptoms suggestive of an atypical or biologic agent, alerts are triggered so that public health professionals are notified of a potential threat.

Surveillance system components

Surveillance systems may range from rudimentary to complex—ie, from manual collection and documentation on sheets of paper to automated real-time data delivery. The steps required for a public health surveillance system include data acquisition on a periodic and ongoing basis, timely data collation and analysis, and the application of these data by the proper public health professionals. The basic components of a surveillance system include equipment, personnel, and the required resources for the personnel to analyze the data, communicate promptly and effectively, and maintain the system adequately.

The ability to amass and analyze large amounts of information has markedly improved with the advent of current computer technology. Therefore, essential equipment for an ED-based public health surveillance system now includes a robust computerized database system with appropriate Internet and networking capabilities, along with sophisticated software to analyze data for areas of interest. The potential applications of data and the requirements for interoperability with collaborators, such as regional, state, or national systems, dictate the necessary degree of complexity.

Fundamental personnel consist of individuals responsible for (1) data collection, (2) information analysis, and (3) timely response to material collected. Thus, many partners are involved, including health care providers in physicians' offices and EDs and public health professionals in local, state, and federal agencies, as well as laboratory workers, researchers, academicians, and information technology (IT) experts. The ability to maintain multidirectional communication flow among these team members is critical for a functional system.

Required additional resources include financial, institutional, and IT (encompassing communication, data management, and data analysis). To be effective, surveillance system development requires full endorsement and involvement from interested public health, political, and private leaders in many fields. Data sources may include standardized clinical databases from hospitals, doctors' offices, EDs, pharmacies, telephone health lines, and others. The integration of these databases into a cohesive system requires significant time and effort to garner support of critical partners and to make the system fully operational.

Definition of syndromic surveillance

Syndromic surveillance describes a dynamic process of collecting real-time or near real-time data on symptom clusters suggestive of a biological disease outbreak. Ideally, these diseases will be detected early in the process—before the definitive diagnosis—to enable a rapid response and mitigate adverse outcomes [4,5]. Syndromic surveillance systems have secondary objectives including determining the size, spread, and tempo of an outbreak, or even providing reassurance that an outbreak has not occurred [4].

Initially, syndromic surveillance systems were designed for the early detection of biological terrorism agents. The focus has evolved subsequent to the 9/11 World Trade Center and anthrax terrorist attacks of 2001. Present emphasis lies on the timely collection, assimilation, and analysis of health care data gathered from existing community systems to provide immediate feedback to decision makers about unexpected disease clusters or sentinel cases [4].

In contrast to the standard diagnosis-based disease surveillance (labs and cultures), syndromic surveillance is prediagnostic—ie, it recognizes a cluster of symptoms, or the onset of a disease, before full-blown illness manifestation. Identifying a peak of unusual symptoms above the background/steady state may allow a few extra days for further observation, evaluation, and treatment before the severe illness becomes apparent by conventional diagnostic methods. Theoretically, early detection equates to earlier treatment and decreased morbidity and mortality.

Syndromic surveillance systems tend to derive their data from two sources: (1) clinical data from health care services (ED visits, clinic visits, or Emergency Medical Services [EMS] records), and (2) alternative sources (work or school absentee rates, pharmaceutical sales, calls to emergency or information hotlines, Internet-based illness reporting systems) [6]. Each data source has advantages. For example, clinical data sources provide the ability to follow patients and, in the case of a public health emergency, to contact infected individuals. These actions, however, would require significant efforts and high-level approvals to override existing privacy and confidentiality safeguards. In addition, clinical data encourages bidirectional communication and fosters improved relationships between community providers and public health staff, which is an important step in a functional public health system. Alternative data sources, such as pharmacy sales including over-the-counter products, may signal the occurrence of events before people seek formal health care and may represent a broader sample of the population at risk.

In one study of 3919 ED visits, Begier and colleagues [5] found good overall agreement (kappa = 0.639) between chief complaint and discharge diagnosis, but substantial variability by specific syndromes. All ED patient encounters were coded via a mutually exclusive algorithm into one of eight syndromes: death, sepsis, rash, respiratory illness, gastrointestinal illness, unspecified infection, neurologic illness, and other. They observed lower agreement among sepsis, neurologic, and unspecified infection. Begier and colleagues concluded that although there is good agreement for most syndromes, the chief complaint better identifies illnesses with nonspecific symptoms (ie, fever), while discharge diagnoses detect illnesses requiring clinical evaluation (ie, sepsis and meningitis).

Another form of syndromic surveillance is "event-based" or "drop-in" surveillance, which lasts for a finite period or event. It relies on health care providers in EDs and large clinics to collect nonroutine data. Such a system was implemented and proved useful during the 2000 Democratic National Convention in California and the 2002 Winter Olympic Games in Utah [7,8].

Although syndromic surveillance may be able to play a key role in early recognition of disease outbreaks, it neither replaces traditional public health surveillance nor supplants the critical role of an astute physician reporting atypical diseases and events.

Why is surveillance important?

General rationales for ED-based public health surveillance

There are a number of rationales for the development of public health surveillance based on ED visits [9]. These include:

1. Improved communication between health departments and emergency departments for addressing ongoing local, regional, and state-level problems.
2. Improved public health response to rapidly developing public health emergencies.
3. Improved ability to correlate environmental events and visits.
4. Improved information on the scope and nature of ED visits for injuries (both minor and major).
5. Improved documentation and evaluation of ED visits for infectious diseases.
6. Improved hospital-based patient record systems.

7. Influence policy discussions and decisions through improved data.

These rationales can be conceptually divided into those designed to improve the health of the public and those designed to improve the security of the population.

Improving public health

Surveillance is an outcome-oriented science that provides information for action. Public health surveillance focuses on health-related issues or their preceding events. It plays a key role in protecting the public by devising ways to improve health and to mitigate morbidity and mortality. In the context of public health, Teutsch and Churchill [10] described multiple ways that surveillance data are useful: to estimate the magnitude of a health problem; to understand the natural history of a disease or injury; to detect outbreaks or epidemics; to document the distribution and spread of a health event; to test hypotheses about etiology; to evaluate control strategies; to monitor changes in infectious agents; to monitor isolation activities; to detect changes in health practice; to identify research needs and facilitate epidemiologic and laboratory research; and to facilitate planning.

Surveillance allows for the monitoring and evaluation of the health of the public. However, it is critical that appropriate public health professionals then translate the information garnered from these efforts into action. A feedback loop is thus developed to produce positive effects within the monitored population. Timely and accurate health-related data, properly collected and analyzed, allow public health leaders, politicians, and others to act appropriately to mitigate disasters or epidemics through judicious allocation of suitable resources.

A current example of ongoing surveillance of a potential public health threat is the actions by national governments in Asia, the CDC, and the World Health Organization (WHO) to monitor the current status of avian influenza (bird flu), especially the influenza A (H5N1) virus [11]. While H5N1 primarily affects fowl, there is concern for the potential person-to-person transmission of the virus leading to a pandemic. Thus the CDC has recommended enhanced surveillance for this disease in the United States to promote its rapid diagnosis and to prevent its dissemination. If bird flu were discovered in a patient in the United States, the CDC could rapidly mobilize resources to limit the spread of infection and panic among the population.

Terrorism response/homeland security

According to the Advisory Panel to Assess Domestic Response Capabilities for Terrorism Involving Weapons of Mass Destruction, "a robust public health system is fundamental to a long-term solution for a variety of health issues, including terrorism" [12]. Public health surveillance systems, such as those based on ED visits, are part of this solution. While it is difficult to assess the magnitude of the threat, there is no question that all societies are at risk from conventional explosives and, potentially, from weapons of mass destruction. Within this global context of increased insecurity, it is important to be able to detect unusual diseases and events. The ongoing, systematic collection of ED data to identify unusual diseases and patterns may help shorten the time required to respond to biological or chemical attacks and thus decrease the morbidity and mortality from these weapons. Recognition on the national level can be seen by the increased federal dollars allocated to public health, much of which has been used for increased disease surveillance and response. Additionally, a number of projects focusing on syndromic surveillance, such as the Electronic Surveillance System for the Early Notification of Community-Based Epidemics (ESSENCE), were developed or tested through funding from the Defense Advanced Research Project Agency (DARPA) and the Department of Defense [13].

Stakeholders in developing surveillance systems

Health care facilities

The ED plays a key role in the development and use of a public health surveillance system. Patients come into EDs 24 hours a day, 7 days a week, every day of the year, making it an appropriate place for data gathering and collation. Health care providers in the ED simultaneously see multiple patients and often have high daily patient volumes. This enables the derivation of the relative prevalence of symptom clusters that may represent worrisome syndromes or epidemics. Outlying clinics frequently refer sicker patients to local EDs, facilitating collection of information on more cases. Emergency physicians are taught to have a high index of suspicion for uncommon diseases, leading to broad differential diagnoses and clinical acumen. They are the first physician contacts for patients in many situations and may detect aberrations in the usual incidence of disease. From these frontline positions, they need to be able to transmit their findings and concerns in a timely and accurate manner to the appropriate public health authority. As a primary participant in the disease recognition process, emergency physicians and other ED staff must be involved in surveillance system development.

The information collecting process should be simple, quick, and easy to implement with minimal or no impact on health care practitioners. Automatic classification of broad symptom categories for chief complaints can be included as a part of triage. Alternatively, a computer can be placed in a kiosk by the registration desk in the ED. Simple questions may identify symptom clusters that the computer can analyze at regular intervals and produce warnings or alerts to hospital personnel or public health agencies.

ED personnel end up participating in the surveillance process to some degree whether they realize it or not. Simply observing patients and assimilating and documenting information (gathering chief complaints, identifying trends, and so forth) contributes. Passing the data to the public health sector may mitigate morbidity and mortality. Automatic data entry from multiple hospitals into a centralized repository may facilitate disease recognition and coordinate findings citywide, similar to a well-run emergency medical services system. Ideally, a large funding source, such as state and federal governments, should support this initiative in the interest of the public's health.

Public health agencies

Public health agencies and their staff play a pivotal role in monitoring and managing the public's health, from scrutinizing for disease outbreaks to implementing quarantine measures. They function as the keystone of a public health surveillance system and their involvement in system development and use is crucial. While EDs and other data sources, such as laboratory personnel and pharmacists, supply the input, public health professionals must accept the collected data, analyze it, and then return recommendations and policy actions to appropriate officials. Timely reporting is critical to allow public health professionals to perform their jobs.

As part of this involvement, bidirectional communication is vital between frontline providers, such as emergency physicians, and public health experts. While it is important that accurate information be sent to the health department in a timely manner, it is of equal significance that informed and authoritative health messages be disseminated to both health care professionals and to the public. The information received by emergency physicians and other practitioners influences the evaluation and treatment of patients. Public health messages can assist in the effective management of the behavior and responses of the community at large, especially in times of crisis.

Of additional consequence in this partnership between health care and public health is the understanding that system development requires the support, financial and otherwise, of health departments and public health professionals. An individual ED is not a surveillance system, although it may function as a monitoring station within one. A public health surveillance system based on ED visits, as well as other potential data sources, requires significant infrastructural support to receive large amounts of health-related data and then to rapidly analyze it for unusual patterns or increased disease frequency.

Information technology

With the increased ability to rapidly collect and analyze data from multiple sources, the involvement and support of experts in information technology are important aspects of the team effort to develop a functional public health surveillance system. In general, data are not transmitted as a continuous stream, but rather at periodic intervals (eg, hourly, daily, weekly). Data can be collected and analyzed manually, but the greater the automation, the more rapid and accurate the results are likely to be. Automation can enhance the data collection and analysis process, minimizing delays and decreasing inaccuracy caused by the need to depend on human interactions. Through the use of software that automatically collects the number of visits (or other data parameter) by category, the amount of effort required by health care providers in data input can be significantly decreased. Advanced logic algorithms can help look for unusual trends through analysis of the data from multiple sources and can be instructed to alert when specific patterns are noted. While these processes can decrease the daily effort required of health care and public health professionals, individuals knowledgeable about the appropriate software and hardware are required for a smoothly functioning, integrated system.

Surveillance implementation

Health data standards and timeliness

An ideal public health surveillance system would be interoperable, universal, automated, real-time, economical, secure, sensitive, and specific. To date, information technology (IT) developers have not created a product to satisfy these parameters. To enhance interoperability between different current systems and between existing and future systems, certain information system standards have been identified. In addition, information systems supported by government funds must comply with federally mandated standards.

Broome and Loonsk [14] discussed three vital justifications for standards-based system development: (1) electronic messaging (ie, Standard Health Level 7, or HL7, interface) provides the most effective and efficient way to collect real-time data from multiple sources; (2) specified standards provide public health departments greater control over previous investments in their IT infrastructures; and (3) standard formats and electronic data delivery reduce the burden on individual providers' reporting practices.

Multiple government agencies have identified important standards integral to improved information exchange between clinicians and health departments [14]. The CDC and its state and local delegates formed the Public Health Information Network that identified standards for data, technology, terminology, and confidentiality. This network named five major functional areas (detection and monitoring, data analysis, knowledge management, alerting, and response) and itemized specifications for nine IT functions that form the basis for interoperable standards-based systems:

1. automated data exchange between public health partners;
2. use of electronic clinical data for event detection;
3. manual data entry for event detection and management;
4. specimen and laboratory result information management and exchange;
5. management of possible case, contacts, and threat data;
6. analysis and visualization;
7. directories of public health and clinical personnel;
8. public health information dissemination and alerting; and
9. IT security and critical infrastructure protection [15].

At the request of the CDC Information Council, the Gartner Group, an independent IT consulting firm, reviewed the Public Health Information Network's specifications and functions and endorsed them as the "foundational road map" for systems integration in public health [16].

Timeliness related to surveillance systems impacts all aspects of the process from data collection, through data transfer and analysis, to returning treatment and policy recommendations. These criteria are ranked among the most important and most often described in published reports [17,18]. The ability to react quickly to public health emergencies depends on rapid recognition and response to possible or actual threats, which is the core issue of timeliness.

Data collection

Two prevailing data-gathering principles in public health surveillance are (1) collect information judiciously, and (2) gather and retain information as locally as possible [6]. Both principles facilitate compliance with the Health Insurance Portability and Accountability Act (HIPAA) of 1996 and also help limit the amount of labor involved in the data input phase. From a pragmatic perspective, it is important to limit the amount of data collection effort required by frontline providers, to achieve high levels of compliance and data fidelity without impacting providers' ability to care for patients.

While most hospitals do not have real-time or near-real-time surveillance systems, some have adapted current systems to achieve this objective. For example, in Hong Kong the hospital authority developed an ED computer system used across the region. For 2 years (1999–2000) they gathered data on common diseases, namely upper respiratory infections and gastrointestinal illnesses, and followed trends and seasonal peaks. They tracked diagnoses, prescriptions, specialty information, and patient demographics monthly. When peaks exceeded two standard deviations of variance, a computer-generated report was sent to the ED director and hospital authority officials for appropriate intervention [19]. Noting the unexpected infectious disease surges, the health authorities alerted the media and educated the public. This may have helped curtail disease transmission.

The simple step of compiling computerized ED records of patient volume, chief complaints, and diagnoses, along with applying a standard statistical program, forms the first step in disease surveillance. Providers, in general, do not prioritize nonclinical responsibilities during clinical hours. In a busy ED, an emergency physician will need to see direct patient care benefit from data collection, otherwise data acquisition will be inconsistent. Much of the data collation can occur in an environment away from the clinical area thereby limiting the impact on the health care providers.

Data transfer

As discussed above, standards are important to ensure timely and accurate transfer of data. Considering the current state of computer technology, electronic data transfer best meets these needs. In addition, data security, such as encryption, is of fundamental importance, especially when considering the increased responsibility of covered entities to securely protect the confidentiality of personal health information. While HIPAA allows for exemptions concerning the use of data for public health purposes, surveillance systems and related stakeholders would have difficulty withstanding public scrutiny if data were mishandled or inappropriately released.

Data analysis

Rapid, accurate analysis of the data is important to develop appropriate and timely policy recommendation. It is the critical step in turning large amounts of seemingly unrelated data into coherent information, and subsequently into action. Individuals may analyze data manually with statistical programs or using automated algorithmic processes. In most instances it will be a combination of both modalities. Automatic algorithms can greatly enhance the speed of analysis and produce predefined alerts, but will still require interpretation and monitoring by those with an in-depth knowledge of the surveillance system.

While there are many similarities between systems designed to collect health data, sources of information vary. Data analysis solutions require modifications for specific circumstances. For example, the detection of an abnormal increase in a disease is dependent on the definition of the baseline incidence of that disease, as seen by syndromic surveillance for flu-like illnesses. The number of cases that would be considered abnormal will be very different in the winter months during the "flu season," as opposed to the summer months when influenza is unlikely. One solution to this problem is to use a progressive baseline derived from the number of flu-like cases in the previous 2 weeks. Thus, when influenza spreads through the community in late fall/early winter, the system would initially produce alerts based on a predetermined variance from baseline but would quickly develop a modified baseline that would be appropriate for a season of increased cases. This baseline would then decrease as the number of flu-like illnesses drop in late winter/early spring leading to an appropriate baseline for a low-incidence season.

Another aspect of data analysis involves investigating specific alerts. For example, signal investigation plays a key role in outbreak detection. Steiner-Sichel and colleagues [20] described their experience with the New York City Department of Health and Mental Hygiene (DOHMH), which has operated a syndromic surveillance system based on ED chief complaints since November 2001. The DOHMH conducted field investigations of suspected outbreaks when the surveillance systems signaled an unexpected increase/excess above the expected rates for respiratory, fever, diarrhea, and vomiting syndromes. They sought to determine if the signals correlated with clinically significant disease outbreaks. In more than 40 signal investigations, none definitively detected an infectious disease outbreak. They also found that none of the localized outbreaks investigated by the traditional methods revealed any syndromic surveillance signal. Steiner-Sichel and colleagues attributed this to the difficulty of proving causality and using a sensitive, but not specific, detection system. The advantage of early detection may be offset by the complexities of field investigation and epidemiologic data acquisition.

At the present time a number of issues need to be addressed to improve data analysis, particularly as it relates to syndromic surveillance. These issues include how to best analyze data from multiple data streams [21,22], improve the linkage of data from different data sources [23], and create flexible space-time shapes in the analysis of disease clusters [24]. While a great deal of energy and resources have been spent to improve public health surveillance, especially as it relates to syndromic surveillance, further work is clearly necessary.

Use and misuse of data

Although there are clear public health and public safety aspects to the use of aggregated health-related data, the potential misuse of data is of significant concern. Misuse and abuse may come in many forms. The ability to contact trace individuals in case of a highly transmissible and deadly infectious disease or a bioterrorism event is critical to decreasing the potential morbidity and mortality. On the other hand, sufficient safeguards must be in place to prevent the inadvertent or malicious release of personal information. HIPAA attempts to address many of the issues related to the use and sharing of individual health records, especially as it is collected from clinical encounters, and mandates the appropriate handling of this personal information.

One way to address the conflict between public health and patient privacy is by releasing only de-identified data to the public health agency collecting the data, thus making inadvertent tracing much less likely. If specific information is needed to prevent a public health emergency, then the appropriate individuals with the proper legal authority could request the specific identifiable information from the data-collecting site, such as the hospital. This multiple-step process may slow the evaluation and possible response by public health officials, but this must be balanced with the need to protect individuals' privacy. The complex interplay between the health needs of the general public and an individual's rights and privacy is placed within an intricate legal setting and leads to one of the great dynamics of public health, namely balancing human rights and public safety.

Barriers to surveillance systems development

General barriers to ED-based public health surveillance

There are a number of barriers to the development of public health surveillance based on ED visits [9]. These include the following:

1. Costs for public health agencies
2. Costs for emergency departments and hospitals
3. Need to improve and standardize data collection
4. Security and confidentiality issues
5. Obtaining acceptance and support from emergency medicine leadership and practitioners

These can be conceptually divided into funding issues, data-related issues, and the need to obtain acceptance and support from key partners.

Funding

Development of the public health surveillance infrastructure requires significant financial investment, especially by public health authorities. Whereas governments can mandate certain actions (especially on the part of large entities such as hospitals), institutions will resist actions that adversely impact their financial status. Since the end users of these systems are public health authorities and ultimately the public, it is the responsibility of the government to bear a significant burden of the cost.

Since the terrorist attacks of September 11, 2001, and the subsequent anthrax letters, a significant amount of federal dollars has gone to public health agencies, especially at the local jurisdiction. Much of this money was designated for terrorism response activities, including improving surveillance and communications. Despite these large sums of money, there is considerable variance in current public health surveillance infrastructure throughout the United States. Additional funding is needed to continue to improve and standardize public health surveillance activities—especially syndromic surveillance. These resources will need to be shared between the data collection entities and those entities analyzing the data and producing public health responses.

Sharing of data

The data that routine surveillance systems collect differ from syndromic surveillance data in that the former are based on diagnostic or culture-positive diseases, whereas the latter are founded in prediagnostic, or clusters of symptoms suggesting potentially infectious disease outbreaks. Health information privacy rules such as HIPAA may apply differently to routine and syndromic surveillance data. The prevailing feeling among some physicians is that reporting and investigating patients with culture-positive diseases do not violate patient privacy, whereas inconclusive disease processes are not certain enough to warrant full disclosure of patient privacy information for further contact [25]. Data collection for syndromic surveillance requires the ability to identify and contact individual patients when a surge in unusual symptoms (signal) occurs.

In a survey sent to state epidemiologists and terrorism preparedness coordinators regarding the effects of HIPAA Privacy Rule requirements on syndromic surveillance system implementation, Drociuk and colleagues [25] found that more than half reported "some" or "substantial" problems. HIPAA's "minimum necessary" stipulation thwarted disease surveillance activities. The "minimum necessary" standard states that health care providers must take reasonable steps to limit the use or disclosure of protected health information (PHI) to the minimum necessary to accomplish the intended purpose [26]. Covered entities (ie, all health care organizations) have the flexibility to make their own assessment of what PHI is reasonably necessary for a particular purpose. Unfortunately, there is no broadly accepted definition for "minimum necessary" in either routine or syndromic surveillance systems.

As noted above, a proper balance must exist between protecting personal health information and the need to protect the general public health. The HIPAA Privacy Rule permits PHI disclosures without individual authorization to public health agents and designees when intended to prevent or control disease, injury, or disability, including public health surveillance, investigation, and intervention [27]. One solution to satisfy patient confidentiality concerns is collecting limited data sets, ie, information that is not directly identifiable. Specific data use agreements must establish who is permitted to use the data. The benefit is fewer problems with HIPAA and potentially better participation from surveillance institutions, but the drawback includes delayed signal investigations. The delays may significantly counter the potential theoretical advantage of early outbreak detection by syndromic surveillance.

Regarding data transfer, 27/32 (87%) respondents reported no security concerns because of the secure transmission measures and off-system data-archiving protocols [25]. Despite the problems with patient confidentiality and data transfer, physicians felt more secure and ready for potential terrorist attacks. Furthermore, the mere fact that surveillance systems exist may serve as deterrence against terrorist strikes since the community may appear poised and ready to act.

Buy-in from collaborators

There are two main groups that are important for a functional public health surveillance system based on ED data: the hospitals (ie, the data sources) and the public health departments (ie, data analyzers and users) [9]. Both groups should be actively involved in the creation and deployment of the final system, since ongoing bidirectional communication and interagency cooperation are critical. The development of the relationship between the hospitals and the health department are as important as the final system structure, since public health professionals need the data to help make informed policy decisions and action recommendations, and medical professionals, such as emergency physicians, may need to implement these recommendations.

Obtaining this buy-in requires a commitment from both sides. Cooperation is developed through working together and developing a shared vision. There needs to be mutual understanding of the goals and expectations for the system and the roles that each participating organization will play. There are a number of potential barriers to the creation of a relationship, including the costs involved for both the data collection and the data analysis. However, a clearer understanding of the importance of the public health–medical collaborations has grown over the past 5 years with the increased awareness of the risks of disease spread, such as from avian influenza, and the potential for bioterrorism.

Criteria for evaluating a surveillance system

Buehler [28], from the CDC 2003 Working Group on Public Health Surveillance Systems, described a comprehensive framework of four categories for evaluating all public health surveillance systems: system description, outbreak detection, experience, and conclusions and recommendations.

In summary, the *system description* should clearly state the system's purpose, including indications for its use, duration, area of emphasis, and the desired sensitivity and specificity. It should identify the stakeholders, meaning those supplying the data and applying the information. Finally, it should provide a detailed description of all operational aspects including data flow, data sources, data processing before analysis, statistical analysis, and epidemiological analysis and interpretation [25].

The second category is *outbreak detection* and discusses factors affecting timely data gathering and processing, data validity, and data aberrancy–detection methods. Timeliness describes a continuum from the onset of symptoms to public health intervention. Establishing the validity of a surveillance system to detect an outbreak requires epidemiological tools like outbreak and case definitions, statistical analysis, and assessment of the data quality.

The third area for system evaluation is documented *experience* with the system. Important factors for system experience include the following: usefulness (impact of its application), flexibility (ability to adapt easily to changing needs and new technology), acceptability (willingness of parties to submit timely and complete data, widespread use), portability (ease of reproduction in other centers), stability (minimal downtime and maximal consistency), and cost (for software and support as well as for false alarms and failed detection).

The final system evaluation category is a summary of the *conclusions and recommendations* of the advantages and disadvantages of each system. A useful approach would include possible modifications of present systems to meet the increasing needs in public health surveillance.

Bravata and colleagues performed a systematic review on surveillance systems for the early detection of bioterrorism-related diseases [15,29]. After reviewing more than 17,000 article citations and 8000 web sites, they found 192 reports on 115 systems that gathered surveillance data, including nine syndromic surveillance systems. Bravata and colleagues evaluated the systems for reports on nine qualities the CDC had defined previously: usefulness, importance, timeliness, flexibility, sensitivity, representativeness, simplicity, acceptability, and specificity [30–32]. Only one article addressed all nine criteria [16]. Usefulness, importance, and timeliness were most commonly described, whereas only three reports of three systems provided actual values for sensitivity and specificity [15]. Clearly, there is little scientific evidence supporting the use of surveillance systems. Future studies are needed to evaluate present and new systems for these nine characteristics of effective surveillance systems. Three of the most important criteria appear to be sensitivity and specificity, timeliness, and the ability of the system to impact decision making.

Sosin and DeThomasis [33], members of the CDC 2003 Working Group on Public Health Surveillance Systems, summarized the group's findings by developing a task list of specific, goal-directed questions for early outbreak detection. Sosin and DeThomasis reviewed 99 abstracts presented at the 2003 National Syndromic Surveillance conference and found limited information on system evaluation. Because a detailed analysis of systems would likely be laborious and expensive, Sosin and DeThomasis proposed emphasizing timeliness, validity, and usefulness to measure the success of detection methods.

Criteria for evaluating surveillance systems are more complex and difficult to assess than originally conceived. Despite rigorous descriptions and defined criteria, few researchers have produced data following the CDC's recommended framework. Perhaps a simplified approach reviewing only timeliness, validity, and usefulness may show the impact and cost of detection methods.

Summary

The development of public health surveillance systems based on ED visits, in conjunction with other health and nonhealth-related data, is an important step to better understanding the health needs of the US population. There are multiple steps required to develop a functional organization, and these actions require the support and involvement of many different partners. In any given jurisdiction a number of obstacles to structure development may exist and will require teamwork to overcome. Yet, the information derived from these systems on the acute health needs and health care usage patterns of the US population can help both to improve the health of the public and to serve as an early warning system for a possible bioterrorism event. Whereas surveillance systems can serve many important functions, it is also critical to maintain the privacy and confidentiality of protected health information while these systems are created and used. Through the establishment of public health surveillance systems, bidirectional communication is developed, strengthening the relationship between clinical and public health practitioners. The ability to (1) analyze data; (2) distribute results; and (3) influence policy, funding, and patients' behavior are important outgrowths of emergency department–based public health surveillance systems.

References

[1] 45 CFR 46.102(d).

[2] McCaig LF, Burt CW. National Hospital Ambulatory Medical Care Survey: 2003 emergency department summary. Advance data from vital and health statistics; No. 358. Hyattsville, MD: National Center for Health Statistics. Available at: http://www.cdc.gov/nchs/data/ad/ad358.pdf. Accessed July 16, 2006.

[3] Centers for Disease Control and Prevention. Comprehensive plan for epidemiologic surveillance. Atlanta, GA: CDC; 1986.

[4] Henning KJ. Overview of syndromic surveillance. What is syndromic surveillance? MMWR 2004;53(Suppl):5–11.

[5] Begier EM, Sockwell D, Branch LM, et al. The national capitol region's emergency department syndromic surveillance system: do chief complaint and discharge diagnosis yield different results? Emerg Infect Dis [serial online] 2003 Mar. Available at: http://www.cdc.gov/ncidod/EID/vol9no3/02-0363.htm. Accessed March 7, 2005.

[6] Buehler JW. Review of the 2003 National Syndromic Surveillance Conference—lessons learned and questions to be answered. MMWR 2004;53(Suppl):18–22.

[7] County of Los Angeles, Department of Health Services, Acute Communicable Disease Control. Special studies report 2000: Democratic National Convention—bioterrorism syndromic surveillance. Los Angeles: County of Los Angeles Department of Health Services, 2000. Available at: http://www.lapublichealth.org/acd/reports/spclrpts/spcrpt00/demonatconvtn00.pdf. Accessed July 16, 2006.

[8] Gesteland PH, Wagner MM, Chapman WW, et al. Rapid deployment of an electronic disease surveillance system in the state of Utah for the 2002 Olympic Winter Games. Proc AMIA Symp 2002;285–9.

[9] Hirshon JM. The rationale for developing public health surveillance systems based on emergency department data. Acad Emerg Med 2001;7:1428–32.

[10] Teutsch SM, Churchill RE. Principles and practice of public health surveillance. 2nd ed. Oxford, NY: Oxford University Press; 2000.

[11] Centers for Disease Control and Prevention: Key Facts About Avian Influenza (Bird Flu) and Avian Influenza A (H5N1) Virus. Available at: http://www.cdc.gov/flu/avian/gen-info/facts.htm. Accessed August 28, 2005.

[12] Third annual report to the president and the Congress of the advisory panel to assess domestic response capabilities for terrorism involving weapons of mass destruction. Dec 15, 2001. p. 25. Available at: http://www.rand.org/nsrd/terrpanel/terror3-screen.pdf. Accessed July 16, 2006.

[13] Burkom HS, Elbert Y, Feldman A, Lin J. Role of data aggregation in biosurveillance detection strategies with applications from ESSENCE. MMWR 2004;53(Suppl):67–73.

[14] Broome CV, Loonsk J. Public health information network—improving early detection by using a standards-based approach to connecting public health and clinical medicine. MMWR 2004;53(Suppl):199–202.

[15] CDC. Public Health Information Network standards, specifications, and functions. Atlanta, GA: US Department of Health and Human Services, CDC, 2003. Available at: http://www.cdc.gov/phin/architecture/index.htm. Accessed.

[16] Gartner, Inc. Technical review of issues related to version 1 of the Public Health Information Network functions and specifications. Stamford, CT: Gartner, Inc.; 2003. Available at: http://wwwcdc.gov/phin/conference_presentations/05-13-03/. Accessed August 29, 2006.

[17] Bravata DM, McDonald KM, Smith WM, et al. Systematic review: surveillance systems for early detection of bioterrorism-related diseases. Ann Intern Med 2004;140:910–22.

[18] Takahashi H, Fujii H, Shindo N, et al. Evaluation of the Japanese school health surveillance system for influenza. Jpn J Infect Dis 2001;54:27–30.

[19] Chan JTK, Cameron PA. A pragmatic approach to timely disease surveillance in the emergency department. Emerg Med J 2003;20(Iss. 5):443–8.

[20] Steiner-Sichel L, Greenko J, Heffernan R, et al. Field investigations of emergency department syndromic surveillance signals—New York City. MMWR 2004;53:184–9.

[21] Burkom HS, Murphy S, Coberly J, et al. Public health monitoring tools for multiple data streams. In: Syndromic surveillance: reports from a national conference, 2004. MMWR 2005;54(Suppl):55–62.

[22] Wong W-K, Cooper G, Dash D, et al. Use of multiple data streams to conduct Bayesian biologic surveillance. In: Syndromic Surveillance: Reports from a National Conference, 2004. MMWR 2005;54(Suppl):63–9.

[23] Magruder S, Henry J, Snyder M. Linked analysis for definition of nurse advice line syndrome groups, and comparison to encounters. In: Syndromic surveillance: reports from a national conference, 2004. MMWR 2005;54(Suppl):93–7.

[24] Iyengar VS. Space-time clusters with flexible shapes. In: Syndromic surveillance: reports from a national conference, 2004. MMWR 2005;54(Suppl):71–6.

[25] Drociuk D, Gibson J, Hodge J. Health information privacy and syndromic surveillance systems. MMWR 2004;53(Suppl):221–5.

[26] United States Department of Health and Human Services. Office of Civil Rights—HIPAA. Last revised 16 Sep 04. Available at: http://www.hhs.gov/ocr/hipaa/. Accessed March 20, 2005.

[27] CDC. HIPAA Privacy Rule and public health: guidance from CDC and the US Department of Health and Human Services. MMWR 2003;52(Suppl):1–20.

[28] Buehler JW. Framework for evaluating public health surveillance systems for early detection of outbreaks: recommendations from the CDC Working Group. MMWR Recomm Rep 2004;53(RR-5):1–11.

[29] Bravata DM, Sundaram V, McDonald KM, et al. Evaluating detection and diagnostic decision support systems for bioterrorism response. Emerg Infect Dis 2004;10(1):100–8.

[30] CDC. Guidelines for evaluating surveillance systems. MMWR 1988;37(No. S-5):1–18.

[31] Sosin DM. Draft framework for evaluating syndromic surveillance systems. J Urban Health 2003;80(2, Suppl 1):i8–13.

[32] CDC. Updated guidelines for evaluating public health surveillance systems. Recommendations from the Guidelines Working Group. MMWR 2001;50(RR13):1–35.

[33] Sosin DM, DeThomasis J. Evaluation challenges for syndromic surveillance: making incremental progress. MMWR 2004;53(Suppl):125–9.

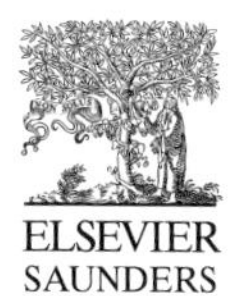

Emerg Med Clin N Am
24 (2006) 1053–1073

The Future of Emergency Medicine Public Health Research

Karin V. Rhodes, MD, MS[a],*,
Daniel A. Pollock, MD[b,c]

[a]Department of Emergency Medicine, School of Social Policy & Practice,
University of Pennsylvania, 3815 Walnut Street, Room 201,
Philadelphia, PA 19104, USA
[b]Healthcare Outcomes Branch, Division of Healthcare Quality Promotion,
National Center for Infectious Diseases, Centers for Disease Control and Prevention,
1600 Clifton Rd, Atlanta, GA 30333, USA
[c]Department of Emergency Medicine, Emory University School of Medicine,
1365 Clifton Road, Suite B6200, Atlanta, GA 30322, USA

The distinguishing feature of public health research is its focus on assessing, measuring, and monitoring the health of *populations*; in contrast, traditional biomedical research focuses on studying disease and treatment for *individual* patients [1]. Compared with most medical specialties, emergency medicine (EM) is well positioned to bridge biomedical and public health approaches for preventing disease and injury and promoting health through population-based strategies targeted at the community [2]. In its strategically vital position at the boundary between the hospital and the surrounding community, the emergency department (ED) is actually the linchpin for multiple systems of care. When all systems are functioning, EM offers access for all patients 24 hours a day, 7 days a week, regardless of their ability to pay. EM provides triage and care for both mental and physical health conditions, and links patients with the most appropriate providers and care settings for their presenting conditions. EM identifies unmet health needs and interfaces with primary care, specialty care, inpatient, outpatient, and community-based social services. The ED also collects data used for surveillance of infectious diseases (eg, sexually transmitted infections, tuberculosis, severe acute respiratory syndrome [SARS]) and environmental emergencies

* Corresponding author.
E-mail address: kvr@sp2.upenn.edu (K.V. Rhodes).

doi:10.1016/j.emc.2006.06.003   *emed.theclinics.com*

(eg, heat waves, toxic spills) and forwards patient-level data to public health departments. However, research advances and practical innovations are needed to enhance surveillance data by enabling "real-time" reporting of more cases and more complete data about each case. In addition, the ED is well positioned to recognize and call attention to major social problems that impact the health of the public (breaches in food safety, homelessness, lack of health insurance or care coordination, child abuse, interpersonal violence). EM has great potential as a public health partner capable of monitoring and providing input into policies affecting the health of populations along a number of dimensions.

Background: EM and public health

The specialty of EM was launched in the 1970s in response to patients' needs for improved access to care. Indeed, the topic of access, particularly for vulnerable populations, pervades much of EM public health research. Before the 1980s, it was both traditionally and federally reinforced through Hill Burton funding that hospitals provided the majority of "charity care" [3]. The original emergency rooms were started in response to unattached patients. At that time, those individuals without primary care physicians who presented to the hospital in acute distress would be evaluated by the charge nurse and, if necessary, the on-call physician. Early EDs were primarily staffed by nurses, rotating residents from various specialties, and physicians trying to build practices [4]. The growth of the specialty of EM was very much consumer driven as the volume increased to the point that overwhelmed existing staff, who were all trying to do other jobs. Finally, small groups of physicians began providing full-time coverage of EDs as attending physicians dedicated to providing emergency care; the Pontiac Plan and the Alexandria Plan were examples. These informal groups soon united to define the scope of EM, develop curriculum and board certification, and lobby organized medicine for specialty status. The new specialty grew exponentially and was amazingly successful both for hospitals and EM physician groups [4]. However, major changes in the financing and delivery of health care in the 1980s resulted in increasing rates of uninsured patients [5]. Many private hospitals started to baulk at absorbing this burden and developed policies of referring or transferring uninsured ED patients to publicly funded county hospitals. Emergency physicians and patients responded to these "patient dumping" policies with research and advocacy [6]. Understanding this close relationship between EM, the needs of health care consumers, and the development of current health care policies gives a framework for a discussion of the past challenges, successes, and potential for future EM public health research.

Monitoring health care access: negotiating emergency care during changes in health policy

Past challenges, research findings, and their impact

Like EM itself, EM *research* has its roots in advocacy efforts by emergency physicians to provide access to care for vulnerable patient populations. Much of this work was composed of descriptive studies designed to document disparities in care for the poor and uninsured. Among these studies were descriptive analyses of "patient dumping," a practice in which private hospitals transferred uninsured patients to public hospital EDs, regardless of medical condition [7]. This analytic work influenced landmark federal legislation, the Emergency Medical Treatment and Active Labor Act (EMTALA), which established a statutory duty for Medicare-participating hospitals with EDs to serve any person seeking emergency care [8].

In the early 1990s, governmental and free market cost-containment strategies, including the penetration of health maintenance organizations, accelerated. Many policy analysts questioned the opportunity costs of paying for the high cost of emergency care. Several researchers, however, reported that the marginal costs of ED care, especially for nonurgent problems, were actually much less than widely believed. Williams [9] provided evidence that the majority of ED costs were fixed because of the necessity of standby capacity for unexpected trauma and acute medical emergencies, and that the excess charges primarily reflected cost shifting to pay for the uninsured. Tyrance and colleagues [10] found that "ED use accounts for a small fraction of medical spending" and suggested that "Attempts to restrict ED use would disproportionately burden minorities and the poor who receive much of their out patient care in EDs." They also recommended that "Strategies that reduce demand for ED services should be pursued to improve health, not because of anticipated cost savings." Nonetheless, many health policy experts and politicians considered "inappropriate ED use" to be an important cause of high medical costs. This led to attempts by managed care organizations to constrain patient access to emergency services. One opinion of primary care specialists is summarized by Dowling [11] from the Department of Family Medicine at the University of California, Los Angeles. He referred to ED care as "fragmented, uncoordinated, incomplete, and inappropriate" and said the real cost of an ED visit was its "missed opportunity for prevention." These criticisms may have had more validity if, at the same time, there hadn't been a lack of access to primary care for a large portion of Americans based on inadequate or lack of health insurance [12–15].

In 1994, a group of emergency physicians formed the multisite Medicaid Access Study Group to study the problems that Medicaid recipients were experiencing when they tried to access primary care. In the nine cities, they trained research assistants to pose as patients seeking care for relatively minor, but physically uncomfortable health problems [16]. Only 44% of Medicaid callers could secure an appointment at any point in time, and only 8% could get an appointment within 2 working days without agreeing to pay a substantial amount of cash at the time of the visit. When callers recontacted the same primary care practices and stated that they had private insurance, twice as many were granted a timely appointment. The authors concluded that Medicaid patients have few options outside of the ED.

Other studies in the mid-1990s focused on the impact of HMO-mediated ED access barriers [17–19].

These research studies and advocacy efforts on the part of organized emergency medicine and health care consumers eventually led to the Healthy People (HP) 2010 objective 1-10, to "reduce the proportion of persons who delay or have difficulty in getting emergency medical care" and the overarching goal to "improve access to high-quality health care services" [18]. Many state governments and the federal Medicare and Medicaid programs adopted the "prudent layperson standard" in defining a medical emergency for purposes of health insurance coverage. The prudent layperson standard also was incorporated into a federal legislative proposal that would make it applicable to emergency care reimbursement decisions by all health care plans nationwide [18]. This standard obligated managed care plans to provide coverage for ED services based on an enrollee's presenting symptoms (including severe pain) rather than the final diagnosis. The test for triggering reimbursement under this standard was whether a prudent layperson (a person who possesses an average knowledge of health and medicine) would reasonably expect that the absence of immediate medical attention could result in harm [6].

Future research: access to care

New research insights into access problems and their solutions can be achieved through studies that focus on patient flow and care processes outside the ED. EM researchers are well positioned to study the most cost-effective and appropriate method of providing for the health care needs of vulnerable populations [19]. EM investigators have already taken the important step of moving from merely observing access problems to measuring and quantifying the factors that keep people from accessing needed care and linking these barriers to adverse patient outcomes [20–22]. Next steps include designing and evaluating interventions to reliably link patients to appropriate services. For some patients, the most efficient gateway to primary and specialty health care services may be through the ED, because of its 24-hour availability. One example might be a system where the ED provides initial triage for all acute ambulatory care and has the capacity to make urgent primary and specialty appointments for patients in an open access framework. On the other hand, it might turn out that other options such as open access systems or allowing patients to make their own appointments on the Internet are more reliable or cost-effective [23,24]. Regardless, creative reengineering of the current health system will allow the ED to function as effectively as possible in delivering care directly and enabling patients to access other health care and social services that may be needed. Ideally, EM will not only be involved in the development of any new system changes but also their evaluation.

One important unresolved conceptual challenge will be for EM to help define the ideal "access"—a term whose meaning has shifted over time along with differing policies and expectations of the American health care system. Consensus on the meaning of access is still lacking: many might consider access to be the provision of medical care that is adequate and timely enough to prevent adverse health outcomes. Others, including consumers, might believe that health care access is not adequate unless it can ensure safe, quality, timely, cost-effective, culturally competent, appropriate care that optimizes mental and physical health outcomes, including satisfaction with care. Keeping in mind that health services are only one of several means to the desired outcome of "health," a public health approach to access would include a consideration of population-based health indicators and outcome measures. Moreover, we need to consider the opportunity costs of the proportion of the gross national product (GNP) and other resources going to health care services versus housing, education, recreation, environmental protection, and other social obligations that impact the health of the public.

Surveillance of diseases, injuries, and health risks

While health departments bear the responsibility for surveillance and monitoring the health of the public, emergency departments are at the front line of any emerging health hazard and, as such, have the potential to play a more immediate and sentinel role [25,26]. Public health surveillance was originally developed as part of local, state, and national efforts to control infectious diseases. Early detection and response are longstanding priorities, and the premium placed on rapid reporting has only increased in recent years. New emerging infectious diseases, which are rapidly spread in our global economy (eg, SARS) [27], and recent acts of bioterrorism [28] have focused attention on the need for real-time reporting from EDs to public health agencies.

More rapid public health reporting from EDs is part of a larger vision of EM's role in public health [29,30]. Previous usage of ED-based data had been largely retrospective and seldom population-based. An early exception was the northeastern Ohio trauma study in the early 1980s [31]. Usage of ED data to describe the scope and nature of specific problems has been limited because of selection biases, retrospective information, and inability to acquire timely data. ED-based surveillance began to receive serious attention and discussion in the 1990s, most notably in the areas of infectious diseases and violence. The Weapon Reporting Injury Surveillance System (WRISS) of Massachusetts collected information on all weapon-related injuries treated in all of the EDs within Massachusetts and proved very useful for the development and evaluation of prevention strategies [32]. EMERGEncy Net ID was established in 1995 to sample ED-based infectious diseases. The network is not population-based and is significantly retrospective in its timeliness, but it provides an important demonstration of the value of ED data for surveillance purposes [33].

Other subjects for ED-based surveillance included intimate partner violence [34] and firearms [35]. As an example of the latter, Atlanta-based EDs were among the first to enroll in a firearm surveillance project with Emory's Injury Control Center that provided timely information to law enforcement and public health officials on the scope and nature of firearm injuries in the metro-Atlanta area [35]. These state and local efforts complement national-level surveillance of ED-treated injuries by the National Electronic Injury Surveillance System (NEISS) of the US Consumer Product Safety Commission. National estimates of nonfatal firearm-related injuries are derived using weighted data for patients treated in a nationally representative, stratified probability sample of US hospital emergency departments [36].

ED encounter databases in which external cause of injury codes are assigned for each injury-related visit are another resource for injury surveillance. Paramedic and emergency medical systems (EMS) can provide additional data for surveillance purposes. However, not all public health departments currently have data in electronic format and there is a noted lack of uniformity among regional and state-based surveillance systems.

Future ED-based surveillance

Currently, most health departments conduct surveillance on a limited set of diseases and injuries. Additional investments are needed to close gaps in existing surveillance capacity and extend surveillance to other conditions. A start in this direction would be the dissemination of uniform data elements for use by ED systems (DEEDS). This was developed by the CDC in collaboration with emergency physicians and other stakeholders with the hope of creating regional linkages between public health departments and EDs. It uses electronic tools to enable the emergence of real-time ED-based surveillance [37]. These efforts will be greatly strengthened by the application of new information technology. Currently, work on uniform data collection systems [38] and ED-based research networks [39,40] is still in its infancy. Real time ED-based surveillance has become an increasingly important concept but is currently limited to sampling EDs in the United States for specific problems: product-related injuries NEISS for the Consumer Product Safety Commission, and The Drug Abuse Working Network (DAWN), an ED-based system for surveillance of drug abuse.

EM researchers have opportunities to help develop more efficient and real-time public health surveillance systems as part of an overall public health strategy [41]. Inherent in this effort is the possibility of EM serving as a coordinator and catalyst of links between hospitals, local governing bodies, public health agencies, and other community organizations whose policies impact the health of the public. Advances in information technology are likely to enable automatic reporting of a variety of health problems from ED electronic health record system to public health agencies. These efforts will require careful attention to the quality of ED data and safeguards for privacy and confidentiality [37,41].

Preventive services in the ED

Historically, in most Western societies, advances in antimicrobials and vaccines and improvements in sanitation have shifted much of the burden of disease morbidity and mortality from infections to injuries and chronic diseases [42]. Clinical preventive services aimed at reducing behavioral antecedents of injuries and chronic diseases (such as excessive use of alcohol, obesity, tobacco use) provide an important way to further reduce morbidity and mortality. Yet risky behaviors have only recently been viewed as potential public health threats that should be monitored and addressed. Initially, chronic diseases such as cancer and heart disease were viewed as hereditary and incurable. It was not until 1957 that the Surgeon General issued a warning against "excessive cigarette smoking" [42]. It still took a tremendous effort on the part of physicians and public health professionals to change the public's perception that smoking cessation, control of blood pressure, improved diet, decreased stress, and greater exercise could increase life expectancy and lead to more quality years of healthy living. However, the success of these efforts on the part of the American Heart Association, American Cancer Society, and the US Preventive Services Task Force is evidenced in the declining age-adjusted mortality rates for several cardiovascular diseases. Likewise, both passive (seatbelts) and active (speed limits, helmets) injury-prevention strategies have been associated with a decline in death rates from motor vehicle crashes. The *Healthy People* initiative began in the late 1970s to increase health promotion and prevent disease [42]. Gradually, prevention became widely regarded as the answer for preventing premature death and prolonging years of healthy life. However, to date, it is recognized that the patients who most need preventive services are those least likely to receive them [43].

The US Preventive Services Task Force (USPSTF) recommended that all physicians take advantage of acute care visits to provide preventive services. However, nearly all the preventive services identified by the USPSTF as efficacious and cost-effective are provided at unacceptably low rates, even to patients who regularly visit traditional primary care settings [44]. Many patients only receive acute episodic care in EDs. Thus, EDs may be in a position to treat those patients with the greatest potential to benefit from preventive services. Nevertheless, there are some concrete and controversial questions about whether the USPSTF recommendations apply to EDs, and if so, which preventive services should be provided. It is perhaps important to clarify that classical primary preventive services are those delivered before onset of a condition, such as education and immunization. Secondary prevention is targeted at high-risk individuals before they suffer the adverse consequences of their behaviors, such as counseling problem drinkers to cut down or those with risky sexual behaviors to use condoms to prevent HIV infection. Tertiary preventive care is targeted at halting progression of clinically apparent conditions, eg, advising individuals with heart disease to quit smoking or referring substance abusers for treatment. While these preventive interventions are provided to individuals, they are generally considered part of an overall public health strategy.

EM's role in delivering clinical preventive services has been a source of controversy [2]. A relatively young specialty, EM has been defined by unscheduled acute care and crisis management, an emphasis that is reflected in the scope of residency curriculum. Emergency physicians in training have little exposure to the assessment of patient psychosocial or behavioral health risks or skills in motivational interviewing. Other impediments to delivering clinical preventive services in the ED involve competing clinical priorities and constraints on time, resources, and reimbursement for prevention. While recognizing the health burden of unhealthy behaviors, even strong advocates for ED prevention recognize that screening and intervention of any kind has been difficult in the ED. Moreover, the EDs that treat the most vulnerable patients are the most stressed. High-volume public hospital EDs with long waits, limited budgets, and insufficient staff, do not have the resources to add to their scope of practice.

As emergency medicine has matured, there has been more focus on the public health implications of being a "safety net" provider for more than 40 million uninsured Americans. In the past 10 years, there has been increasing recognition of the potential role of EDs in injury surveillance and population-based public health strategies [2], including the need to address the behavioral health risks that put individuals and their communities at risk of adverse health outcomes.

In 1998, the Society of Academic Emergency Medicine's (SAEM) Board of Directors directed the SAEM Public Health Task Force (PHTF) to develop recommendations for prevention, screening, and counseling activities to be conducted in emergency departments. This action followed several initiatives to increase EM's involvement in national public health planning and in helping to define the national health priorities of "increasing quality and years of healthy life" and "eliminating health disparities," as a participating organization in the Healthy People 2010 Consortium. Following the lead of the USPSTF, the SAEM PHTF developed a list of candidate prevention services recommended by the USPSTF for traditional primary care settings that appeared to be effective, inexpensive, and potentially feasible and in the ED. They used a systematic approach to collect evidence from published clinical research and to judge the quality of individual studies. Given the very few high-quality studies of preventive services in the ED setting, they also accepted high-quality studies from primary care, where there was evidence for feasibility of the intervention in the ED setting. Using this criterion, the PHTF identified only five preventive services with sufficient evidence of effectiveness to support a recommendation in the ED setting: alcohol screening and intervention, HIV screening and referral (in high-risk populations), hypertension screening and referral, pneumococcal vaccinations (age > 65), and smoking cessation counseling [45].

While not fully addressed by the PHTF, episodes of trauma care are widely recognized as unique opportunities to identify injury risk factors and initiate interventions aimed at breaking the cycle of injury recidivism [46,47]. Although emergency physicians and nurses have been increasingly involved in injury control and prevention efforts, the ED remains a clinical setting where the primary focus is treatment of the physical manifestations of emergency medical conditions. Screening for underlying injury risk factors and counseling and other forms of risk reduction are not consistently performed and often neglected [25]. To reduce injury morbidity and mortality, it may be imperative to capitalize on the opportunities that the ED presents for injury prevention [48]. Moreover, attention to injury epidemiology will help in the development and evaluation of intervention programs. ED-based injury surveillance will need to be strengthened and integrated into local, state, and national prevention strategies.

Some have advocated that screening all ED patients for injury risk behaviors, such as intoxicated driving and seatbelt use, should become the routine practice [47,49,50]. One of the most controversial questions is whether emergency physicians should screen all women for intimate partner violence (IPV). Recognizing that intimate partner violence is a major cause of morbidity and mortality, medical organizations [51,52] and the Joint Commission on Accreditation of Healthcare Organizations (JCAHO) recommended that all EDs implement protocols for screening and intervention of this high-risk group [53]. However, most articles from the ED setting have reported on the system's failure to identify IPV and the barriers involved in universal screening [54,55]. The feasibility issues combined with a lack of an evidence-basis that IPV screening in a health care setting leads to a reduction in morbidity and mortality [56] have resulted in general discouragement regarding universal screening for IPV [57]. Currently, the USPSTF and others suggest that we should not engage in any screening or intervention that lacks an evidence basis [58]. While IPV screening is a low-risk, low-cost procedure with reliable screening tools [59], time spent on screening or counseling for non-evidence-based conditions is costly and infringes on other physician tasks of proven benefit [60]. Indeed, reimbursement for such activities will need to be prefaced by studies show-ing improvement in outcomes [46]. Studying the effectiveness of ED-based interventions will require careful consideration of particular outcomes and valid measurements of these outcomes.

Clearly there are knowledge gaps that need to be addressed before evi-dence-based recommendations can be made in favor of screening for health risks in the ED setting. One of these gaps is a lack of well-defined, desirable, and measurable outcomes related to the screening process itself. For exam-ple, any understanding of the value of identifying IPV in a health care setting is confounded by the psychosocial and biological complexity of violence. Using "incidence of violence" as an outcome measure for the effect of a brief intervention in health care setting involves measuring the behavioral out-comes of a third party, something that is not necessarily under the control of either the physician or the patient. Establishing a direct link between phy-sician screening and incidence of violence is not feasible under that condition.

The most appropriate outcomes for evaluating screening interventions in a health care setting may involve measuring the direct effect of screening on the outcomes of care. For example, information about abuse histories may influence assessment and treatment of other health problems. Nonetheless, it is time to expand the vision of potential outcomes to be measured from screening and counseling interventions in a health care setting, including identification of patient-desired outcomes. One example from the substance abuse literature might be to measure the impact of an ED intervention on a patient's stage of readiness to change the risky health behavior [61]. Another way to conceptualize ED screening for adverse health behaviors would be to think of ED screening as just one component of an overall pub-lic health strategy to influence health behaviors. Acknowledging that this is the case means that we must also evaluate the value of ED interventions in proportion to other population-based strategies such as public service announcements and other educational interventions.

Future research on providing preventative care in the ED

There are several arguments to support expanding our research in the area of prevention. First, EDs are already doing a significant amount of prevention, screening, and counseling. Most emergency physicians order tetanus immunizations for patients with lacerations. We should know if this is a good use of ED provider time. Perhaps it would make more sense to immunize the large numbers of patients at risk for more common infec-tions such as pneumococcal pneumonia and influenza, as both of these immunizations have been shown to be effective and feasible in the ED set-ting [62]. Many ED physicians write, "Stop drinking" or "Stop smoking" on discharge instructions. A fruitful area of research would be to identify effective, efficient methods of how the ED staff might provide such advice and to identify if it is indeed helpful and linked to desired outcomes [63].

Second, to the extent that EDs serve as "safety nets" treating patients without other sources of care, we are the only potential source of prevention services for a highly vulnerable portion of the US population. Over 40 million uninsured Americans have limited access to medical care outside of the ED. These Americans are particularly likely to have unmet needs for prevention services. Smokers, drinkers, drug users, and motor vehicle crash victims presenting to the ED could benefit the most from behavioral interventions. Homeless people at risk for tuberculosis and patients with sexually transmitted diseases in need of HIV counseling and testing commonly use the ED for health care. ED physicians are frequently the only health care providers for these patients. ED use has been found to be a marker for under-vaccination [64,65] as well as lack of other preventive services. Many of our patients may not receive prevention services at all if they do not receive them in the ED [66].

Third, it is likely that unmet preventive health needs will result in ED visits for more serious problems. A retrospective review by Stack and colleagues [67] found that 55% of their patients admitted with pneumococcal bacteremia had been seen in the ED an average of 3.4 times during the 72 months before their bacteremic episode; 88% of those patients were at high risk for pneumococcal disease by CDC criteria and 10% of them died during their admission. A large multisite study of ED patients by Lowenstein and colleagues [68] found very high prevalence rates of injury-prone behaviors as well as risk factors for chronic disease. High proportions of these patients were deficient in recommended preventive services. This was true even among the patients with access to primary care. It has long been acknowledged that ED visits are frequently the result of a failure of prevention and that public health problems such as substance abuse, sexually transmitted disease (STD) treatment, and violence have placed a major burden on EDs. One area of future research is to document the extent and costs of these patients recycling back to the ED if there is no attempt at intervention.

Last, patients in the ED may experience a "teachable moment." The ED patient treated for an injury following a motor vehicle collision may be more receptive to advice about seatbelts than he was a month earlier in his internist's office. The teenager with an STD may be more receptive to safe-sex counseling than she was in a high school lecture the week before. There is evidence that ED patients have both a need and a desire for preventive services to be initiated in the ED setting [69]. There is some evidence that ED interventions targeted at high-risk populations can be very effective [63,70]. Parents trained about adolescent suicide risks during an ED visit for an adolescent behavior problem were four times more likely to take steps to limit their child's access to guns and prescription drugs than parents without the training [71]. However, the hypothesis that the ED visit is a "teachable moment" has yet to be rigorously tested.

There are also reasons *not* to provide preventive services in the ED. What most constrains us from instituting preventive programs in the ED is a concern about lack of time and resources. The EDs that treat the most vulnerable patients (where prevention, screening, and counseling activities should be focused) are the most stressed. High-volume public hospital EDs with long waits, limited budgets, and insufficient staff do not have the resources to add to their scope of practice. In these settings, coordinating follow-up for screening lab test results, determining what immunizations a patient has had previously, and so forth, may render many preventive and screening services much more difficult and potentially less effective than in primary care settings. The worse scenario would be if the provision of preventive services detracted from our ability to provide critical care. So perhaps the appropriate research questions are not should we be doing prevention, but what prevention should we be doing, what resources do we need to do to perform these services, and how well does it work?

Policy-relevant research on health services systems, social welfare, and social determinants of health

Current and future EM public health researchers wishing to engage in policy-relevant research will need to take a broad "big picture" approach to studying health. In the process they can study not only the micro- and macro-factors related to quality in the health system but whether our current health system actually impacts health. They will need to reach outside the clinic walls and consider the opportunity costs of our current high-priced high-tech health system and finally study the social determinants of health itself.

Research on the quality of emergency medical care:
addressing the quality chiasm

The Institute of Medicine (IOM) outlined six aims to improve the quality of care in the United States [72]. The implication of each of these for future EM research was presented at an SAEM 2002 consensus conference [73]. These suggestions are very applicable to EM public health research. They suggest identifying whether ED care is *effective* ("based on the use of systematically acquired evidence to determine whether an intervention, such as a preventive service, diagnostic test, or therapy, produces better outcomes than alternatives—including the alternative of doing nothing") [72,74], *efficient* (avoids the waste of equipment, supplies, money, ideas, or energy) [72], *timely* (able to avoid delays caused by patient, provider, or system factors), *safe* ("when patients [can] avoid injury from the care that is intended to help them") [72,75], *patient-centered* (care that promotes patient involvement in medical decision making and helps care providers "in attending to their patients' physical and emotional needs, and maintaining or improving their quality of life") [72], and *equitable* (free of bias). To identify opportunities for research within each of these six quality domains, the authors classify current research into four research steps that build upon each other: (1) evidence does not exist and there is a need to generate rigorous research studies, (2) evidence exits but there is a need for synthesis of existing evidence into guidelines and quality measures, (3) there are existing evidence-based clinical guidelines and measures and a need for assessment of the quality of clinical practice compared with evidence-based guidelines and quality measures, and (4) there is a need to design and evaluate new interventions to improve clinical quality of care.

EM public health research on health disparities

As an important part of the safety net for vulnerable populations, the ED is ideally positioned to conduct studies on health disparities [76]. ED physicians see the results of inadequate education, social services, and health care. Multiple studies have demonstrated inequities in the delivery of health services attributable to gender, race, and age [77–79]. There is a need, however, for investigation into the causes of these differences and interventions to correct the disparities. Moreover, inequities in health care do not only exist outside of emergency medicine: we also need to examine our own practice. While most emergency physicians agree that the same high quality of care should be available to all patients, prior research suggests that this may not always be the case [80]. For instance, African Americans and Hispanics are less likely to receive analgesics for painful conditions [81]. Research is needed to assess the degree to which such disparities exist for other emergency conditions. When inequities in care are documented, there is need for investigation into the patient and provider factors that may contribute to differences so that interventions to close these gaps can be designed and evaluated. As an example, we can explore the influence of time pressure and complex cognitive tasks on medical decision making to see if bias exists in the treatment of critical conditions (eg, chest pain, respiratory failure, end-of-life care, pain management) in need of immediate assessment and treatment. It has been suggested that these conditions increase the likelihood that providers will use stereotypes or prejudice as they provide clinical care [80]. When systematic health disparities are identified by race or socioeconomic status, there is a need to look at the broader educational, health, and social welfare systems to identify the sources and mechanisms of these disparities, not only to document these inequities but to help develop and assess new polices designed to ameliorate such disparities.

Future research on the functioning of the health system and the fraying safety net

The ED can be a unique resource for gaining knowledge that will strengthen the safety net. In its position as "a window on the safety net" and as "the last hole that patients fall through in the fraying health care safety net," EDs can monitor the performance of the entire system [82]. We see the patients who "fall through the cracks," and can study where those patients come from, where they get resources, and who provides their primary care. We can learn what patients want, how they use the system, and how nonhealth factors affect their choices [82]. A broad system-level approach suggests that EM public health research will need to study how the social service, primary care, and referral systems are working and help identify how the entire system might improve. Gordon [83] suggested that one model for remediating health disparities would be to think of the ED as a vital component of the social welfare system and to begin to embrace and study that role.

Currently, EM sits at the hub of a number of governmental and market forces that both regulate and threaten our ability to provide quality care. Since the late 1990s, we have been living in an era of failed health care reform where cost containment strategies have created additional nonprice barriers to care. Americans are faced with an increasingly complex health care system and the barriers to care are more pervasive and subtle than previously identified barriers because of unfavorable insurance status. While earlier legislative initiatives such as EMTALA and the prudent layperson standard provided important safeguards for managed care plan enrollees and the larger community, many emergency providers eventually came to resent the legislation as an unfunded federal mandate for universal access to health care via emergency departments [14]. The resultant combination of regulatory and fiscal pressures on hospitals resulted in increasingly stressed and crowded conditions in many EDs [3]. Regulatory extensions of EMTALA have held health systems liable for providing not only emergency care, but also any needed care. With decreases in reimbursement for the care of publicly insured patients, the ED has become a medical-legal and financial liability for many hospital systems, as the primary portal of entrance for uninsured and publicly insured patients who compete with privately insured patients for scarce inpatient beds [15].

ED crowding

Several recent national reports find that this competition for inpatient beds has contributed to ED crowding and prolonged wait times to see an ED physician [84,85]. EM research began to focus on the implications and patient outcomes associated with the failing safety net [86–88]. A March 2003 report from the US General Accounting Office (GAO) found that measures of ED crowding varied widely across hospitals and communities, with hospitals in urban areas (with populations greater than 2.5 million) and cities with greater proportions of uninsured people experiencing the most severe crowding conditions [84]. The National Hospital and Ambulatory Medical Care Survey (NHAMCS) found average 2001 ED waiting times for nonurgent conditions had increased 33% in a 3-year period [89]. The current widespread occurrence of long waiting times for hospital beds, ambulance diversion, and high percentages of patients leaving EDs without being seen calls into question the amount of progress being made toward the Healthy People 2010 objective 1-10, which is to "reduce the proportion of persons who delay or have difficulty in getting emergency medical care" [90]. In addition, an overburdened emergency care system cannot be expected to adequately serve the country's need for emergent care, public health, or surveillance. The terrorist attack on September 11, 2001, further called attention to the need for coordinated community responses to disasters and the role of EM in mass casualty intervention. However, many emergency physicians point out that the current capacity of the emergency response system is already exceeded on a daily basis.

A recent analysis of the National Health Interview Survey (NHIS) found that a substantial number of adults report delay or difficulty in accessing needed emergency care. Moreover, there appear to be significant disparities in rates of problems encountered by adults seeking emergency medical care, with younger, lower income, uninsured patients, and those reporting poorer health being at greatest risk of experiencing delays or difficulty [91]. Future work is needed to examine whether the same groups that are experiencing lack of access to primary care are experiencing problems accessing emergency care as well. Work also needs to be done to explore whether the financing of the US health care system has contributed to current health care disparities. For public health research, it will be important to identify baseline population-based measures such as the NHIS for tracking access to both the primary care and emergency care system. The value of establishing baseline measures is that they can be used for tracking the effects of policies designed to remedy health disparities and ensure equal access to timely emergency care. Further work will be necessary to assess the impact of access barriers on actual health outcomes.

Future research on ED crowding

Although ED crowding as a concept has a lot of "face validity," uniform definitions or valid measures of the problem are currently lacking. More importantly, the causal links between crowded conditions and adverse patient outcomes have not been well established. Asplin and colleagues [92] focused this discussion on the larger supply and demand mismatches in the health care system. They point out that ED crowding is the end result of a cascade of system characteristics that adversely affect the supply of and demand for emergency care. Thus, the problem cannot be solved by examining the ED in isolation. To find solutions, the entire delivery system must be examined using reliable methods to describe, measure, and monitor system capacity. Therefore, they have proposed a conceptual framework to explain ED crowding that includes input, throughput, and output factors [92]. Use of such a conceptual model can highlight specific areas of study to identify the places where the system is failing.

The importance of methodological rigor in EM public health research

Future EM public health research requires a higher degree of methodological rigor. Quantitative research should focus on hard outcomes. For example, health promotion research should go beyond prevalence studies to design new interventions, follow morbidity and mortality, and document the health consequences of lack of access to preventive care. However, descriptive studies of previously undescribed phenomena will continue to be important. With its wealth of patient stories, EM lends itself well to rigorous qualitative research—a methodological approach that has yet to be adequately developed in this setting. Studies of interventions should ideally use randomized designs and minimize selection bias by using systematic rather than convenience samples. When experimental design and randomization are not feasible, the analysis for comorbidity and confounders should be controlled so that our nonexperimental studies have more validity. Increasingly, EM researchers are beginning to realize the value of exploring EM questions through the use of population-based databases. Collaborations with other disciplines can also bring new methods to bear on common EM problems. For example, the disciplines of economics, sociology, and anthropology can provide new perspectives on the culture of emergency medicine and the communities we serve. A greater depth of understanding of the problems we are seeing is needed. For example, we need to go beyond describing health disparities and try to identify the mechanisms and individual, provider, and system-level issues that are contributing to disparities in health and health outcomes. Geographic Information Systems analysis along with census measures of poverty and race can help identify and provide a picture of health disparities.

Last, the focus of EM public health research needs to reach out beyond the clinic walls to the surrounding neighborhoods and community members. Involvement in community-based participatory research will improve the understanding of patient barriers to healthy behavior and the role that family members, religion, social support, and neighborhood factors play in health.

Summary

With more than 110 million patient visits annually, EDs can provide information on the health care needs of a diverse population and serve as a unique research laboratory for studying the functioning of the health care system. As the only provider mandated by federal law to provide universal health care, the ED is uniquely qualified to work at the interface of medicine, public health, social services, and the community. With the advent of uniform data collection systems and ED-based surveillance systems, EM has the potential to play a powerful role in measuring and improving the health of the population. Much of past EM public health research has focused on three large areas, all of which continue to have major relevance as topics of public health research: access to systems of care; the identification of the unmet medical and behavioral health needs of ED populations and the potential for meeting these needs during an ED visit; and the need for surveillance for infectious diseases, behavioral health risks, and injuries. The future potential for EM public health research will involve expanding into more policy-relevant work that takes into account larger system issues and the social determinants of health. In helping to ensure the health of the public, a multidisciplinary framework of population-based systems of care is needed. Fulfilling this function includes conducting rigorous research studies to monitor and ensure that the public's needs are met, as well as continuing to advocate for high-quality universal health care for all Americans.

References

[1] Lasker RD. Medicine & public health: the power of collaboration. New York: NY Academy of Medicine; 1997.

[2] Clancy CM, Eisenberg JM. Emergency medicine in population-based systems of care. Ann Emerg Med 1997;30:800–3.

[3] Weissman J. Uncompensated hospital care: Will it be there if we need it? JAMA 1996;276: 823–8.

[4] Krome R. Twenty-five years of evolution and revolution: how the specialty has changed. Ann Emerg Med 1997;30:689–90.

[5] Nadel V. Emergency departments: unevenly affected by growth and change in patient use. US General Accounting Office: Report to the Chairman, Subcommittee on Health for Families and the Uninsured, Committee on Finance, US Senate. Washington, DC: US Government Printing Office; 1993.

[6] Li J, et al. The 'prudent layperson' definition of an emergency medical condition. Am J Emerg Med 2002;20:10–3.

[7] Schiff R, Ansell DA, Schlosser JE, et al. Transfers to a public hospital: A prospective study of 467 patients. N Engl J Med 1986;314:552–7.

[8] Rothenberg KH. Who cares? The evolution of the legal duty to provide emergency care. Houston Law Rev 1989;26:21–76.

[9] Williams RM. The cost of visits to emergency departments. N Engl J Med 1996;334:642–6.

[10] Tyrance PH, Himmelstein DU, Woolhandler S. US emergency department costs. No emergency. Am J Public Health 1996;86:1527–31.

[11] Dowling PT. Emergency department costs. Am J Public Health 1996;87:1866.

[12] Young, Wagner MB, Kellerman AL, et al. Ambulatory visits to hospital emergency departments. JAMA 1996;276(6):460–5.

[13] Cunningham, Clancy CM, Cohen JW, Wilets M. The Use of Hospital Emergency Departments for Nonurgent Health Problems: A National Perspective. Med Care Res & Rev 1995;52:453–74.

[14] Lewin-Epstein N. Determinants of regular source of health care in Black, Mexican, Puerto Rican and Non-Hispanic White populations. Med Care 1991;29:543–57.

[15] Franks, Clancy CM, Gold MD. Health insurance and mortality. JAMA 1993;270:737–41.

[16] Medicaid Access Study Group. Access of Medicaid recipients to outpatient care. New Engl J Med 1994;330:1426–30.

[17] Lippman H. The games plans play with ER bills. Bus Health 1996;14(6):20–8.

[18] Cardin BL. We need Federal standards for managed care plans. Acad Med 1997;72:706–7.

[19] Aday LA. At risk in America: The health and health care needs of vulnerable populations in the United States. San Francisco, CA: Jossey-Bass; 1993.

[20] Baker DW, Stevens CD, Brook RH. Patients who leave a public hospital emergency department without being seen by a physician. Causes and consequences. JAMA 1991;266: 1085–90.

[21] Bindman AB, Grumbach K, Keane D, et al. Consequences of queuing for care at a public hospital emergency department. JAMA 1991;266:1091–6.

[22] Young GP, Lowe RA. Adverse outcomes of managed care gatekeeping. Acad Emerg Med 1997;4:1129–36.

[23] Stoddart H, Evans M, Peters TJ, et al. The provision of 'same-day' care in general practice: an observational study. Fam Pract 2003;20(1):41–7.

[24] Institute for Healthcare Improvement. Available at: http://www.ihi.org. Accessed March 14, 2003.

[25] Hargarten SW, Olson L, Sklar D. Emergency medicine and injury control research: past, present, and future. Acad Emerg Med 1997;4:243–4.

[26] Scott BC. Emergency departments: an important component of public health. J Natl Med Assoc 1995;87:181–3.

[27] Riley S, Fraser F, Donnelly CA, et al. Transmission dynamics of the etiological agent of SARS in Hong Kong: impact of public health interventions. Science 2003;300(5627):1961–6.

[28] Henderson DA. The looming threat of bioterrorism. Science 1999;283:1279–82.

[29] Martinez R. New vision for the role of emergency medical services. Ann Emerg Med 1998;32: 5:594–9.

[30] Garrison H, Runyan CW, Tintinalli JE, et al. Emergency department surveillance: an examination of issues and proposal for a national strategy. Ann Emerg Med 1994;24(5): 849–56.

[31] Barancik JI. Northeastern Ohio Trauma Study: I. magnitude of the problem. Am J Public Health 1983;73:746–51.

[32] Barber CW, Ozonoff VV, Schuster M, et al. Massachusetts weapon-related injury surveillance system. Am J Prev Med 1998;15(3S):57–66.

[33] Talan D, Moran GJ, Mower WR, et al. EMERGEncy ID Net: an emergency department-based emerging infections sentinel network. Ann Emerg Med 1998;32:5:703–11.

[34] Michigan Intimate Partner Violence Surveillance System. A profile of 2000 prosecuting attorneys' data. Report produced for the Center for Collaborative Research in Health Outcomes and Policy at the Michigan Public Health Institute under a contract with the Michigan Department of Community Health; 2004.

[35] Kellerman A, Bartolomeos K. Firearm injury surveillance at the local level: from data to action. Am J Prev Med 1998;15(3S):109–12.

[36] Available at: http://www.cdc.gov/mmwr/preview/mmwrhtml/ss5002a1.htm. Accessed August 16, 2006.

[37] Pollock DA. DEEDS Writing Committee: data elements for emergency department systems, Release 1.0 (DEEDS): A summary report. Ann Emerg Med 1998;31:264–7.

[38] National Center for Injury Prevention and Control. Data elements for emergency department systems, Release 1.0. Atlanta, GA: Centers for Disease Control and Prevention; 1997.

[39] Emergency Department 24-hour Research Network (ED24). Available at: http://www. emnet-usa.org/background.html. Accessed March 14, 2005.

[40] Multicenter Airway Research Collaboration. Available at: http://www.emnet-usa.org/ Marc_25/M25.cfm. Accessed March 14, 2005.

[41] Pollock DA, Lowery DW, O'Brien PM. Emergency medicine and public health: new steps in old directions. Ann Emerg Med 2001;38:675–83.

[42] Richmond JB, Kotelchuck M. Coordination and development of strategies and policy for public health promotion in the United States. In: Holland WW, Detels R, Knox G, editors. Oxford textbook of public health. 2nd edition. New York: Oxford University Press; 1991.

[43] Vogt TM, Hollis JF, Lichtenein E, et al. The medical care system and prevention: the need for a new paradigm. HMO Pract 1998;12:5–11.

[44] Putting prevention into practice. Available at: http://www.ahcpr.gov/. Accessed August 16, 2006.

[45] Rhodes KV, Gordon JA, Lowe RA, for the SAEM Public Health Task Force. Clinical preventive services: are they relevant to emergency medicine? Acad Emerg Med 2000;7: 1036–41.

[46] Madden C, Cole TB. Emergency intervention to break the cycle of drunken driving and recurrent injury. Ann Emerg Med 1995;26:177–9.

[47] Soderstrom CA, Cowley RA. A national alcohol and trauma center survey: missed opportunities, failures of responsibility. Arch Surg 1987;122:1067–71.

[48] Burt CW. Injury-related visits to hospital emergency departments: United States, 1992. Advance data from vital and health statistics; no. 261. Hyattsville, MD: National Center for Health Statistics; 1995.

[49] Vinson DC, Mabe N, Leonard LL, et al. Alcohol and injury: a case crossover study. Arch Fam Med 1995;4:505–11.

[50] Cherpitel CJ. Alcohol and injuries: a review of international emergency room studies. Addiction 1993;88:923–37.

[51] American Medical Association, Council on Scientific Affairs. Violence against women: relevance for medical practitioners. JAMA 1992;267:3184–9.

[52] American College of Emergency Physicians. Domestic violence. Approved October 1999. Policy No. 400286. Available at: http://www.acep.org/1, 2194, 0.html. Accessed March 3, 2005.

[53] Joint commission. Tighter domestic abuse standards should improve assessment. Aids Alert 1993;8(10):152–4.

[54] Larkin GL, Hyman KB, Mathias SR, et al. Universal screening for intimate partner violence in the emergency department: important patient and provider factors. Ann Emerg Med 1999; 33(6):669–75.

[55] Gremillion DH, Kanof EP. Overcoming barriers to physician involvement in identifying and referring victims of domestic violence. Ann Emerg Med 1996;27:769–73.

[56] Neilson HD, Nygren P, McInerney KJ. Screening women and elderly adults for family and intimate partner violence: a review of the evidence for the US Preventive Services Task Force. Ann Intern Med 2004;140(5):387–96

[57] Ramsay J, Richardson J, Carter H, et al. Should health professionals screen women for domestic violence? Systematic review. BMJ 2002;325:314–8.

[58] Ramsay J, Richardson J, Carter YH, et al. Should health professionals screen women for domestic violence? Systematic review. BMJ 2002;325(7359):314.

[59] Koziol-McLain J, Coates CJ, Lowenstein SR. Predictive validity of a screen for partner violence against women. Am J Prev Med 2001;21(2):93–100.

[60] Neilson HD, Nygren P. McInerney, Klein J. Screening Women and Elderly Adults for Family and Intimate Partner Violence: A Review of the Evidence for the US Preventive Services Task Force. Ann Intern Med 2004;140(5):387–96.

[61] Prochaska JO, Velicer WF, Rossi JS. Stage of change and decision balance for 12 problem behaviors. Health Psych 1994;13(1):39–46.

[62] Slobotkin D, Zielske PG, Kitlas JL, et al. Demonstration of the feasibility of emergency department immunization against influenza and Pneumococcus. Ann Emerg Med 1998; 32:537–43.

[63] Bernstein E, Bernstein J, Levenson S. Project ASSERT: An ED-based intervention to increase access to primary care, preventative services, and the substance abuse treatment system. Ann Emerg Med 1997;30(2):181–9.

[64] Rodewald LE, Szilagyi PG, Humiston SG, et al. Is an emergency department visit a marker for undervaccination and missed opportunities among children who have access to primary care? Pediatrics 1993;91:605–11.

[65] Rodrigues RM, Baraff LJ. Emergency department immunization of the elderly with pneumococcal and influenza vaccines. Ann Emerg Med 1993;22:1729–32.

[66] Bernstein E, Bernstein J. Case studies in emergency medicine and the health of the public. Boston: Jones and Barlett Publishers; 1996.

[67] Stack SJ, Martin DR, Plouffe JF. An emergency department-based pneumococcal vaccination program could save money and lives. Ann Emerg Med 1999;33:299–303.

[68] Lowenstein SR, Koziol-McLain J, Thompson M, et al. Behavioral risk factors in emergency department patients: a multisite survey. Acad Emerg Med 1998;5:781–7.

[69] Rodrigues RM, Kreider WJ, Baraff LJ. Need and desire for preventive care measures in emergency department patients. Ann Emerg Med 1995;26:615–20.

[70] Ernst AA, Romolo R, Nick T. Emergency department screening for syphilis in pregnant women without prenatal care. Ann Emerg Med 1993;22:781–5.

[71] Kruesi M, Grossman J, Pennington JM. Suicide and Violence Prevention: Parent Education in the Emergency Department. J Am Acad Child Adolesc Psychiatry 1999;38:250–5.

[72] Committee on Quality on Health Care in America, Institute of Medicine. Crossing the quality chasm: a new health system for the 21st century. Washington, DC: National Academy Press; 2001.

[73] Magid DJ, Rhodes KV, Asplin BR, et al. Designing a research agenda to improve the quality of emergency care. Acad Emerg Med 2002;9:1124–30.

[74] Callaham M. Quantifying the scanty science of prehospital emergency care. Ann Emerg Med 1997;30(6):785–90.

[75] Institute of Medicine. To err is human: building a safer health system. Washington, DC: National Academy Press; 2000.

[76] Aday LA. At risk in America: the health and health care needs of vulnerable populations in the United States. San Francisco, CA: Jossey-Bass; 1993.

[77] Yarzebski J, Col N, Pagley P, et al. Gender differences and factors associated with receipt of thrombolytic therapy in patients with acute myocardial infarction: a community-wide perspective. Am Heart J 1996;131:43–50.

[78] Allison JJ, Kiefe CI, Centor RM, et al. Racial differences in the medical treatment of elderly Medicare patients with acute myocardial infarction. J Gen Intern Med 1996;11: 736–43.

[79] Gurwitz JH, Gore JM, Goldberg RJ. Recent age-related trends in the use of thrombolytic therapy in patients who had had acute myocardial infarction. Ann Intern Med 1996;124: 283–91.

[80] VanRyn M. Research on the provider contributions to race/ethnicity disparities in medical care. Med Care 2000;40(1):I140–51.

[81] Todd KH, Lee T, Hoffman JR. The effect of ethnicity on physician estimates of pain severity in patients with isolated extremity trauma. JAMA 1994;271(12):925–8.

[82] Gordon JA, Billings J, Asplin BR, et al. Safety net research in emergency medicine. Proceedings of the Academic Emergency Medicine Consensus Conference on "The Unraveling of the Safety Net." Acad Emerg Med 2001;8:1024–9.

[83] Gordon JA. The hospital emergency department as a social welfare institution. Ann Emerg Med 1999;33:321–5.

[84] Derlet R, Richards J. Overcrowding in the nation's emergency departments: complex causes and disturbing effects. Ann Emerg Med 2000;35:63–8.

[85] US General Accounting Office. Hospital emergency departments: crowded conditions vary among hospitals and communities. Washington, DC: GAO; 2003.

[86] Kellerman AL. Too sick to wait. JAMA 1991;266:1123–4.

[87] Bindman AB, Grumbach K, Keane D, et al. Consequences of queuing for care at a public hospital ED. JAMA 1991;266:1091–6.

[88] Barlas, Homan CS, Rakowski J, et al. How well to patients obtain short-term follow-up after discharge from the ED. Ann EM 1999;34:610–4.

[89] McCaig LF, Burt CW. National Hospital Ambulatory Medical Care Survey: 2001 Emergency Department Summary. Adv Data 2003;335:1–36.

[90] US Department of Health and Human Services. Healthy people 2010: understanding and improving health. 2nd edition. Washington, DC: US Government Printing Office; 2000.

[91] Kennedy J, Rhodes KV, Walls C, et al. Access to emergency care: restricted by long wait times and cost/coverage concerns. Ann Emerg Med 2004;43:567–73.

[92] Asplin BR, Magid DJ, Rhodes KV, et al. Conceptual model of emergency department crowding Annals of EM 2003;42:173–80.

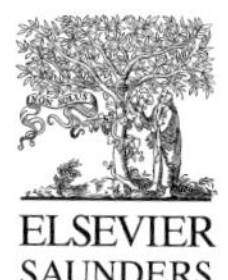

ELSEVIER
SAUNDERS

Emerg Med Clin N Am
24 (2006) 1075–1080

EMERGENCY
MEDICINE
CLINICS OF
NORTH AMERICA

Index

Note: Page numbers of article titles are in **boldface** type.

United States Postal Service

Statement of Ownership, Management, and Circulation

1. Publication Title	2. Publication Number	3. Filing Date
Emergency Medicine Clinics of North America	0 0 0 - 7 1 4	9/15/06

4. Issue Frequency	5. Number of Issues Published Annually	6. Annual Subscription Price
Feb, May, Aug, Nov	4	$175.00

7. Complete Mailing Address of Known Office of Publication (*Not printer*) (*Street, city, county, state, and ZIP+4*)

Elsevier Inc.
360 Park Avenue South
New York, NY 10010-1710

Contact Person
Sarah Carmichael
Telephone
(215) 239-3681

8. Complete Mailing Address of Headquarters or General Business Office of Publisher (*Not printer*)

Elsevier Inc., 360 Park Avenue South, New York, NY 10010-1710

9. Full Names and Complete Mailing Addresses of Publisher, Editor, and Managing Editor (*Do not leave blank*)

Publisher (*Name and complete mailing address*)

John Schrefer, Elsevier Inc., 1600 John F. Kennedy Blvd., Suite 1800, Philadelphia, PA 19103-2899

Editor (*Name and complete mailing address*)

Karen Sorensen, Elsevier Inc., 1600 John F. Kennedy Blvd., Suite 1800, Philadelphia, PA 19103-2899

Managing Editor (*Name and complete mailing address*)

Catherine Bewick, Elsevier Inc., 1600 John F. Kennedy Blvd., Suite 1800, Philadelphia, PA 19103-2899

10. Owner (*Do not leave blank. If the publication is owned by a corporation, give the name and address of the corporation immediately followed by the names and addresses of all stockholders owning or holding 1 percent or more of the total amount of stock. If not owned by a corporation, give the names and addresses of the individual owners. If owned by a partnership or other unincorporated firm, give its name and address as well as those of each individual owner. If the publication is published by a nonprofit organization, give its name and address.*)

Full Name	Complete Mailing Address
Wholly owned subsidiary of	4520 East-West Highway
Reed/Elsevier Inc., US Holdings	Bethesda, MD 20814

11. Known Bondholders, Mortgagees, and Other Security Holders Owning or Holding 1 Percent or More of Total Amount of Bonds, Mortgages, or Other Securities. If none, check box ► None

Full Name	Complete Mailing Address
N/A	

12. Tax Status (*For completion by nonprofit organizations authorized to mail at nonprofit rates*) (*Check one*)

The purpose, function, and nonprofit status of this organization and the exempt status for federal income tax purposes:

Has Not Changed During Preceding 12 Months

Has Changed During Preceding 12 Months (*Publisher must submit explanation of change with this statement*)

(*See Instructions on Reverse*)

PS Form **3526**, October 1999

---

13. Publication Title	14. Issue Date for Circulation Data Below
Emergency Medicine Clinics of North America	August, 2006

15. Extent and Nature of Circulation			Average No. Copies Each Issue During Preceding 12 Months	No. Copies of Single Issue Published Nearest to Filing Date
a.	Total Number of Copies (*Net press run*)		2,925	2,800
b. Paid and/or Requested Circulation	(1)	Paid/Requested Outside-County Mail Subscriptions Stated on Form 3541. (*Include advertiser's proof and exchange copies*)	1,726	1,606
	(2)	Paid In-County Subscriptions Stated on Form 3541 (*Include advertiser's proof and exchange copies*)		
	(3)	Sales Through Dealers and Carriers, Street Vendors, Counter Sales, and Other Non-USPS Paid Distribution	383	422
	(4)	Other Classes Mailed Through the USPS		
c.	Total Paid and/or Requested Circulation [*Sum of 15b. (1), (2), (3), and (4)*] ►		2,109	2,028
d. Free Distribution by Mail (*Samples, complimentary, and other free*)	(1)	Outside-County as Stated on Form 3541	137	126
	(2)	In-County as Stated on Form 3541		
	(3)	Other Classes Mailed Through the USPS		
e.	Free Distribution Outside the Mail (*Carriers or other means*)			
f.	Total Free Distribution (*Sum of 15d. and 15e.*) ►		137	126
g.	Total Distribution (*Sum of 15c. and 15f.*) ►		2,246	2,154
h.	Copies not Distributed		679	646
i.	Total (*Sum of 15g. and h.*) ►		2,925	2,800
j.	Percent Paid and/or Requested Circulation (*15c. divided by 15g. times 100*)		93.90%	94.15%

16. Publication of Statement of Ownership

Publication required. Will be printed in the **November 2006** issue of this publication.　　Publication not required

17. Signature and Title of Editor, Publisher, Business Manager, or Owner　　Date

[signature] Joel Fanucci – Executive Director of Subscription Services　　9/15/06

I certify that all information furnished on this form is true and complete. I understand that anyone who furnishes false or misleading information on this form or who omits material or information requested on the form may be subject to criminal sanctions (including fines and imprisonment) and/or civil sanctions (including civil penalties).

Instructions to Publishers

1. Complete and file one copy of this form with your postmaster annually on or before October 1. Keep a copy of the completed form for your records.
2. In cases where the stockholder or security holder is a trustee, include in items 10 and 11 the name of the person or corporation for whom the trustee is acting. Also include the names and addresses of individuals who are stockholders who own or hold 1 percent or more of the total amount of bonds, mortgages, or other securities of the publishing corporation. In item 11, if none, check the box. Use blank sheets if more space is required.
3. Be sure to furnish all circulation information called for in item 15. Free circulation must be shown in items 15d, e, and f.
4. Item 15h., Copies not Distributed, must include (1) newsstand copies originally stated on Form 3541, and returned to the publisher, (2) estimated returns from news agents, and (3), copies for office use, leftovers, spoiled, and all other copies not distributed.
5. If the publication had Periodicals authorization as a general or requester publication, this Statement of Ownership , Management, and Circulation must be published; it must be printed in any issue in October or, if the publication is not published during October, the first issue printed after October.
6. In item 16, indicate the date of the issue in which this Statement of Ownership will be published.
7. Item 17 must be signed.
   Failure to file or publish a statement of ownership may lead to suspension of Periodicals authorization.

PS Form **3526**, October 1999 (*Reverse*)

Moving?